Hypertension Pearls

Hypertension Pearls

Daniel W. Jones, MD
Vice Chancellor for Health Affairs
Dean, School of Medicine
University of Mississippi Medical Center
Jackson, Mississippi

Deborah S. King, PharmD
Assistant Professor of Pharmacy Practice and Medicine
University of Mississippi Medical Center
Jackson, Mississippi

Marion R. Wofford, MD, MPH
Associate Professor of Medicine
Director, Division of Hypertension
University of Mississippi Medical Center
Jackson, Mississippi

Hanley & Belfus
An Affiliate of Elsevier

HANLEY & BELFUS, INC.
An Affiliate of Elsevier Inc.

The Curtis Center
Independence Square West
Philadelphia, Pennsylvania 19106-3399

Notice

Primary Care Medicine is an ever-changing field. Standard safety precautions must be followed, but as new research and clinical experience broaden our knowledge, changes in treatment and drug therapy may become necessary or appropriate. Readers are advised to check the most current product information provided by the manufacturer of each drug to be administered to verify the recommended dose, the method and duration of administration, and contraindications. It is the responsibility of the treating physician, relying on experience and knowledge of the patient, to determine dosages and the best treatment for each individual patient. Neither the Publisher nor the authors assume any liability for any injury and/or damage to persons or property arising from this publication.

The Publisher

Library of Congress Control Number: 2003115700

HYPERTENSION PEARLS
ISBN: 1-56053-583-0

Printed in the United States of America.

Last digit is the print number: 9   8   7   6   5   4   3   2   1

CONTENTS

CONTRIBUTORS

Kim G. Adcock, PharmD
Assistant Professor of Pharmacy Practice and Pediatrics, University of Mississippi Medical Center, Jackson, Mississippi

Betsy Andrews
Student, University of Mississippi School of Pharmacy, Collierville, Tennessee

Bryan N. Batson, MD
Physician, Department of Internal Medicine, Hattiesburg Clinic, Hattiesburg, Mississippi

K. Lindsey Batte, BA
Student, School of Medicine, University of Mississippi Medical Center, Jackson, Mississippi

Joseph W. Blackston, MD, JD
Medical Director, Mississippi Department of Corrections, Jackson, Mississippi

George Joshua Blair, MD
Resident, Department of Medicine, University of Mississippi Medical Center, Jackson, Mississippi

Barbara Boss, RN, CFNP, PhD
Professor, School of Nursing, University of Mississippi Medical Center, Jackson, Mississippi

C. Andrew Brown, MD, MPH
Associate Professor of Medicine, Director, Division of General Internal Medicine, Department of Medicine, University of Mississippi Medical Center, Jackson, Mississippi

Nancy L. Campbell, MD
Resident, Department of Medicine, University of Mississippi Medical Center, Jackson, Mississippi

Jonathan S. Caudill, MD
Resident, Departments of Internal Medicine and Pediatrics, University of Mississippi Medical Center, Jackson, Mississippi

LeAnn Causey, PharmD
Pharmacist, Causey's Pharmacy, Natchitoches, Louisiana

Christopher Christensen, MD
Resident, Department of Medicine, University of Mississippi Medical Center, Jackson, Mississippi

James A. Cloy, MD
Assistant Professor of Family Medicine, Department of Family Medicine, University of Mississippi Medical Center, Jackson, Mississippi

Brenda M. Davy, PhD, RD, LD
Assistant Professor, Department of Human Nutrition, Foods, and Exercise, Virginia Polytechnic Institute and State University, Blacksburg, Virginia

Sharon Dickey, PharmD
Drug Information Specialist, Department of Pharmacy, University of Mississippi Medical Center, Jackson, Mississippi

Hal Dillon, PharmD
Pharmacist, Department of Pharmacy, University of Mississippi Medical Center, Jackson, Mississippi

Karen Dillon
Student, School of Medicine, University of Mississippi Medical Center, Jackson, Mississippi

Audwin Fletcher, RN, CFNP, MSN
Assistant Professor, School of Nursing, University of Mississippi Medical Center, Jackson, Mississippi

Chris Friedrich, MD, PhD
Associate Professor of Medical Genetics, Department of Preventive Medicine, Division of Medical Genetics, University of Mississippi Medical Center, Jackson, Mississippi

James K. Glisson, MD, PharmD
Resident, Department of Internal Medicine, University of Mississippi Medical Center, Jackson, Mississippi

George E. Habeeb, Jr., MD
Assistant Professor of Medicine, Division of Hypertension, University of Mississippi Medical Center, Jackson, Mississippi

Kimberly G. Harkins, MD
Assistant Professor of Medicine, Division of Hypertension, University of Mississippi Medical Center, Jackson, Mississippi

Spencer E. Harpe, PharmD, MPH
Graduate Research Fellow, The Ohio State University, College of Pharmacy, Columbus, Ohio

Thomas Kristopher Harrell, PharmD
Assistant Professor of Pharmacy Practice, University of Mississippi School of Pharmacy, Jackson, Mississippi

Pamela Helms, RN, CFNP, MSN
Assistant Professor, School of Nursing, University of Mississippi Medical Center, Jackson, Mississippi

Honey East Holman, MD
Assistant Professor of Medicine, Division of General Internal Medicine, University of Mississippi Medical Center, Jackson, Mississippi

Michelle M. Horn, MD
Resident, Departments of Internal Medicine and Pediatrics, University of Mississippi Medical Center, Jackson, Mississippi

Jon Hubanks
Student, University of Mississippi School of Pharmacy, Jackson, Mississippi

Dena W. Jackson, MD
Assistant Professor of Medicine, Division of General Internal Medicine, Department of Medicine, University of Mississippi Medical Center, Jackson, Mississippi

Peter N. Johnson
Student, University of Mississippi School of Pharmacy, Ridgeland, Mississippi

Daniel W. Jones, MD
Vice Chancellor for Health Affairs, Dean, School of Medicine, University of Mississippi Medical Center, Jackson, Mississippi

Kevin Lee Keeton
Student, School of Medicine, University of Mississippi Medical Center, Jackson, Mississippi

Kristi W. Kelley, PharmD, BCPS
Assistant Clinical Professor, Auburn University School of Pharmacy, Carraway Medical Foundation, Birmingham, Alabama

Deborah S. King, PharmD
Assistant Professor of Pharmacy Practice and Medicine, University of Mississippi Medical Center, Jackson, Mississippi

Fleetwood Loustalot, RN, NP-C, MSN
Instructor, School of Medicine, University of Mississippi Medical Center, Jackson, Mississippi

Anderson Mehrle, MD
Cardiology Fellow, Deparatment of Medicine, University of Mississippi Medical Center, Jackson, Mississippi

Trenika Mitchell
Student, University of Mississippi School of Pharmacy, Ridgeland, Mississippi

Michael Mohundro, PharmD
Resident, University of Mississippi Medical Center, Jackson, Mississippi

Michael Shoemaker-Moyle, MD
Instructor in Medicine, Division of General Internal Medicine, University of Mississippi Medical Center, Jackson, Mississippi

Sara L. Noble, PharmD
Clinical Associate Professor, Department of Family Medicine, University of Mississippi Medical Center, Jackson, Mississippi

Leigh Ann Ramsey, PharmD
Assistant Professor, School of Pharmacy, University of Mississippi Medical Center, Jackson, Mississippi

Holly E. Rogers, PharmD
Assistant Professor, Pharmacy Practice and Medicine, University of Mississippi Medical Center, Jackson, Mississippi

James T. Samuel, PharmD
Clinical Instructor, Department of Pharmacy Practice, University of Mississippi Medical Center, Jackson, Mississippi

Jinna M. Shepherd, MD
Assistant Professor of Medicine, Division of General Internal Medicine, University of Mississippi Medical Center, Jackson, Mississippi

Michael Shoemaker-Moyle, MD
Instructor in Medicine, Division of General Internal Medicine, University of Mississippi Medical Center, Jackson, Mississippi

Jimmy L. Stewart, MD
Assistant Professor of Medicine and Pediatrics, Division of Hypertension, University of Mississippi Medical Center, Jackson, Mississippi

Angela Stubbs, RN, CFNP, MSN
Instructor, School of Medicine, Department of Ambulatory Services, University of Mississippi Medical Center, Jackson, Mississippi

Caryl Sumrall, RN, CFNP, MSN
Instructor, School of Medicine, University of Mississippi Medical Center, Jackson, Mississippi

Gary D. Theilman, PharmD
Consultant, University of Mississippi School of Pharmacy, Department of Pharmacy Practice, University of Mississippi Medical Center, Jackson, Mississippi

Jennifer Rea Thomas, PharmD
Clinical Instructor, Department of Pharmacy Practice, University of Mississippi Medical Center, Jackson, Mississippi

Keith Thorne, MD
Resident, Department of Medicine, University of Mississippi Medical Center, Jackson, Mississippi

Steve A. Watts, MD
Assistant Professor of Family Medicine and Orthopedics, Department of Family Medicine, University of Mississippi Medical Center, Jackson, Mississippi

Amanda James Wilburn, PharmD
Resident, Bennett's Apothecary, Corinth, Mississippi

Karen Winters, RN, MSN
Assistant Professor, School of Nursing, University of Mississippi Medical Center, Jackson, Mississippi

Marion R. Wofford, MD, MPH
Associate Professor of Medicine, Director, Division of Hypertension, University of Mississippi Medical Center, Jackson, Mississippi

Rebecca L. Wood, PharmD
Pharmacist, G.V. (Sonny) Montgomery VA Medical Center, Jackson, Mississippi

Sharon B. Wyatt, RN, CANP, Phd
Professor, School of Nursing, Medicine, Division of Hypertension, University of Mississippi Medical Center, Jackson, Mississippi

Alexander Zubkov, MD, PhD
Resident, Department of Neurology, University of Mississippi Medical Center, Jackson, Mississippi

PREFACE

Learning comes from many sources, and medical education is no exception. Students of medicine at any stage and any age depend on many sources for improving their knowledge base. We are grateful to experienced medical educators, our teachers, who have shared their wisdom. We benefit from textbooks, which collect known concepts and facilitate understanding. And we learn from the medical literature, that body of knowledge accumulated through research.

We have found our patients to be a source of unmatched knowledge. The "practice" of medicine—repetitive contact with patients—is responsible for the honing of our skills as clinicians more than any other learning experience.

From the very beginning of our clinical exposure, the most productive and pleasurable learning experiences come through case-based learning. Whether it is from direct contact with the patient, hearing a colleague describe a case on rounds or in a conference setting, or a written presentation, the "case approach" offers learning opportunities unmatched by any other educational tool.

Hypertension Pearls is intended for use by students from multiple healthcare disciplines who aspire to provide patient care. It is a practical approach to expanding the learner's knowledge base about the management of hypertensive patients. The cases are taken from years of experience by a broad range of authors with varying clinical backgrounds, including hypertension specialists, specialty-trained physicians and pharmacists, generalist physicians, nurse practitioners, and others. The cases range from the common to the unusual. Though each case may present the reader with a number of opportunities for learning, the "Pearls" are the focal learning points. It is hoped that these pearls of wisdom will stay with you and improve your clinical skills.

This book is not intended to be comprehensive. Every clinical problem in hypertension cannot be covered in a book of this scope. For each case, the material should be sufficient for a satisfying learning experience. However, if you are inspired to explore a topic further, then we have fulfilled our mission.

We are grateful to the authors for their contributions and to the publishers for their guidance. We are grateful to our families for sharing the time needed for this work. We are grateful to our teachers and colleagues who have contributed to our knowledge of hypertension management. We reserve our deepest gratitude to those who have unselfishly taught us the most, our patients.

DANIEL W. JONES, MD
DEBORAH S. KING, PHARMD
MARION R. WOFFORD, MD, MPH
EDITORS

Acknowledgement

The editors wish to thank and acknowledge the significant contributions of our colleagues who assisted with editing these cases and discussions. Dr. George Habeeb, Dr. Kimberly Harkins, Dr. Jimmy Stewart, and Dr. Sharon Wyatt were instrumental in the preparation of this book. As with all of our work, this book has been improved by the collaborative efforts within the University of Mississippi Medical Center, Division of Hypertension.

DANIEL W. JONES, MD
DEBORAH S. KING, PHARMD
MARION R. WOFFORD, MD, MPH

Anderson Mehrle, MD
Kimberly G. Harkins, MD

PATIENT 1

A 66-year-old woman with dyspnea

A 66-year-old female smoker with hypertension presents to the emergency department complaining of dyspnea on exertion of several-month duration. Her symptoms are progressive, and she is now dyspneic with minimal activity. Over the last week she has developed two-pillow orthopnea and a dry cough. She has been admitted to the hospital three times in 2 years for similar symptoms, once requiring mechanical ventilation. During each admission her symptoms responded quickly to diuresis. She reports a diagnosis of congestive heart failure, but her most recent echocardiogram (see page 2) demonstrates normal left ventricular systolic function.

Physical Examination: Temperature 98.2°F, pulse 100, respiratory rate 22, blood pressure 176/90. Oxygen saturation 93% on 40% FiO_2 by face mask. General: moderate respiratory distress, appears fatigued. Cardiac: regular rhythm, prominent S_4 gallop, no murmur or S_3. Jugular Venous Pressure: 9 cm pulses normal in all extremities. No peripheral edema. Pulmonary: bilateral rales to mid-lung fields.

Laboratory Findings: WBC 8900/μl with a normal differential. Hct 30%. Electrolytes and glucose normal, BUN 12 mg/dl, creatinine 1.3 mg/dl. EKG: sinus tachycardia with left ventricular hypertrophy (see figure). Chest x-ray: bilateral patchy infiltrates, mildly enlarged cardiac silhouette.

Question: Does her history support a diagnosis of congestive heart failure?

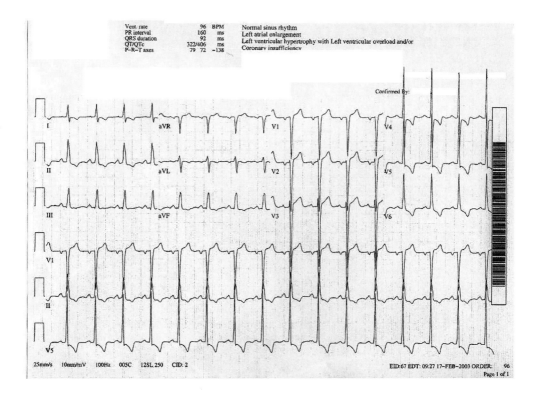

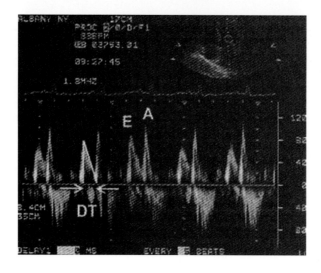

Diagnosis: Diastolic dysfunction

Discussion: Diastolic heart failure is a clinical syndrome characterized by signs and symptoms of classic systolic heart failure with or without systolic left ventricular (LV) dysfunction. The abnormalities in mechanical function are present during the "filling period." The ventricle is unable to accept volume of blood during diastole sufficient to maintain adequate stroke volume. Relaxation of the contracted myocardium normally occurs at the onset of diastole, causing a rapid pressure drop due to the elasticity of the ventricle. This creates a suction effect that increases the left-atrium-to-left-ventricle pressure gradient, augmenting diastolic filling. During late diastole, a normal left ventricle offers minimal resistance. Very low filling pressures in the left atrium are required, and pulmonary capillary pressure is < 12 mmHg. The contribution of atrial contraction to ventricular filling is relatively small.

The left ventricle becomes less compliant, and a higher filling pressure is required with LV hypertrophy or ischemia. The higher left atrial pressure and pulmonary capillary pressure create a shift of ventricular filling to later diastole with a greater dependence on atrial contraction. Symptoms related to pulmonary edema can occur with any condition that shortens filling time, such as tachycardia. This patient's symptoms may have been caused by her anemia and resultant tachycardia. Atrial fibrillation can also lead to symptoms, due to the loss of atrial contraction.

Diastolic dysfunction most often affects elderly patients with hypertension. As in this patient, dyspnea on exertion and reduced exercise tolerance are the earliest symptoms. As the disease progresses, dyspnea at rest and orthopnea may occur. Paroxysmal nocturnal dyspnea is a late manifestation. Pulmonary edema is common and often responds much more quickly to diuresis than does the edema of systolic heart failure.

The most common physical examination finding is elevated blood pressure with diastolic dysfunction. This patient had elevated blood pressure, a prominent S_4, and evidence of pulmonary congestion. The S_4 is often heard in patients with diastolic dysfunction as the left ventricle's ability to relax during diastole is impaired, due to more filling via atrial contraction and less by passive relaxation. An audible S_3 may be present due to stiffness of the ventricle, particularly in the later stages of the illness.

As LV end-diastolic pressure and left atrial pressure rise, pulmonary venous and microvascular pressure become elevated. Filtration of protein-poor liquid into the pulmonary interstitium and alveolar spaces leads to decreased diffusing capacity, hypoxemia, and dyspnea. Concomitant systemic illness such as anemia, fever, sepsis, or tachycardia can create "flash" pulmonary edema in patients with diastolic dysfunction.

Our patient's EKG demonstrated LV hypertrophy. LV hypertrophy, although the most common electrocardiographic finding in diastolic dysfunction, has a poor predictive value due to low sensitivity and specificity. Evidence of left atrial enlargement may be seen as well. Early in the disease state, the chest X-ray will be normal. The initial radiographic evidence of diastolic dysfunction is frequently a normal cardiac silhouette with pulmonary venous congestion. Later in the disease process, evidence of LV enlargement with or without left atrial enlargement may be seen.

The diagnosis of diastolic dysfunction is made by observing the signs and symptoms of heart failure in the setting of normal systolic function. It is difficult to differentiate between systolic and diastolic heart failure without the aid of ancillary testing. Cardiac catheterization, long considered the gold standard for diagnosis, has been replaced by **echocardiography** as the diagnostic modality of choice. Echocardiography can measure relaxation intervals and Doppler inflow to detect filling abnormalities consistent with diastolic dysfunction for this patient (see figure). In a normal heart, the inflow pattern across the mitral valve is characterized by a **large E wave** (representing passive filling in early diastole) and a **smaller A wave** (representing flow created by atrial contraction in late diastole). The E wave is dramatically reduced and the A wave becomes much larger (indicating the important role of atrial contraction in filling a stiff left ventricle) with diastolic dysfunction.

A second pattern of mitral inflow in diastolic dysfunction is **pseudonormalization**. As the diastolic function worsens, the LV pressure increases to the point that atrial contraction can contribute little to LV filling. The left atrial pressure is increased beyond the elevated LV end-diastolic pressure, and filling is primarily during early diastole; therefore, the E wave again becomes the predominant wave seen by Doppler. Restrictive physiology is diagnosed when the E wave velocity is more than twice the A wave velocity.

Pulmonary vein flow may also be used. Pulmonary vein flow is normally greater during systole. With elevated atrial pressure, pulmonary vein flow occurs predominantly during diastole when the mitral valve is open. This patient's echocardiogram might show a pseudonormal or impaired filling pattern as well as diastolic-dominant pulmonary vein flow.

The prognosis of diastolic heart failure is difficult to assess due to the variety of causes. Morbidity overall remains quite high and is nearly equal to the morbidity associated with systolic dysfunction. Hospital admission and readmission rates are high. Treatments aimed at modification of pathophysiology have been evaluated by few studies.

Treatment of diastolic heart failure, and of hypertension in the patient with diastolic dysfunction, is empiric, including judicious use of diuretics to reduce volume for symptomatic relief. As LV filling is the root of the problem, medications that slow the heart rate should be beneficial. Calcium channel blockers and beta-blockers have been shown to improve exercise tolerance and reduce mortality in small studies. Angiotensin-converting enzyme inhibitors (ACEI) and angiotensin receptor blockers (ARBs) are currently being evaluated in a number of studies. In the Losartan Intervention for Endpoint Reduction Study (LIFE), the ARB losartan reduced cardiovascular complications in patients with hypertension and LV hypertrophy, compared to the beta-blocker atenolol. Blocking angiotensin II will aid in afterload reduction and may aid in regression of LV hypertrophy. Spironolactone, which has been shown to reduce mortality in systolic heart failure, is under investigation in diastolic heart failure.

Hypertension remains the strongest risk factor for developing heart failure, whether diastolic or systolic. Aggressive blood pressure control remains the cornerstone of treatment of diastolic dysfunction. When the diagnosis is made, an evaluation for coronary artery disease should also be promptly initiated. Ischemia can not only cause diastolic dysfunction, but repeated ischemia can cause hospitalization due to flash pulmonary edema from impaired relaxation.

Diastolic heart failure plays a major role in cardiovascular disease in the United States, but remains under-recognized. The presence of heart failure signs and symptoms with preserved systolic function by echocardiography should prompt the caregiver to consider diastolic dysfunction. The patient in this case had been diagnosed with heart failure in the past, but the differentiation of diastolic heart failure had not been made. Further treatment should be focused on volume reduction, heart rate control, myocardial ischemia evaluation, and, most importantly, blood pressure reduction.

Clinical Pearls

1. Diastolic dysfunction is common, particularly among elderly hypertensive patients.
2. Diastolic dysfunction is caused by impaired ventricular relaxation from a variety of causes.
3. Signs and symptoms are similar to systolic heart failure but with preserved systolic function.
4. Echocardiography is the modality of choice for evaluating diastolic dysfunction.
5. Mortality and morbidity in diastolic heart failure are similar to those in systolic heart failure.
6. Blood pressure reduction is the cornerstone of treatment, through diuresis, rate-limiting agents, and agents that block the renin-angiotensin-aldosterone system.

REFERENCES

1. Angeja BG, Grossman W: Evaluation and management of diastolic heart failure. Circulation. 107:659–663, 2003.
2. Dahlof B, Devereux RB, Kjeldsen SE, et al: Cardiovascular morbidity and mortality in the Losartan Intervention for Endpoint Reduction Study (LIFE): A randomised trial against atenolol. Lancet 359:995–1003, 2002.
3. Zile MR, Brutsaert DL: New concepts in diastolic dysfunction and diastolic heart failure. Part I: Diagnosis, prognosis, and measurements of diastolic function. Circulation 105:1387–1393, 2002.
4. Zile MR, Brutsaert DL: New concepts in diastolic dysfunction and diastolic heart failure. Part II: Causal mechanisms and treatment. Circulation 105:1503–1508, 2002.

Marion R. Wofford, MD, MPH

PATIENT 2

A 23-year-old woman with new-onset hypertension

A 23-year-old woman presents upon referral to the hypertension clinic for evaluation of elevated blood pressure. She had been seen 2 weeks prior by a cardiologist who conferred the diagnosis of hypertension. An electrocardiogram and echocardiogram were performed and reported to be normal. Atenolol 50 mg was prescribed, and the patient was referred for further evaluation. She has been experiencing fatigue and headaches for several months. Her blood pressure has been checked on several occasions, with readings in the range of 150–170/90–100 mmHg. The patient has taken oral contraceptives for the last 5 years and has had regular follow-ups with her gynecologist. She denies the use of tobacco, alcohol, or over-the-counter medications. She has no significant family medical history.

Physical Examination: Pulse 90, blood pressure 170/90 mmHg, body mass index 19. General: thin, appears uncomfortable due to headache. Neck: no bruits or masses. Retinae: no papilledema, arteriolar narrowing. Cardiac: regular rhythm without murmurs. Lungs: normal breath sounds bilaterally. Abdomen: flat, normal bowel sounds, no palpable masses.

Laboratory Findings: Complete blood count: normal. K^+ 4.2 mEq/L, HCO_3^- 24 mEq/L, BUN 13 mg/dl, creatinine 0.8 mg/dl. Urinalysis: no red blood cells, blood, or protein.

Question: Should an evaluation for secondary hypertension be conducted?

Diagnosis: Early age of onset of hypertension necessitates evaluation for secondary causes.

Discussion: Ninety-five percent of the 50 million adults in the United States with hypertension have **primary (essential hypertension)**. The remaining 5% of adults with hypertension have an identifiable or "secondary" disorder responsible for the elevated blood pressure. Although **secondary hypertension** seems relatively rare, these disorders occur in a great number of people, given the overall prevalence of hypertension. The diagnosis of secondary hypertension is important, as specific treatments based on the underlying pathophysiology are available and the conditions causing blood pressure elevation are potentially curable. Detection and treatment are critical to prevent end-organ damage and to achieve control of elevated blood pressures.

The causes of secondary hypertension are numerous. In general, these causes are categorized into one of three etiologies including renal, endocrine, and miscellaneous causes. Renal parenchymal disease is believed, by some, to be the most common cause. Renovascular disease, although rare, is the most common surgically correctable form of secondary hypertension. Among the endocrine causes, primary hyperaldosteronism, once thought to be very uncommon, is now recognized with increasing frequency. Other causes that deserve consideration include pheochromocytoma, thyroid disease, and miscellaneous causes such as obstructive sleep apnea and drug interactions and abuse.

The diagnostic approach to secondary hypertension is not always straightforward and may require a complex investigation to determine (or exclude) a cause. A thorough history and physical examination, careful observation, and proper laboratory studies give important clues to the presence of the underlying disease. Patients often do not present with classic characteristics of secondary hypertension. Therefore, the practitioner must maintain some level of suspicion. An important historical clue is that there is no family history of hypertension. Patients whose onset of hypertension occurs either before the age 20 or after age 50, who have severe diastolic hypertension defined as a diastolic blood pressure above 110 mmHg, and/or who are refractory to therapy should raise the suspicion for secondary hypertension. Other features that suggest secondary hypertension include grade III or IV retinopathy, evidence of peripheral vascular disease, abdominal bruits, absent pulses, truncal obesity with abdominal striae as seen in Cushing's disease, or exophthalmos due to hyperthyroidism. Biochemical tests related to specific disorders include hypokalemia, an elevated creatinine level, proteinuria, or hypercalcemia. These may provide clues for underlying secondary causes of hypertension.

The Joint National Committee (JNC) for Prevention, Detection, Evaluation, and Treatment of High Blood Pressure recommends that the initial biochemical testing on all hypertensive patients include a hematocrit, chemistry profile (glucose, creatinine, potassium), lipid profile, calcium, and urinalysis. An electrocardiogram is recommended to determine evidence of end-organ damage such as left ventricular hypertrophy or ischemic heart disease. Additional tests such as renin, aldosterone, thyroid functions, or 24-hour urines for metanephrines should be used only when a specific secondary cause is suspected. The JNC further recommends that referral to a hypertension specialist be considered for patients with resistant hypertension, defined as poor control of blood pressure on full doses of three antihypertensive agents of which one is a diuretic.

An evaluation for secondary causes in all hypertensive patients is *not* necessary or cost-effective. Clinical clues obtained from a careful history, physical, and laboratory assessment guide the clinician through an appropriate evaluation for identifiable causes. A combination of the clinician's index of suspicion and interpretation of data provide guidance in the choice of diagnostic tests and therapies to target the mechanisms contributing to poor blood pressure control.

Clinical Pearls

1. Secondary hypertension refers to an identifiable cause for elevated blood pressure, which is often correctable.
2. The initiation of an evaluation for secondary hypertension is dependent on a careful history and physical, biochemical evidence, and a clinical suspicion for secondary causes.
3. Clues that suggest secondary hypertension include: age of onset of hypertension, poor response to therapy, significant target-organ injury, a lack of family history of hypertension, and findings on physical or laboratory testing that suggest a secondary cause.

REFERENCES

1. Chobanian AV, Bakris GL, Black HR, et al: National Heart, Lung, and Blood Institute Joint National Committee on Prevention, Detection, Evaluation, and Treatment of Blood Pressure; National High Blood Pressure Education: The Seventh Report of the Joint National Committee on Prevention, Detection, Evaluation, and Treatment of High Blood Pressure: the JNC VII report, JAMA 289(19):2560–2572, 2003.
2. Kaplan NM: Clinical Hypertension, 8th ed. Baltimore, Lippincott Williams & Wilkins, 2002.

Amanda James Wilburn, PharmD
K. Lindsey Batte, BA
Deborah S. King, PharmD

PATIENT 3

A 37-year-old woman self-treated with fish oil for hypertension

A 37-year-old woman comes to the clinic for a follow-up visit. She reports an increase in home blood pressure readings over the last several months. No other complaints are expressed. Her past medical history is significant for hypertension, which was previously controlled with hydrochlorothiazide 12.5 mg daily, a low-sodium diet, and a regular exercise regimen. The patient claims to be compliant with her diet and exercise regimen. She admits to the substitution of fish oil for her diuretic for the past 3 months.

Physical Examination: Temperature 98.2°F, pulse 87, respiratory rate 17, blood pressure 150/95, height 5 feet 9 inches, weight 69.9 kg. General: well-developed, well-nourished. HEENT: unremarkable. Cardiac: regular rate and rhythm with no murmurs, rubs, or gallops. Chest: clear to auscultation. Abdomen: nontender, nondistended. Extremities: no edema.

Laboratory Findings: Blood chemistry: normal.

Question: Why is the patient suddenly experiencing a rise in blood pressure?

Diagnosis: Uncontrolled hypertension due to noncompliance with prescribed regimen and self-treatment with dietary supplements.

Discussion: Appropriately treating hypertension is important for reduction of cardiovascular, cerebrovascular, and renovascular complications associated with elevated blood pressure. Often patients do not perceive the importance of keeping hypertension under control. Nonadherance is a very common problem in hypertension management. Poor compliance may be due to many reasons. Patients may lack the financial means to pay for medications. Others may find it difficult to have prescriptions refilled in a timely fashion. Some may be unwilling to make necessary lifestyle changes, or they may simply not want to take medication. Many hypertensive patients may feel worse clinically while taking antihypertensives as compared to living with symptom-free hypertension.

The public is continuously exposed to information concerning dietary supplements. Oftentimes, marketing practices may be misleading. For example, dietary supplements are usually marketed as "completely natural" and therefore "100% safe." Health care providers must be aware that these products do carry potential risks and sometimes provide no benefit in the treatment of hypertension.

Dietary supplements are readily available to the public. Individuals may purchase these products in pharmacies, health food stores, grocery stores, or on the Internet. Easy access, as well as misleading marketing practices, are probably responsible for the recent surge in utilization of these products by the public.

Although patients may consider dietary supplements to be effective, appealing alternatives to prescription medications, it is the responsibility of health care professionals to educate the public about risks associated with dietary supplements, as well as potential benefits and proper dietary supplement utilization.

There are several problems associated with self-treatment with dietary supplements. There have been very few clinical trials determining the efficacy of dietary supplements. Of the studies conducted, much of the data is controversial. In the area of hypertension, there have been studies providing evidence that vitamin C, garlic, fish oil, and coenzyme Q10 (CoQ10) may have some benefit in moderately reducing blood pressure. For example, fish oil has been effective in lowering both systolic and diastolic blood pressure at a dose of 3.7 g per day. The American Heart Association has recently advocated the addition of fish oil supplements for patients at increased risk for coronary heart disease. It is important to note that dietary supplements should be taken under the close supervision of a health care provider.

Additional problems arise because natural products are not standardized. Unlike conventional prescription medications, dietary supplements are not regulated by the U.S. Food and Drug Administration (FDA). Healthcare professionals must be aware that dietary supplements may vary according to composition and amount of supplement present in each individual dose.

As with any medication, one must be careful about pharmacological interactions and associated adverse effects. It is imperative that healthcare providers educate patients that "natural" products are not necessarily "safe."

Some dietary supplements, including fish oil, may moderately decrease blood pressure when taken in conjuction with traditional lifestyle changes. Dietary supplements are not meant to replace prescription medications, proper diet, or exercise regimens. The patient in the present case did not understand the importance of taking dietary supplements under the supervision of a health care provider. In addition, she made the mistake of assuming that fish oil would be an effective alternative to taking hydrochlorothiazide.

There are both risks and benefits associated with fish oil supplementation. Although moderate blood pressure reduction has been observed with the consumption of fish oil, it also has the potential to increase bleeding, decrease renal function, and cause a lingering "fishy taste." To date, no long-term safety and efficacy studies have been conducted using fish oil. Hence, there is much knowledge to be desired concerning the use of these substances.

It is imperative that healthcare professionals keep abreast of new information available to the public. It is also very important for healthcare professionals to ask patients specifically about dietary supplement utilization. Many patients are uncomfortable revealing such information. Others simply do not consider dietary supplements to be drugs, so when asked if they take any over-the-counter medications they omit mentioning the dietary supplements.

Dietary supplements do play a role in the treatment of hypertension. In mild cases of hypertension, dietary supplements along with proper lifestyle modifications may provide adequate blood pressure control. In the treatment of higher blood pressures, dietary supplements may be used in addition with conventional medications. Many supplements are marketed to "support a healthy cardiovascular system," but for many of these supplements there is little or no evidence to support efficacy. There are studies supporting the efficacy of vitamin C, garlic, fish oil, and CoQ10 in the treatment of hypertension.

This patient admitted to finding information on the Internet claiming that fish oil radically lowers blood pressure "the natural way." She read that fish oil provided the same benefits, as prescription medications, but unlike the medications fish oil had absolutely no side effects. After reading the website, she happened to see fish oil while in her local grocery store and purchased a bottle. It was much more convenient for her to buy the supplement while grocery shopping than to wait in line at the pharmacy for the hydrochlorothiazide. The healthcare provider informed the patient of the frequently misleading marketing associated with dietary supplements. She was told that although dietary supplements have shown benefit in the treatment of hypertension, they are not meant to substitute for prescription medications. The importance of taking dietary supplements under the supervision of her healthcare provider was also stressed. The hydrochlorothiazide was resumed and she was encouraged to continue her good diet and exercise practices. The patient was told that although it would be appropriate to continue the fish oil in addition to her medication, it probably would not be necessary, since she was previously controlled with hydrochlorothiazide and lifestyle modifications alone. After resuming the hydrochlorothiazide, her blood pressure returned to normal.

Clinical Pearls

1. Patients must be educated about the potential risks associated with dietary supplementation. A "natural" product is not necessarily a "safe" product.
2. Dietary supplements are not regulated by the FDA, and no standardization protocols are in place.
3. Health care providers should ask patients specifically about their use of dietary supplements, since patients are not always apt to disclose such information.
4. Vitamin C, garlic, fish oil, and CoQ10 have shown benefit in the treatment of hypertension. Other dietary supplements have shown little or no potential benefit.

REFERENCES

1. Wilburn AJ, King DS, Glisson J, et al: Dietary supplements in the treatment of hypertension: An evidence-based review. Journal of Clinical Hypertension (in press)
2. Kris-Etherton PM, Harris WS, Appel LJ: Omega-3 fatty acids and cardiovascular disease: New recommendations from the American Heart Association. Arterioscler Thromb Vasc Biol 23:151–152, 2003.
3. Kaplan NM, Rose BD: Fish oil in treatment of hypertension. In Rose BD (ed): UpToDate pp. 1–5, 2002, http//www.updateonline.com
4. Kaplan NM: Kaplan's Clinical Hypertension, 8th ed. Philadelphia, Lippincott Williams & Wilkins, 2002.

C. Andrew Brown, MD, MPH
Marion R. Wofford, MD, MPH

PATIENT 4

A 58-year-old man with long-standing, poorly controlled hypertension and hypokalemia

A 58-year-old man with a 25-year history of poorly controlled hypertension presents to your office for consultation and treatment of his hypertension. Over the years he has been on multiple medication regimens without achieving goal blood pressure. Currently he is on three medications taken once daily: Hyzaar 50/12.5 mg, atenolol 100 mg, and Norvasc 10 mg. He recalls being told several times in the past by his primary care physician that his potassium was low and he has required oral supplementation on occasion. He relates having occasional muscle weakness and cramps, usually following bouts of strenuous physical exertion. He denies chest pain, shortness-of-breath, or palpitations. He smokes a pack of cigarettes per day and denies alcohol use.

Physical Examination: Pulse 68, blood pressure 178/96, respiratory rate 16. BMI 30. General: moderate obesity. Funduscopic: arteriovenous nicking noted. Skin: normal. Cardiac: no murmurs. Abdomen: obese, no masses or bruits. Extremities: normal strength, trace pretibial edema.

Laboratory Findings: WBC normal with normal differential, Hgb 18 g/dL. Electrolytes: potassium 3.1, bicarbonate 30; BUN and creatinine normal. Plasma aldosterone 38 ng/dL (normal 3–31 ng/dL), plasma renin activity < 0.2 ng/mL/hr (normal, 1.3–4.0 ng/mL/hr)

Question: What do the laboratory findings suggest as an underlying diagnosis?

Answer: Primary hyperaldosteronism

Discussion: This patient should be evaluated for the presence of inappropriate levels of aldosterone that may be the cause of resistant hypertension and hypokalemia.

In 1955, Conn first detailed a disorder characterized by resistant hypertension, hypokalemia, alkalosis, suppressed plasma renin activity (PRA), and excessive aldosterone production. He named this disorder primary hyperaldosteronism (PA). Conn estimated the prevalence of the disorder to approach approximately 1% and suggested PA was the most "curable" form of secondary hypertension.

Previously thought to be very rare, this disorder is the most common endocrine cause of secondary hypertension, with prevalence rates of 10–15% among hypertensive patients. Given the number of patients with hypertension in the United States and around the world, screening for this disorder may result in identifying many patients that could benefit from early detection and treatment of this form of secondary hypertension.

In 1981, Hiramatsu suggested calculating the ratio of plasma aldosterone to PRA as a screening tool for the disorder. The ratio can be calculated from a single blood sample and is less influenced by medication use, diet, posture, or time of day. A suppressed renin and an elevated aldosterone are critical to the recognition of PA. A ratio greater than 75 is a sensitive indicator for aldosterone-producing adenomas. Patients with essential hypertension have ratios < 20. Those individuals with ratios between 20 and 75 probably have bilateral zona glomerulosa hyperplasia.

Two major classifications of PA exist. These two forms, aldosterone-producing adrenal adenomas (APA) and zona glomerulosa hyperplasia (IHA), are based on histologic characteristics and physiological response. Distinguishing between these two pathologic abnormalities is important clinically, since removal of a unilateral APA may result in correction of elevated blood pressure and hypokalemia. However, in some cases, both conditions occur concomitantly; or the patient may have PA and essential hypertension. The severity of hypertension and hypokalemia may provide some clue to the underlying pathologic condition leading to the syndrome of PA. The incidence of APA is higher in those with more severe forms of the disease (e.g., severe resistant hypertension and marked unprovoked hypokalemia), whereas IHA is more common in those with milder forms of PA.

Primary aldosteronism should be suspected in patients with moderate-to-severe hypertension, in those with hypertension refractory to standard treatment, or in hypertensive patients with disease onset at an early age. It should also be suspected in those individuals with low normal potassium, as seen in this patient, or in whom low-dose diuretics causes hypokalemia. Furthermore, hypertensive individuals with left ventricular hypertrophy should also be screened. The aldosterone-to-renin ratio is an easy, inexpensive and rapid means to screen for the disorder.

Although the ratio is a reliable means of screening for PA, there are some caveats that may influence its predictive value. PRA less than 1 ng/dL is seen in virtually all PA patients but also in 20–25% of patients with essential hypertension. Thus, obtaining the ratio while the patient is in the upright position enhances the predictability of the ratio and generally should be performed after 2 hours in the upright position. Production of aldosterone is reduced in the hypokalemic state, so potassium should be repleted prior to measuring the ratio.

The following laboratory results were obtained from our patient after potassium supplementation: plasma aldosterone 28 ng/dl, plasma renin activity < 0.2 ng/ml/hr. The ratio of 140 and aldosterone level > 15 ng/dl is a positive screening test.

Although most medications do not affect the ratio, some antihypertensives may potentially cloud the interpretation. Therefore, they should be considered in the interpretation of the aldosterone-PRA ratio. Spironolactone should be held at least 6 weeks prior to measuring the ratio. Beta-blockers may result in false-positive tests by lowering the PRA, and calcium channel blockers may result in false-negative results. Alpha-blockers and vasodilators appear to have no affect on the ratio.

Although plasma aldosterone-PRA ratio is the screening test of choice, further confirmatory testing is required to clinch the diagnosis. Several tests are used to demonstrate the autonomous production of aldosterone. Aldosterone production can be suppressed with oral or intravenous sodium, and, historically, the most commonly employed test to detect PA was the abnormal urinary excretion of aldosterone following 3 days of high salt intake (> 200 mEq/day). Another confirmatory test relies on the lack of suppression of aldosterone after saline infusion. After the patient has been upright for 2 hours, blood for a plasma aldosterone level is drawn. The level is repeated 4 hours later, during which time the individual has received 2 liters of 0.9% saline. Plasma aldosterone levels above 5–10 ng/dL are considered abnormal.

The most sensitive test to confirm the diagnosis of PA is the fludrocortisone suppression test.

After repleting potassium levels, patients are placed on a high-salt diet (> 200 mEq sodium) and fludrocortisone. Two standard doses of fludrocortisone are used for 3 days: 0.1 mg every 6 hours or 0.2 mg twice a day. In patients without aldosteronism, plasma aldosterone levels will suppress to < 5 ng/dL; a level of > 5 ng/dL is considered confirmatory.

Saline or oral salt loading and fludrocortisone should be used cautiously, if at all, as many patients with PA have very poor control of hypertension even on multiple medications.

For those individuals with elevated ratios and positive confirmatory testing, consideration should be given to the underlying pathology of the disorder. The majority of people with the disorder either have APA or IHA. Both high-resolution CT scans and MRI (see figure) appear to have similar ability to differentiate between APA and IHA, although comparison data are limited in delineating the diagnostic accuracy of the two imaging procedures. Both imaging studies can ascertain adrenal adenomas > 5 mm in size, but cannot assess the physiologic, or rather, the biochemical output of the adenoma. Several nuclear scans are available to ascertain the physiologic function of an adrenal adenoma, but all have limited reliability. In those instances where scans detect a solitary nodule > 1 cm in a patient with clinical and biochemical PA, and the contralateral adrenal appears normal, surgical resection should be considered. For this subgroup of patients, adrenal vein sampling may be necessary to assure physiologic functioning of the adenoma and to exclude concomitant IHA. Also, an imaging study suggestion of IHA does not preclude the need for adrenal vein sampling and the possibility of surgical intervention, since marked unilateral overproduction of aldosterone can occur. Although cure is less likely, significant improvement in the clinical manifestations of the disorder are possible.

As with essential hypertension, the goal of treatment is to prevent the long-term sequelae of hypertension and to avoid the long-term consequences of PA itself. The underlying pathology

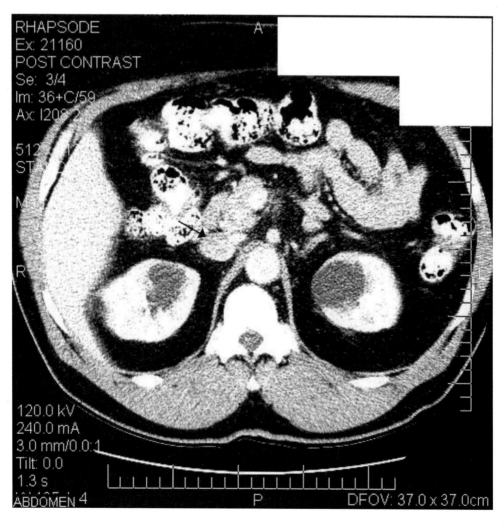

resulting in PA dictates the treatment strategy. Patients with APA should be investigated for potential surgical resection and possible cure. Regrettably, patients with IHA are limited to medical management.

All patients with PA should be educated about lifestyle interventions such as ideal body weight, exercise, smoking cessation, and excessive alcohol avoidance. Strict sodium intake (< 100 mEq/day) is necessary. Supplementation of potassium is typically of little benefit. The drug of choice is spironolactone, an aldosterone-receptor antagonist. Patients should be educated about potential adverse effects of spironolactone such as impotence, decreased libido, gynecomastia, and menstrual irregularities. For those patients who develop untoward effects of spironolactone, amiloride or triamterene are alternatives. The U.S. Food and Drug Administration (FDA) recently approved eplerenone, a selective aldosterone antagonist. Patients with PA should respond favorably to this agent. Additional agents may be necessary in some patients who do not achieve target blood pressure despite therapeutic doses of these potassium-sparing diuretics.

Surgical intervention should be entertained in those patients with PA in whom imaging studies suggest an adenoma. Also, some patients with IHA may have disease that is amenable to surgical intervention. The patient should be advised that surgical intervention may not achieve complete benefit. Some patients may have both IHA and APA or, more likely, PA and essential hypertension. Those with the most to benefit from surgery tend to be younger, have lower PRA values, and have lateralization of aldosterone secretion.

The evaluation and management of patients with PA is an area of much debate. Some advocate a much less invasive, and less expensive, approach employing a trial of lifestyle and medical management. Others champion a rigorous pursuit of potential surgical candidates. To date, no large-scale clinical trials exist to affirm one approach over the other. Until then, patients should be advised of their therapeutic options and become active participants in the decision-making process.

A conservative approach was taken in the current patient. A very high aldosterone-PRA ratio and a suppressed renin is highly suggestive of PA. Spironolactone 25 mg was initially added to his current regimen. On return, the blood pressure was much improved, although not optimal, so the medication was increased. The patient did not desire to pursue surgical intervention, so imaging studies were not performed. His blood pressure continued to decrease, making discontinuation of other antihypertensive drugs a desirable option in his continued care.

Clinical Pearls

1. Primary aldosteronism has a prevalence rate of 10–15% among patients with hypertension.
2. Patients with resistant hypertension should be screened for PA using the plasma aldosterone–plasma renin activity ratio.
3. Some patients with PA have normokalemia.
4. The medical management of PA includes the use of potassium-sparing diuretics.
5. Positive confirmatory tests for PA are followed by imaging of the adrenal glands.
6. Aldosterone-producing adenomas and adrenal hyperplasia are two major subtypes of PA.

REFERENCES

1. Young WF Jr: Primary aldosteronism: Management issues. Ann N Y Acad Sci 970:61–76, 2002.
2. Fardella CE, Mosso L, Gomez-Sanchez CE, et al: Primary hyperaldosteronism in essential hypertensives: Prevalence, biochemical profile, and molecular biology. J Clin Endocrinol Metab 85:1863–1867, 2000.
3. Gordon RD: Primary aldosteronism. J Endocrinol Invest 18:495–511, 1995.
4. Gordon RD, Stowasser M, Tunny TJ, et al: High incidence of primary aldosteronism in 199 patients referred with hypertension. Clin Exp Pharmacol Physiol 21:315–318, 1994.
5. Weinburger MH, Fineberg NS: The diagnosis of primary aldosteronism and separation of two major subtypes. Arch Intern Med 153:2125–2129, 1993.
6. Hiramatsu K, Yamada T, Yukimura Y, et al: A screening test to identify aldosterone-producing adenoma by measuring plasma renin activity. Results in hypertensive patients. Arch Intern Med 141:1589–1593, 1981.
7. Conn JW: Primary aldosteronism, a new clinical syndrome. J Lab Clin Med 45:3–7, 1955.

PATIENT 5

A 42-year-old man with high-normal blood pressure

A 42-year-old African American man presents with high-normal blood pressure. The patient has no physical complaints and is not sure why his family physician sent him to the hypertension clinic, except that his blood pressure has been "creeping up" over the past 5 years. He is a nonsmoker and abstains from alcohol, has no significant past medical history, and takes no medications other than occasional ibuprofen for muscle aches and pains. His mother and maternal grandmother died from strokes in their early 60s.

Physical Examination: Temperature 98.9°F, pulse 72, respiratory rate 16, seated blood pressure (average of two readings obtained after a 5-minute rest using a large adult cuff) 138/88. General: slightly overweight. Chest: clear. Cardiac: without murmurs. Abdomen: protruding. Extremities: without edema. Eyes: normal funduscopic. Height: 5 feet 10 inches. Weight: 202 Pounds. BMI: 29. Waist circumference: 102 cm. Arm circumference: 35 cm.

Laboratory Findings: CBC: normal. Glucose, BUN, and creatinine normal. Total cholesterol 205 mg/dl (normal < 200 mg/dl), LDL-C 140 mg/dl (normal < 130 mg/dl), HDL-C 29 mg/dl (normal 35–59 mg/dl), fasting triglycerides 180 mg/dl. TSH normal. Urinalysis normal. 24-hour sodium excretion 260 mEq/24 hr (normal 40–217 mEq/24 hr). EKG: normal.

Question: How should this patient be medically treated?

Answer: Prehypertension, requiring life style intervention

Discussion: According to current guidelines, this patient has prehypertension with two major risk factors for hypertension (dyslipidemia, and possible family history of cardiovascular disease). According to the Seventh Report of the Joint National Committee on the Prevention, Detection, Evaluation, and Treatment of High Blood Pressure (JNC VII), he would be classified as prehypertensive, which advises lifestyle modification as the initial treatment approach.

Lifestyle modifications that would be recommended for this patient include weight reduction to reduce his abdominal obesity, increased physical activity (e.g., walking 30–45 minutes each day), and a reduction in dietary sodium intake to 2.4 g per day (6 g NaCl). African Americans as a group may be more sensitive to changes in sodium intake than the general population. A diet rich in fruits, vegetables, and low-fat dairy products such as that used in the Dietary Approaches to stop Hypertension (DASH) trials should be encouraged (see table).

The pharmacologic treatment of mildly elevated blood pressure has been the subject of some debate and controversy. It has been suggested that individuals with prehypertension pressure may benefit from early treatment with antihypertensive medication. Many individuals with blood pressure above optimal levels (120/80 mmHg) but not considered hypertensive (140–159/90–99 mmHg) have cardiovascular disease (CVD). All-cause mortality and death from CVD is increased not only in those with high blood pressure, but also in those with "high-normal" blood pressure, or prehypertension. Vascular changes associated with elevated blood pressure may occur prior to the diagnosis of hypertension, and may be reversed with early treatment.

African Americans have a higher incidence of hypertension-related morbidity and mortality than other racial and ethnic groups—hypertension develops earlier in life and average blood pressures are higher in African Americans as compared to Caucasians. Individuals who argue for early pharmacologic treatment of hypertension might suggest that in this patient, elevated blood pressure is a precursor to future hypertension and early treatment may produce normotension after the discontinuation of drug treatment.

If antihypertensive drug therapy is selected, a diuretic may be the initial drug of choice. In African Americans and in Caucasians, diuretics may reduce hypertension-related morbidity and mortality. In addition, results from the Antihypertensive and Lipid-Lowering Treatment of Prevent Heart Attack Trial (ALLHAT) indicate that a thiazide diuretic is more effective than a calcium channel blocker and an angiotensin-converting enzyme inhibitor in preventing one or more major forms of CVD. Thus, due to their lower cost, and, possibly, better effectiveness in preventing CVD, a diuretic may be the optimal first-step antihyper-

The DASH Diet

Food Group	Daily Servings	Serving Sizes	Example
Grains and grain products	7–8	1 slice bread	Whole wheat bread, oatmeal, cereals
		½ c. dry cereal	
		½ c. cooked rice, pasta or cereal	
Vegetables	4–5	1 c. raw vegetables	Tomatoes, spinach, carrots, broccoli
		½ c. cooked vegetables	
Fruits	4–5	6 oz. fruit juice	Bananas, oranges, melons, peaches, strawberries,
		1 med fruit	
		½ c. fresh, frozen, or canned fruit	
Low-fat or nonfat dairy foods	2–3	8 oz. milk	Skim or 1% milk, nonfat or low-fat yogurt
		1 c. yogurt	
		1.5 oz. cheese	
Meats, poultry, and fish	2 or less	3 oz. cooked meats, poultry or fish	Chicken breast, salmon, lean beef, and pork
Nuts, seeds, and legumes	4–5 per week	1.5 oz. or 1/3 c. nuts	Almonds, walnuts, kidney beans, lentils
		½ oz. or 2 T. seeds	
		½ c. cooked legumes	

tensive drug choice. Regardless of whether or not drug therapy is initiated, lifestyle modification is an essential component of treatment.

The present patient is an abdominally obese African American man with prehypertension, which will likely continue to rise if untreated. He was advised to begin a low-sodium weight-reduc- tion diet and a daily walking program. A repeat 24-hour urine collection 6 months after the initial visit indicated a significant reduction in urinary sodium excretion accompanied by a 6 mmHg reduction in systolic blood pressure. He will fol- low up again in 6 months for consideration of pharmacologic therapy.

Clinical Pearls

1. Individuals with prehypertension (120–139/80–89 mmHg) who have chronic kidney dis- ease or diabetes should consider antihypertensive drug therapy. Otherwise, lifestyle mod- ification is recommended as the initial approach for a period of 6 months to 1 year.
2. Even a small reduction in body weight (e.g., 10 pounds) reduces blood pressure in over- weight individuals. Weight reduction also has a beneficial effect on other cardiovascular risk factors such as blood lipids/lipoproteins.
3. Consider initiating drug treatment if lifestyle modification does not adequately manage blood pressure, or if the patient is thought to be a likely candidate for a future diagnosis of hypertension.

REFERENCES

1. ALLHAT officers and coordinators for the ALLHAT collaborative research group: Major outcomes in high-risk hypertensive patients randomized to angiotensin-converting enzyme inhibitor or calcium channel blocker vs. diuretic: The Antihypertensive and Lipid-Lowering Treatment of Prevent Heart Attack Trial. JAMA 288(23):2981–2997, 2002.
2. Nesbitt SD, Julius S: Prehypertension: A possible target for antihypertensive medication. Curr Hypertens Rep 2:356–361, 2000.
3. Chobanian AV, Bakris GL, Black HR, et al: National Heart, Lung, and Blood Institute Joint National Committee on Prevention, Detection, Evaluation, and Treatment of Blood Pressure; National High Blood Pressure Education: The Seventh Report of the Joint National Committee on Prevention, Detection, Evaluation, and Treatment of High Blood Pressure: the JNC VII report, JAMA 289(19):2560–2572, 2003.
4. Appel LJ, Moore TJ, Obarzanek E, et al: A clinical trial of the effects of dietary patterns on blood pressure (DASH). N Engl J Med 336:1117–1124, 1997.
5. Stamler J: Blood pressure and high blood pressure. Aspects of risk. Hypertension 18(3 suppl):I195–107, 1991.

Leigh Ann Ramsey, PharmD
Marion R. Wofford, MD, MPH

PATIENT 6

A 55-year-old man who is agitated, hypertensive, tachycardic, and hyperthermic

A 55-year-old man, disoriented and agitated, presents to the local emergency department with his wife. He becomes increasingly agitated in the waiting area and is unable to complete the necessary paperwork due to a hand tremor. His wife reports that he arrived at their home last evening "smelling of alcohol." She states that he has been anxious and irritated all day, and that he experienced two episodes of vomiting. She also noticed that he has been sweating most of the day. It was not until this evening that she became aware that he was having visual hallucinations, at which point she immediately brought him in for evaluation. The patient's wife provides a history of alcoholism and states he recently enrolled in a treatment program but did not complete it.

Physical Examination: Temperature 100.6°F, pulse 130, respirations 22, blood pressure 182/106. General: diaphoretic and pale. Neck: supple. Chest: clear to auscultation. Cardiac: regular rhythm without mumur, rub, or gallop. Abdomen: benign, no organomegaly. Extremities: no edema. Neurological: fine tremor at rest, level of consciousness full, not lethargic, pupils midsize and reactive, awake and confused, oriented to person only, responds to pain in all four extremities. Skin: not jaundiced.

Laboratory Findings: Electrolytes, BUN, creatinine, phosphorus, magnesium, calcium: normal. Lipid Panel: triglycerides 330; total cholesterol, low density lipoprotein (LDL), high density lipoprotein (HDL) normal. Arterial blood gases: normal. Creatine kinase: normal. Liver panel: ALT 82, AST 174. Amylase and lipase: normal. Coagulation studies: normal. Toxicologic screen: negative. Urinalysis: normal. Blood alcohol level (initial assessment) 179 mg/dl, blood alcohol level (2 hours after initial assessment) 105 mg/dl.

Question: What diagnosis best describes this symptom complex?

Diagnosis: Alcohol withdrawal syndrome

Discussion: Alcohol is the most widely abused drug throughout the world. Alcohol-use disorders are a significant cause of morbidity and mortality in the United States. More than 110 million people over the age of 12 are current alcohol users, with 22 million being alcohol abusers. Alcohol abuse is defined as a pattern of drinking resulting in health consequences, social problems, or both. Alcohol dependence, often referred to as alcoholism, is a disease in which the person exhibits abnormal alcohol-seeking behavior and loss of control over drinking. When a person who is dependent on alcohol stops drinking, withdrawal symptoms occur within 6 to 48 hours, peaking about 24 to 35 hours after the last drink. This is termed alcohol withdrawal syndrome (AWS) and may range in severity from mild to severe based on the complexity of symptoms.

Alcohol withdrawal syndrome can consist of a range of symptoms, from hand tremor to delirium tremens. In mild alcohol withdrawal, symptoms may include tremor, anxiety, nausea, vomiting, diaphoresis, hyperreflexia, and minor autonomic hyperactivity, which usually arise within 24 hours of the decrease or complete discontinuation of alcohol intake. Moderate alcohol withdrawal consists of symptoms the previously described; however, the patient may also exhibit hallucinations, which usually occur 24 hours to several days after cessation of drinking. Severe alcohol withdrawal is characterized by disorientation, agitation, hallucinations, and severe autonomic derangement. Severe alcohol withdrawal may progress to delirium tremens (DTs). The development of DTs is characterized by increasing disorientation, agitation, and autonomic stimulation with hypertension, tachycardia, and significant diaphoresis. This is a life-threatening condition, occurring in approximately 5% of alcoholic patients during withdrawal. In this state, motor activity is increased, and volume can be depleted which may lead to hyperthermia, with temperatures exceeding 104°F. Onset of DTs is not immediate, typically occurring 48 hours or more after last alcohol consumption. The development of seizures is a central nervous system complication that occurs in approximately 10% of adults during alcohol withdrawal, with 60% of these patients experiencing multiple seizures. A seizure may emerge at any level of severity of the alcohol withdrawal syndrome and is commonly the reason the patient seeks medical attention.

The initial assessment upon presentation to the emergency department includes a thorough history from the patient or family member to investigate the amount of alcohol consumed; the time since last drink; previous episodes of alcohol withdrawal; and any history of gastrointestinal bleeding, pancreatitis, hepatitis, or seizures. Vital signs demonstrating hypertension, tachycardia, tachypnea, and fever further support the diagnosis of alcohol withdrawal syndrome. A blood alcohol level should be obtained upon presentation to establish a baseline. A urine toxicology screen will assist in establishing the presence of other medications with a separate withdrawal syndrome. The chemistry panel is drawn to assess possible electrolyte disorders or acid-base derangements, and decreased blood glucose. Liver function tests are obtained, looking for parameters suggestive of hepatic dysfunction. A complete blood count may provide evidence of anemia, thrombocytopenia, leukopenia, or leukocytosis. Amylase and lipase levels are needed to evaluate for acute pancreatitis. A lipid panel, particularly the triglyceride level, provides insight as to this patient's risk for development of pancreatitis. Magnesium levels may decrease during alcohol withdrawal, and, therefore, should be included in the initial assessment. Given the symptom complex described by this patient and the results of the laboratory parameters obtained, the diagnosis of alcohol withdrawal syndrome is established.

The goal of pharmacologic management of alcohol withdrawal syndrome is to prevent the development of symptoms and seizures and the progression to delirium tremens. Benzodiazepines have been used in the treatment of alcohol withdrawal since the 1950s, and after many years of study, remain the mainstay of therapy. Benzodiazepines act upon the inhibitory GABA receptors, replacing the depressant effects of alcohol in the central nervous system. This therapeutic class has the ability to decrease autonomic stimulation, while preventing seizures during alcohol withdrawal. The choice of agents is dependent upon several factors, such as patient age or hepatic function. Longer-acting benzodiazepines, such as diazepam or chlordiazepoxide, may be more likely to prevent seizures while providing less breakthrough withdrawal symptoms. However, some patients may experience excess sedation. A shorter-acting agent, such as lorazepam, may be more appropriate in an elderly patient or in a patient with hepatic impairment.

Patients undergoing alcohol withdrawal may continue to experience autonomic hyperstimulation, including increased blood pressure, despite therapy with a benzodiazepine. Evidence suggests that the addition of a beta-adrenergic antagonist (beta blocker), such as atenolol or propranolol, may be effective in lowering the blood pressure and decreasing the heart rate in this setting. Clonidine, a centrally acting alpha$_2$-adrenergic agonist, is also an option for control of hypertension associated with alcohol withdrawal syndrome. Although beta-blockers and clonidine may decrease risk of cardiovascular sequelae associated with autonomic hyperstimulation, particularly hypertension, they do not prevent central nervous system complications, such as seizures. Therefore, a beta-blocker or clonidine is not recommended as monotherapy, but considered as an adjunct to benzodiazepine therapy.

In the acute management of alcohol withdrawal syndrome, one must consider administration of thiamine prior to intravenous fluid containing dextrose to prevent Wernicke's encephalopathy. Folate supplementation and addition of a multivitamin are recommended, given the poor nutritional status of most patients undergoing alcohol withdrawal. In addition to addressing these nutritional deficiencies in our patient, aggressive hydration was initiated. Pharmacologic intervention of intramuscular lorazepam, given four times daily and tapering over 7 days, was initiated. The patient's blood pressure remained greater than 170/105 mmHg, with a pulse of 120 despite benzodiazepine therapy. Atenolol therapy was initiated with subsequent control of his blood pressure and heart rate.

Clinical Pearls

1. Alcohol withdrawal syndrome may present with symptoms of tremor, anxiety, nausea, vomiting, diaphoresis, hyperreflexia, autonomic hyperactivity, hallucinations, seizures, and delirium tremens, depending on the severity of withdrawal.
2. Benzodiazepines are the mainstay in pharmacologic management of alcohol withdrawal syndrome, demonstrating efficacy in treating symptoms such as autonomic hyperactivity, as well as in preventing seizures and progression to delirium tremens.
3. Beta-adrenergic antagonists (beta-blockers) and clonidine, a centrally acting alpha$_2$-adrenergic agonist, are options for adjunctive therapy for blood pressure management in patients with alcohol withdrawal syndrome not responsive to therapy with a benzodiazepine.
4. Beta-blockers or clonidine are not recommended as monotherapy in alcohol withdrawal.

REFERENCES

1. Chang PH, Steinberg MB: Postoperative medical complications: Alcohol withdrawal. Med Clin North Am 85(5):1191–1212, 2001.
2. Olmedo R, Hoffman RS: Psychiatric emergencies: Withdrawal syndromes. Emerg Med Clin North Am 18(2):273–288, 2000.
3. Carromgtpm RM, Fiellin DA, O'Connor PG: Hazardous and harmful alcohol consumption in primary care. Arch Intern Med 159(15):1681–1689, 1999.
4. Myrick H, Anton RF: Treatment of alcohol withdrawal. Alcohol Health & Research World 22:38–43, 1998.
5. Mayo-Smith MF, Cushman P, Hill AJ, et al: American Society of Addiction Medicine, Committee on Practice Guidelines, Working Group on Pharmacological Management of Alcohol Withdrawal. Pharmacologic management of alcohol withdrawal: A meta-analysis and evidence-based practice guideline. JAMA 278(2):1–24, 1997.
6. Lieber CS. Medical disorders of alcoholism. N Engl J Med 333(16):1058–1065, 1995.

Kim G. Adcock, PharmD
Jimmy L. Stewart, MD

PATIENT 7

A 12-year-old girl with a mild elevation in blood pressure and frequent headaches

A 12-year-old girl is referred for elevation in blood pressure detected during a health fair at school. She complains of no other symptoms except for frequent headaches. Her mother reports heavy snoring by the child during sleep and occasional letters from school complaining of lack of energy and somnolence, which is interfering with her schoolwork. The child is not involved in any school or after-school sports activities and admits to spending significant time watching TV at night and on weekends. There is a family history of hypertension and diabetes.

Physical examination: Blood pressure 125/83 (95th percentile), pulse 80, height 5 feet 1 inch (75th percentile), weight 60.8 kg (95th percentile), BMI 25.3 (95th percentile). General: well developed, well-nourished obese adolescent who appears older than her stated age. Skin: acanthosis nigricans. HEENT: normal. Cardiac: regular rate and rhythm without murmur. Chest: clear. Abdomen: obese with very slight striae, nontender, nondistended, positive bowel sounds. Extremities: slightly limited range of motion in both hips.

Laboratory Findings: CBC: normal. Electrolytes, glucose, BUN, creatinine: normal. Total cholesterol 195 mg/dl, triglycerides 118 mg/dl, LDL-C 129 mg/dl, HDL-C 41 mg/dl (fasting).

Question: What is a major contributing factor to this patient's hypertension?

Diagnosis: Obesity

Discussion: Pediatric obesity is on the rise in the United States, with a dramatic increase since the 1970s. The prevalence of childhood obesity is estimated to be 13–14%, whereas approximately 25–30% of children are considered overweight. Obesity affects all racial and ethnic groups and all ages and sexes. However, it tends to be more prevalent among non-Hispanic African Americans and Mexican Americans than among non-Hispanic Caucasians.

Pediatric obesity is defined as a body mass index (BMI) at the 95th percentile or more according to age and sex. BMI measurements between the 85th and 95th percentile cutoffs are considered at risk values for becoming overweight. Because BMI changes during childhood and differs between boys and girls, age-and sex-specific reference data are necessary to interpret the measurement. In the above case example, the patient's weight and height were 60.8 kg and 1.549 meters, respectively. The calculated BMI was 25.3. Plotting this value on the Centers for Disease Control and Prevention (CDC) Body Mass Index-For-Age Percentiles Growth Chart places this patient at the 95th percentile, thereby giving her a diagnosis of obesity.

Weight gain in general is a result of an imbalance between energy input and output. Children who are obese, however, do not tend to consume more calories than normal-weight children. On the other hand, obese children do have an increase in the size and number of adipocytes.

Obesity in children can be associated with a hormonal or genetic defect, but the majority of cases appear to be environmental in nature. Obese children often have a family history of obesity, have normal mental function, are tall for their age (> 50th percentile), have advanced bone age and can have early onset puberty. Sedentary lifestyle has also been associated with obesity. Even though a family history of obesity was not elicited from this patient, she was in the 75th percentile for height, has an otherwise normal physical examination except for a slight decrease in range of motion in her hip, and has very limited physical activity.

Because pediatric obesity often begins early in life and may persist into adulthood contributing to adult morbidity and mortality, these children need to be evaluated further for other complications. For example, this patient presented with an elevated blood pressure and an abnormal lipid profile, two common consequences of obesity. Evidence correlates childhood obesity with increased risk of acquiring obesity-related medical conditions such as hypertension, diabetes mellitus, respiratory disease, orthopedic disorders, and psychological disorders. Obesity has also been related to an increased risk for dyslipidemia and coronary heart disease.

The mainstay of therapy for childhood obesity is identification of environmental factors that lead to obesity. In addition, the support of the patient and parents is crucial to implementing a successful plan of behavioral changes, weight control, and medical management. A general approach to therapy includes education, family involvement, positive reinforcement, and frequent follow-up appointments. Behavior modification should include identification of problem behaviors, developing an awareness of current eating habits and activity, implementing small permanent changes over time, and continued monitoring. These skills will assist in changing behavior and maintaining those changes.

Many children may benefit from a program of prolonged weight maintenance. Maintaining weight during growth (i.e., growth spurt of adolescence) can lead to effective weight reduction by gradually decreasing the BMI as the child grows in height. However, for those children with a secondary complication and a BMI of > 95th percentile, a weight-loss program may be more appropriate. Older children and adolescents with BMIs between the 85th and 95th percentile with a secondary complication should also institute a weight-loss program. This program should emphasize changes in eating habits and activity to achieve weight loss of approximately one pound per month. An appropriate weight goal to establish for obese children is a BMI of > 85th percentile. Several therapeutic approaches have been successful including individual diet counseling, an exercise prescription, diabetic exchange programs, and the "Traffic Light" program. For those patients with morbid obesity, a more aggressive approach may be tried with the protein-sparing modified fast diet. Surgical therapy and pharmacotherapy are not currently supported as appropriate treatment options for weight loss in children.

This patient's initial presentation with mild hypertension and abnormal lipid profile was concluded to be a consequence of her obesity. Based on her age, a BMI in the 95th percentile, and signs of obesity-related medical conditions, initiating a weight-loss program was deemed appropriate. She was prescribed dietary counseling and an appropriate exercise program with monthly follow-up appointments.

Clinical Pearls

1. Prevention is the best way to deal with pediatric obesity. Goals should be individualized based on race (ethnicity), age, and sex.
2. Diagnosis of childhood obesity is based on the BMI, which is now incorporated into the new CDC growth charts.
3. Due to the increased risk for obesity-related medical conditions in adolescence and adulthood, overweight children should be evaluated for other complications.
4. Identification of environmental factors that lead to obesity is crucial in designing a successful treatment plan.
5. Treatment plans should include an appropriate diet and exercise program. Drug therapy and surgery are not currently supported as appropriate treatment in pediatric obesity.

REFERENCES

1. Curran JS, Barness LA: Obesity. In Behrman RE, Kliegman RM, Jenson HB (eds): Nelson Textbook of Pediatrics, 16th ed. Philadelphia, W.B. Saunders, 2000.
2. Moran R: Evaluation and treatment of childhood obesity. Am Fam Physician 59:861–868, 1999.
3. Barlow SE, Dietz WH: Obesity evaluation and treatment: Expert committee recommendations. Pediatrics 102:e29, 1998.
4. Troiano RP, Flegal KM: Overweight children and adolescents: description, epidemiology and demographics. Pediatrics 101:497–504, 1998.
5. Epstein LH, Myers MD, Raynor HA, Saelens BE: Treatment of pediatric obesity. Pediatrics 101:554–570, 1998.
6. Dietz WH: Health consequences of obesity in youth: Childhood predictors of adult disease. Pediatrics 101:518–525, 1998.

George E. Habeeb, Jr., MD
Kimberly G. Harkins, MD

PATIENT 8

A 67-year-old woman with hypertension and headaches

A 67-year-old woman presents to a clinic for evaluation of uncontrolled hypertension. Although she has had hypertension for about 20 years, she has noticed that recently the readings obtained with her home monitor are much higher than usual. The patient has had headaches with these elevations in blood pressure. She does not use tobacco, alcohol, or nonsteroidal anti-inflammatory drugs. Two brothers have end-stage renal disease. She has been taking propranolol monotherapy for her hypertension for many years.

Physical Examination: Vital Signs: temperature 98.6°F, pulse 70, respiratory rate 18, blood pressure 210/90. General: obese. Neurologic: normal. Funduscopic: stage II hypertensive retinopathy. Neck: no goiter or bruits. Cardiac: normal. Chest: clear. Abdomen: soft, nontender, no audible bruits. Extremities: bilateral pitting ankle edema, normal pulses.

Laboratory Findings: Hemogram: hematocrit 34%. Electrolytes: normal; BUN 38 mg/dl, creatinine 2.9 mg/dl, glucose 130 mg/dl, thyroid stimulating hormone normal. Urinalysis: protein 100 mg/dl. Fasting lipid profile: total cholesterol 240 mg/dl, triglycerides 300 mg/dl, HDL cholesterol 37 mg/dl, LDL cholesterol 170 mg/dl. Renal ultrasonography: left kidney 8 cm long, right kidney 11.5 cm long.

Question: Why has the patient's blood pressure become difficult to control?

Diagnosis: Atherosclerotic renal artery stenosis

Discussion: Atherosclerosis is the most common cause of renal artery stenosis (RAS), a narrowing of the renal artery lumen of >60%. The anatomic lesion produces the pathophysiological response of renovascular hypertension. The prevalence of renovascular disease in the hypertensive population is about 10%. Renovascular hypertension and other causes of nephropathy may coexist, with a synergistic effect leading rapidly to renal insufficiency and failure. RAS generally affects patients older than 45 years, and men are affected more commonly than women. Patients may present with acute, severe, or refractory hypertension. As in this patient, previously well-controlled blood pressure may rapidly become quite severe.

Physical findings in patients with RAS may include hypertension, evidence of peripheral vascular disease, and systolic–diastolic abdominal bruits. Risk factors include dyslipidemia, tobacco use, and known atherosclerosis such as carotid artery disease, coronary artery disease, or peripheral arterial disease. Relapsing "flash" pulmonary edema, particularly in elderly patients, is an important clue suggesting ischemic nephropathy.

Stages of progression of renal arterial atherosclerosis include additional vascular lesions, decreased renal mass, decreased glomerular filtration rate (GFR), and renovascular hypertension (RVH). Lesions are at the aortic orifice or within the proximal third of the renal artery, and may progress gradually or rapidly to total occlusion. Some patients may present with acute renal failure 5 to 7 days after initiation of an angiotensin-converting enzyme (ACE) inhibitor. This clinical presentation suggests bilateral RAS or a solitary kidney with RAS, and is usually reversible with discontinuation of the ACE inhibitor.

Several noninvasive testing options are available for patients with a history and physical examination consistent with bilateral RAS. Renal nuclear imaging following administration of an ACE inhibitor demonstrates renal function and predicts ischemia, but sensitivity and specificity decrease with bilateral renal artery stenosis or renal parenchymal disease. Duplex Doppler ultrasonography of renal arteries can have a sensitivity and specificity of >90%, but the procedure is time-consuming, difficult in obese patients, and highly operator-dependent. Spiral computed tomographic angiography requires iodinated contrast with a risk of contrast nephropathy. With three-dimensional techniques, the sensitivity is 89% and the specificity is 84%. Magnetic resonance angiography (MRA) of renal arteries is safe and nontoxic to the kidneys. Sensitivity ranges from 87% to 100%; specificity is 97%.

The gold standard for diagnosing RAS is renal arteriography. Revascularization should be considered for better blood pressure control, and to potentially delay progression of renal insufficiency. Options for revascularization include percutaneous transluminal angioplasty (PTA) with stent placement and surgical aortorenal bypass. For ostial lesions, PTA alone has a 50% success rate; with stent placement the success rate is higher with stable-to-improved renal function in 66% to 96%. Restenosis rates are 10–18% in the first year. Even with successful revascularization, patients may require anti-hypertensive medications.

This patient had a renal arteriogram revealing a proximal left RAS of 85%, which was reversed to 10% by PTA with stent placement. One month after the procedure, her blood pressure was 160/90 mmHg and her creatinine level was 3.4 mg/dl. With medications including an angiotensin receptor blocker (ARB), loop diuretic, and beta-blocker, over the next 6 months her blood pressure improved to 140/80 mmHg.

In patients who are poor candidates for revascularization, medical management is an option. ACE inhibitors or ARBs in combination with diuretics are particularly effective. In two-kidney, unilateral RAS (a renin-dependent system), an ACE inhibitor produces the most dramatic effect, preserving function in the contralateral kidney while the ipsilateral kidney worsens with ischemic atrophy. In bilateral RAS or solitary-kidney RAS (a sodium-volume dependent system), an ACE inhibitor can precipitate acute renal failure (ARF). Other classes of drugs such as beta-blockers or calcium channel blockers can be useful add-on agents.

Clinical Pearls

1. Patients with resistant hypertension, renal insufficiency, and peripheral vascular disease are at risk for RAS and renovascular hypertension.
2. RAS is the anatomical narrowing of the arterial lumen; renovascular hypertension is the pathophysiological effect of the stenosis.
3. Underlying renal parenchymal disease can coexist with RAS and can produce persistent hypertension, even after revascularization.
4. In two-kidney unilateral RAS the ipsilateral kidney can develop ischemic nephropathy and the contralateral kidney can develop hypertensive nephrosclerosis.
5. Recurrent flash pulmonary edema in the elderly is a clue for and predictor of RAS.

REFERENCES

1. Muray S, Martin M, Amoedo ML, et al: Rapid decline in renal function reflects reversibility and predicts the outcome after angioplasty in renal artery stenosis. Am J Kidney Dis 39:60–66, 2002.
2. Alcazar JM, Rodicio JL: Ischemic nephropathy: Clinical characteristics and treatment. Am J Kidney Dis 36:883–893, 2000.
3. Tullis MJ, Caps MT, Zierler RE, et al: Blood pressure, antihypertensive medication, and atherosclerotic renal artery stenosis. Am J Kidney Dis 33:675–681, 1999.
4. Ghantous VE, Eisen TD, Sherman AH, Finkelstein FO: Evaluating patients with renal failure for renal artery stenosis with gadolinium-enhanced magnetic resonance angiography. Am J Kidney Dis 33:36–42, 1999.

Sara L. Noble, PharmD
Steve A. Watts, MD
Kimberly G. Harkins, MD

PATIENT 9

An 80-year-old woman with chronic knee pain

An 80-year-old woman with hypertension presents to a clinic with a complaint of bilateral knee pain, worse on the left. She has had pain in both knees for many years, and is often able to control her discomfort with acetaminophen. Her hypertension is well-controlled on enalapril, hydrochlorothiazide, and atenolol. At the time of her last clinic visit her blood pressure was 138/62 mmHg. For the past week she has been taking over-the-counter ibuprofen, up to 1000 mg daily.

Physical Examination: Temperature 96.2°F, pulse 80, respiratory rate 18, blood pressure 152/86. Height 5 feet 2 inches, weight 160 pounds, body mass index (BMI) 29. Funduscopic: normal. Lungs: clear bilaterally. Cardiac: regular rhythm; no gallops or murmurs. Abdomen: soft, nontender, no masses or bruits. Musculoskeletal: slight effusion of left knee, discomfort and crepitus with passive range of motion bilaterally. Neurological: normal.

Laboratory Findings: Hemogram: hematocrit 36%. Electrolytes, glucose: normal. BUN 20 mg/dl, creatinine 1.8 mg/dl.

Question: Why is her blood pressure now uncontrolled?

Diagnosis: The patient has uncontrolled hypertension related to nonsteroidal anti-inflammatory drug (NSAID) use.

Discussion: This patient's blood pressure has increased significantly since her last visit. The NSAID she is taking for her osteoarthritis could cause the elevated blood pressure. Meta-analyses of trials designed to evaluate the effect of NSAIDs on blood pressure control have confirmed an average increase in mean arterial pressure of 5.5 mmHg. The postulated mechanism of this increase in blood pressure is inhibition of prostaglandin synthesis.

Renal prostaglandins have several effects on blood pressure. Vascular smooth muscle is relaxed by prostacyclin (PGI_2), with resultant natriuresis through reduction of renal vascular resistance. Prostaglandin E2 (PGE2) can inhibit renal tubular reabsorption of sodium and chloride and tubular responsiveness to vasopressin. Intrarenal vasodilatory prostaglandins effectively diminish the renal response to vasoconstrictor stimuli such as angiotensin II and norepinephrine. NSAIDs can alter blood pressure and complicate the management of hypertension by blunting this counter-regulatory process, thereby increasing sodium reabsorption and water retention.

NSAIDs can affect the mechanism of action of thiazide and loop diuretics, beta-adrenergic blockers, alpha-adrenergic blockers, and angiotensin-converting enzyme (ACE) inhibitors. Calcium channel blockers and angiotensin II receptor antagonists are less susceptible to interaction with NSAIDs.

An alternative to nonselective NSAID use for arthritis pain is the use of COX-2 inhibitors: celecoxib, rofecoxib, and valdecoxib. Two distinct forms of the cyclooxygenase enzyme exist: COX-1 and COX-2. COX-1 mediates production of thromboxane and prostaglandins and is expressed in the gastrointestinal tract, kidneys, and platelets. It is postulated to play a significant role in normal renal function, gastric mucosal integrity, hemostasis, and certain hormonal responses. COX-2 is nearly undetectable in most tissues under normal physiologic conditions; however, expression of COX-2 increases during inflammatory responses. In theory, selective inhibition of the COX-2 isoform decreases inflammation while minimizing the risk of adverse effects. The effects of COX-2 inhibitors on blood pressure are not as well defined as those of nonselective NSAIDs, but are under investigation.

This patient was prescribed celecoxib, and encouraged to use acetaminophen if her pain was not well controlled. She was warned not to take other over-the-counter medications. At her 2-week follow up office visit she was pain free. Her blood pressure was improved with a reading of 139/82 mmHg. Due to the relief of pain, the celecoxib was discontinued and acetaminophen was recommended for recurring pain.

Clinical Pearls

1. Elderly patients with hypertension are at high risk for developing blood pressure increases with NSAID use.
2. The hypertensive effect of NSAIDs varies depending on the specific agent and the antihypertensive regimen.
3. Blood pressure should be monitored when an NSAID is used, particularly in patients treated with diuretics, beta-blockers, or ACE inhibitors.
4. Studies are investigating the risk of cardiovascular events in patients treated with COX-2 inhibitors.

REFERENCES

1. Whelton A, Fort JG, Puma JA, Normandin D: Cyclooxygenase-2-specific inhibitors and cardiorenal function: A randomized, controlled trial of celecoxib and rofecoxib in older hypertensive osteoarthritis patients. Am J Ther 8:85–95, 2001.
2. Perazella MA, Eras J: Are selective COX-2 inhibitors nephrotoxic? Am J Kidney Dis 35:937–940, 2000.
3. Grossman E, Messerli FH. Management of drug-induced and iatrogenic hypertension. In Izzo JL, Black H (eds). Hypertension Primer 2nd edition: The Essentials of High Blood Pressure. Baltimore, Lippincott, Williams, and Wikins, 1999.
4. Johnson A, Nguyen TV, Day DO: Do nonsteroidal anti-inflammatory drugs affect blood pressure? A meta-analysis. Ann Intern Med 121:289–300, 1994.
5. Pope JE, Anderson JJ, Felson DT: A meta-analysis of the effects of nonsteroidal anti-inflammatory drugs on blood pressure. Arch Intern Med 153:477–484, 1993.

PATIENT 10

A 52-year-old woman with a history of panic disorder

A 52-year-old woman has a 5-year history of panic disorder. The episodes have become increasingly severe, requiring admission to the emergency department on multiple occasions over the last 2 years. She admits that the panic attacks are likely related to stress. Her blood pressure during the panic attacks is elevated, but on follow-up with her primary care provider she was not found to be hypertensive. She was referred to psychiatry for further treatment after daily use of propranolol and lorazepam, taken as needed failed to control her symptoms. She denies night sweats, weight loss, constipation, and diarrhea. She has a sensation that her heart is racing during the episodes of panic. She has occasional headaches, which she attributes to stress. She is divorced, unemployed, and is caring for three children. Her mother died of complications from a stroke at the age of 40. Her sister had thyroid surgery.

Physical Examination: Pulse 80, blood pressure 135/80. BMI 35. General: obese, no apparent distress. HEENT: no lid lag. Neck: no goiter. Cardiovascular and neurological examinations normal. Extremities: no pedal edema, normal skin.

Laboratory Findings: Fasting plasma glucose 153 mg/dl, otherwise blood chemistries normal. Thyroid function tests normal.

Question: What form of secondary hypertension should be considered?

Answer: Consider pheochromocytoma.

Discussion: This patient has a number of symptoms that suggest the diagnosis of pheochromocytoma, yet she has been treated for a primary panic disorder for several years. The signs and symptoms of pheochromocytoma are related to the presence of excess catecholamines and may mimic other conditions resulting in misdiagnosis or delayed confirmation. Pheochromocytomas, although rare, may result in dramatic and devastating events. Further evaluation should be conducted if the diagnosis is even remotely possible.

The classic symptoms of headache, sweating, and palpitations suggest pheochromocytoma, although the presentation is variable. Only 48% of patients with these tumors have paroxysmal hypertension. Others have refractory hypertension or may be normotensive. There may be a history of a hypertensive response to beta-blockers, anesthesia, tricyclic antidepressants, metaclopramide, intra-arterial contrast media, or glucagon. Unexpected hypertension during pregnancy, surgery, invasive testing such as colonoscopy, or micturition should prompt the investigation for pheochromocytoma.

Patients with pheochromocytoma may be tremulous, nervous, anxious, or have a feeling of impending death. These symptoms may be paroxysmal or sustained. Hyperthyroidism may cause similar symptoms. The thyroid function studies were normal in this patient.

In addition to hypertension, this patient has hyperglycemia. Elevated fasting plasma glucose may be present, most commonly during paroxysms of catecholamine excess. The elevated glucose is related to low plasma insulin and stimulation of hepatic glucose output, both related to catecholamine excess. Other abnormalities of standard laboratory tests seen in pheochromocytoma include polycythemia, hypercalcemia, or evidence of mild dehydration.

The mother's history of a stroke and the sister's thyroid disease should not be dismissed as non-contributory. Familial syndromes account for 10–15% of pheochromocytomas. These are associated with von Hippel-Lindau (VHL) disease, multiple endocrine neoplasms (MEN), or neurofibromatosis. VHL disease is associated with tumors of the central nervous system or neuroendocrine system (including pheochromocytoma), or with renal cell carcinoma. The MEN type 2A syndrome is characterized by medullary thyroid carcinoma, parathyroid hyperplasia, and pheochromocytoma. von Recklinghausen's disease, neurofibromatosis, is associated with pheochromocytoma, and the presence of mucocutaneous lesions such as café au lait spots or neuromas is consistent with neurofibromatosis.

Biochemical testing to determine excess catecholamines should be conducted in this patient. Plasma-free metanephrines is the test of choice to exclude or confirm the presence of a pheochromocytoma. The use of 24-hour urinary catecholamine studies has a lower sensitivity, which may result in a false-negative result. In some patients, catecholamine secretion is episodic, so repeated measures of plasma metanephrines may be necessary. An oral clonidine suppression test may be used to determine whether the catecholamine excess is neurogenic in mediation. A glucagon stimulation test may be considered if there is high clinical suspicion for the presence of a pheochromocytoma, but biochemical assays of plasma and urine are not confirmatory. The clonidine suppression test and glucagon stimulation test are rarely needed.

The patient described did have an abdominal pheochromocytoma as demonstrated by ^{123}I-meta-iodobenzylguanidine scan (see Figure). Following a complicated perioperative period, she remains free of panic attacks 3 years after her surgery. She now has consistent and optimal control of her blood pressure with monotherapy.

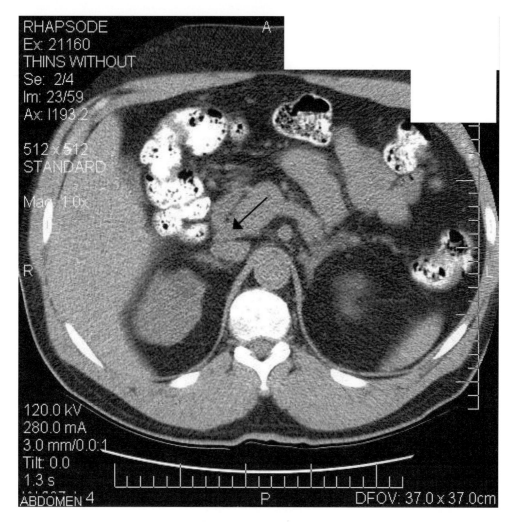

Clinical Pearls

1. The classic presentation of pheochromocytoma is paroxysmal hypertension, headaches, and diaphoresis, but there are a number of other symptoms and signs.
2. The signs and symptoms of this tumor result from catecholamine excess. Failure to consider this disease may result in devastating consequences such as stroke, myocardial dysfunction, or congestive heart failure.
3. Familial syndromes that are related to pheochromocytoma include von Hippel-Lindau disease, multiple endocrine neoplasms, and von Recklinghausen's neurofibromatosis.
4. Plasma-free metanephrines is the test of choice to exclude or confirm the presence of a pheochromocytoma.

REFERENCES
1. Lenders JW, Pacak K, Walther MM, et al: Biochemical diagnosis of pheochromocytoma: Which test is best? JAMA. 287(11):1427–34, 2002.
2. Bravo EL: Evolving concepts in the pathophysiology, diagnosis, and treatment of pheochromocytoma. Endocr Rev 15(3):356–368, 1994.
3. Neumann HP, Berger DP, Sigmund G, et al: Pheochromocytomas, multiple endocrine neoplasia type 2, and von Hippel-Lindau disease. N Engl J Med 329(21):1531–1538, 1993.

Joseph W. Blackston, MD, JD
Marion R. Wofford, MD, MPH

PATIENT 11

A 41-year-old man with poor medical adherence

A 41-year-old man presents to the outpatient clinic with only vague symptoms of palpitations and diaphoresis for the last 2 days. He reports a history of "blood pressure" problems for several years. He is unsure of the names of his medications but one is taken three times a day. He does not have a primary care physician, and his last medical encounter was a few months ago in the local emergency department for a minor trauma. At that time he was prescribed the same "blood pressure pills" that he had taken for the last year and advised to seek the care of a primary care provider.

The patient denies visual disturbance, shortness of breath, dyspnea, or chest pain. There have been no neurologic abnormalities with the exception of the headache. Past medical history is otherwise negative, and there is a family history of hypertension, diabetes mellitus, and premature cardiac disease. The patient drinks beer on weekends, but he does not smoke cigarettes. He works intermittently as a painter.

After consulting his pharmacist the medication regimen was found to be hydrochlorothiazide 12.5 mg a day and clonidine 0.2 mg three times daily.

Physical Examination: Temperature 98.9°F, pulse 96 and regular, respiratory rate 14, blood pressure 180/100. General: well-developed, well-nourished, slightly diaphoretic, alert, in no distress. HEENT: pupils equal, 5 mm, reactive, funduscopic without papilledema; arteriovenous nicking noted. Neck: supple, normal jugular venous pressure, no thyromegaly. Chest: clear. Cardiac: heart sounds normal, no murmur, no gallop. Abdomen: benign. Extremities: no clubbing, cyanosis, or edema. Neurologic: without focal deficit.

Laboratory Findings: Hemoglobin normal, blood chemistries normal. Creatinine 1.6 mg/dl. Urinalysis 1+ protein. EKG: left axis deviation with left ventricular hypertrophy. Sinus Mechanism: no ST elevation or T-wave inversion.

Question: What is the most likely etiology of this man's elevated blood pressure?

Diagnosis: Rebound hypertension

Discussion: This patient may be experiencing "rebound hypertension" secondary to medical nonadherence with clonidine. However, his medical history suggests that his hypertension is likely to be under-treated and longstanding. The patient's creatinine level, urinalysis results, and EKG are more consistent with hypertension of a lengthy duration. He does exhibit some physical signs of increased sympathetic activity, which are seen with rebound hypertension or "antihypertensive withdrawal syndrome." Manifestations of the acute withdrawal syndrome classically include diaphoresis, blood pressure elevation (occasionally greater than pre-treatment levels), agitation or anxiety, and tachycardia.

Clonidine is a centrally acting alpha-adrenergic agonist. By stimulation of pre-synaptic alpha-2 receptors in the central nervous system (CNS), it reduces systemic blood pressure via decreasing vascular sympathetic tone. Clonidine readily crosses the blood brain barrier and is known for CNS side effects such as drowsiness, occurring in up to a third of patients. It is short acting in the oral formulation, but transdermal forms are available, applied once weekly. The transdermal patch enhances compliance for obvious reasons, but is relatively costly, with no generic transdermal delivery form currently available. Generic oral clonidine is very inexpensive, which is probably why it was prescribed in this patient.

Rebound hypertension, also known as "antihypertensive (or acute) withdrawal syndrome" (AWS) or "overshoot hypertension," is probably overdiagnosed as a clinical entity. The syndrome is associated with elevated blood pressure in excess of pre-treatment levels generally with increased sympathetic CNS activity. Clinically, these patients can present with tachycardia, sweating, and anxiousness. Because clonidine acts to reduce sympathetic tone centrally, abrupt cessation of therapy with this drug has been linked to cases of rebound hypertension, ostensibly via increased norepinephrine secretion in response to prior suppression by the drug. Many other agents, including methyldopa (an analog of clonidine) and beta-blockers, especially the shorter-acting forms, are associated with the rebound hypertension phenomenon. Abrupt cessation of therapy when clonidine and beta-blockers are used together is associated with a significant incidence of acute withdrawal syndrome.

True rebound hypertension is unlikely at low doses, but the incidence increases with a larger total daily dose. The risk of rebound hypertension also increases in cases where clonidine and beta-blockers are used concomitantly, occasionally seen at moderate doses of each. There is seldom a need for prescribing central-acting alpha agonists for hypertension management, since the development of more favorable medications including angiotensin-converting enzyme inhibitors, angiotensin receptor blockers agents, long-acting calcium channel and beta-blockers. Cost appears to be the major reason for the use of clonidine, and was likely the reason it was prescribed for this patient. Current hypertension guideline recommendations do not indicate these drugs for routine first-line use, although methyldopa still remains a common agent for pregnant patients or women of child-bearing age, because of its well-known safety profile in pregnancy.

Treatment for antihypertensive withdrawal syndrome or rebound hypertension is generally simple. Blood pressure generally responds to re-institution of the previous antihypertensive agent, where it is known. Aggressive measures to lower the blood pressure are rarely needed. Labetalol, because of its alpha-and beta-receptor properties, is also a useful and safe initial form of treatment, especially if the patient's medication regimen cannot be readily identified.

Although the patient presented in this case could not recall the name of the medication he had been prescribed, the dosing regimen and the clinical picture are consistent with rebound hypertension due to clonidine withdrawal. Clinicians must consider this diagnosis in patients with such presentations to effectively manage the blood pressure.

Clinical Pearls

1. Withdrawal syndrome can occur with rapid cessation of clonidine.
2. True antihypertensive withdrawal syndrome is marked by elevation of blood pressure above pre-treatment levels, and by increased sympathetic activity.
3. Incidence of withdrawal syndrome increases with dose. Small or starting doses are much less likely to result in withdrawal syndrome.
4. Treatment is with re-institution of the discontinued agent or labetalol.

REFERENCES

1. Kaplan NM, Rose BD: Withdrawal syndromes with antihypertensive therapy. UpToDate online; Version 10.2, 2002.
2. Morrison AR: Hypertension. The Washington Manual of Medical Therapeutics, 30th ed. New York, Lippincott, 2001.
3. Chobanian AV, Bakris GL, Black HR, et al: National Heart, Lung, and Blood Institute Joint National Committee on Prevention, Detection, Evaluation, and Treatment of Blood Pressure; National High Blood Pressure Education: The Seventh Report of the Joint National Committee on Prevention, Detection, Evaluation, and Treatment of High Blood Pressure: the JNC VII report, JAMA 289(19):2560–2572, 2003.
4. Metz SA, Klein C, Morton N: Rebound Hypertension after Discontinuation of Transdermal Clonidine Therapy. Am J Med 82:17, 1986.
5. Houston, MC: Abrupt cessation of treatment in hypertension: Consideration of clinical features, mechanisms, prevention, and management of the discontinuation syndrome. Am Heart J 102:415, 1981.

Alexander Zubkov, MD, PhD
Marion R. Wofford, MD, MPH

PATIENT 12

A 62-year-old man with right-sided weakness

A 62-year-old man was found in a public parking lot and brought to the emergency department. The patient was having sudden difficulty speaking and acute right-sided weakness had developed. His past medical history was pertinent for hypertension.

Physical Examination: Blood pressure 230/100. Neurological: reactive pupils 3 mm each eye; right-sided facial weakness, associated with right hemiparesis more pronounced in the right upper extremity, somnolence, left gaze preference, dysarthria with preserved comprehension. Babinski reflex on the right.

Laboratory Findings: CT head scan: 3.5 × 3.5 cm hyperdensity located lateral to thalamus in the region of extreme capsule, with some effacement of right lateral ventricle (see figure).

Question: What is the etiology of this patient's right-sided weakness?

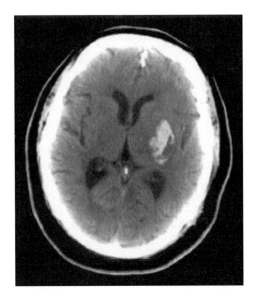

Discussion: Fifteen to thirty percent of all strokes are spontaneous intracerebral hemorrhages (ICHs). More than 50% of the patients die and one half of survivors are left severely disabled. The incidence is higher in African Americans and individuals of asian descent as compared to Caucasians. Risk factors include age, hypertension, history of coronary artery disease, previous strokes, cigarette smoking, and alcohol consumption.

ICH due to chronic hypertension accounts for about one half of the cases. The underlying pathology is the hemodynamic injury to perforating arteries, which arise directly from the large cerebral arteries at right angles. Those arteries include lenticulostriate arteries, thalamoperforating arteries, and paramedian perforating arteries originating from the basilar artery, as well as superior and anterior-inferior cerebellar arteries. The pathological changes in these arteries include hyalinosis, lipohyalinosis or focal necrosis and Charcot-Bouchard (miliary) aneurysm formation.

In a series reported by Weiner, locations of hypertensive ICHs were as follows: 65% were in the basal ganglia, 15% were in the subcortical white matter, 10% were cerebellar, and 10% were pontine. A number of other conditions are known to cause ICH: coagulopathies, cerebral amyloid angiopathy, abuse of illicit drugs (cocaine, amphetamine, phencyclidine, and phenylpropanolamine).

The clinical presentation of ICH usually depends on the location of hemorrhage:

- Hemorrhage in the **basal ganglia** usually presents with initial loss of consciousness, followed by hemiparesis, hemianesthesia, hemianopia, aphasia, or impaired awareness of disorder, as seen in this patient.
- Symptoms of **lobar** ICH depend on location of the hemorrhage, but the majority of lobar ICHs occur in parietal lobes and present with hemiparesis and hemianopia, associated with aphasia or neglect (depending on the side of the lesion).
- **Pontine** hemorrhage usually presents with coma, followed by hemi/quadriparesis and disconjugate gaze.
- **Cerebellar** hemorrhage usually begins abruptly with vomiting and severe ataxia. It is usually accompanied by paralysis of conjugate lateral gaze on one side. These symptoms might not be accompanied by loss of consciousness unless there is compression of the brainstem. Hemiparesis might not be present.

It is important to establish the underlying etiology of ICH. A history of hypertension, drug abuse, or coagulopathy/anticoagulant treatment are important factors.

A CT scan is a rapid and widely available test that can demonstrate blood as a high density image immediately after hemorrhage. Clot volume can be estimated by a modified ellipsoid volume $(a \times b \times c)/2$, where a, b, and c are the diameters of the clot in the three dimensions. Routine laboratory evaluation should include coagulation studies. Magnetic resonance imaging is gaining popularity in the initial evaluation of ICH, but it is not yet universally available around the clock. MRI is not only sensitive to early hemorrhage, but also can reveal causes of a hemorrhage, such as arteriovenous malformation or tumor. Cerebral angiography should be performed if there is any suspicion of vascular lesion, as in the case of ICH with subarachnoid hemorrhage.

It is still controversial whether ICH should be managed medically only or with surgical removal of hematoma. Surgical intervention is not indicated in the cases of ICH when the hemorrhage is very small and does not cause major deficits, or opposite a very large hemorrhage, which is associated with very poor neurological status of the patient.

Medical management of this patient should include the following:

1. Blood pressure management. Blood pressure is always significantly elevated in patients with ICH. This might be a result of previous poorly controlled hypertension or a secondary rise of blood pressure due to increased intracranial pressure (Cushing response). Increased blood pressure will increase risks for rebleeding/extending of the hemorrhage and subsequent deterioration of the patient. Severely increased blood pressure should be managed with intravenous nitroprusside in intensive care units. It is very important to maintain blood pressure at the level of the patient's baseline, otherwise relative hypotension might cause ischemic changes. In addition, over-treatment might compromise cerebral perfusion pressure (CPP = MBP–ICP), which would also cause ischemic changes in the brain. It has been suggested that the mean arterial pressure should be reduced to premorbid level if known or by approximately 20% if unknown. In addition, patients should be treated with beta-blockers, Calcium channel-blockers, or ACE inhibitors for long-term management of hypertension.

2. Increased intracranial pressure management. Mannitol (1 g/kg) is very useful in reducing brain edema in some patients. No benefit has been demonstrated from the use of steroids in ICH.

3. Surgical treatment. Ongoing studies are evaluating the benefits of surgical versus conservative medical management. Patients with (1) clot volume between 20 and 80 mg; (2) superficial/lobar hemorrhages; and (3) worsening conscious/neurological deficits should be considered a candidates for the surgical treatment. Surgical options consist of conventional craniotomy, stereotactic aspiration through a burr hole, and endoscopic surgery.

Clinical Pearls

1. Acute onset of headache, nausea/vomiting, loss of consciousness, and hemiparesis are early signs of ICH.
2. Blood pressure management is the key in the medical management of such patients. Mean arterial pressure should be reduced to the premorbid level if known, or by approximately 20% if unknown.
3. There is still controversy over the benefits of surgical evacuation of the clot. It is probably indicated in the cases of acute deterioration of the patient's level of consciousness or neurological examination.

REFERENCES

1. Siddique MS, Mendelow AD: Surgical treatment of intracerebral hemorrhage. Br Med Bull 56:444–456, 2000.
2. Wolf PA: Epidemiology of intracerebral hemorrhage. In Kase CS, Caplan LR (eds.) Intracerebral Hemorrhage. Boston, Butterworth-Heinemann, 1994.
3. Weiner H, Cooper P: The management of spontaneous intracerebral hemorrhage. Contemp Neurosurg 14:1–8, 1992.

PATIENT 13

A 54-year-old man with primary hypertension and poor
lifestyle choices

A 54-year-old man with a 3-year history of hypertension treated with a combination beta-blocker and thiazide diuretic (bisoprolol/hydrochlorothiazide 5/6.25 mg, two pills daily) comes in to discuss other options for managing his blood pressure. Although the medication does keep his blood pressure under control, he notes that he is fatigued much of the time and has some sexual dysfunction, both of which began when he started on medication. He would like to get off all medications and wants to know if and how he can accomplish this goal.

He gives a history of a 20-pound weight gain prior to the onset of hypertension. He has smoked a pack of cigarettes a day for the past 30 years, but has recently quit and is worried about additional weight gain. Once an avid participant in sports activities, he admits that he has not engaged in any physical activity for the past several years because of the stress of his job and raising teenagers. He skips breakfast and consumes five or more cups of coffee instead, eats fast food most days for lunch, and he and his family eat out at least twice a week at "family style" restaurants to save time. He drinks moderately during the week (two beers per night or two shots of scotch), but he does binge drink (12–15 beers) at least one weekend and smokes one half pack of cigarettes per day. He has never had his cholesterol checked but does report that his father is now taking cholesterol-lowering medication. Both of his parents are on blood pressure medication. His grandfather died of a stroke at age 62.

Physical Examination: Temperature 98.4°F, pulse 78, respiratory rate 16, blood pressure both arms 134/86 sitting, 140/88 standing, height 6 feet, weight 205 pounds, BMI 29, waist circumference 42 inches Eyes: normal funduscopic findings. Neck: thyroid normal. Lungs: clear. Cardiac: normal. Abdomen: obese. Neurological: normal. Extremities: no edema.

Laboratory Findings: Hemogram, blood chemistry, urinalysis and microalbuminuria, thyroid and uric acid test results all normal. Lipids: total cholesterol 241, HDL 41, triglycerides 300, LDL 140. EKG: nonspecific ST-T changes.

Question: What lifestyle interventions might be successful in reducing the dosage of medication or stopping pharmacotherapy in this gentleman?

Topic: Hypertension well-controlled on pharmacotherapy, but inadequate self-care practices

Discussion: Lifestyle modifications that reduce blood pressure are advocated in all major guidelines. For example, the Joint National Commission (JNC) on Prevention, Detection, Evaluation and Treatment of High Blood Pressure calls for lifestyle intervention in four explicit circumstances: (1) as a way to prevent hypertension, (2) as initial therapy in newly diagnosed hypertensive patients, (3) as adjuvant therapy in persons on antihypertensive medications, and (4) as a way to facilitate medication cessation or step-down in persons with well-controlled hypertension who are on pharmacological therapy. Clearly this patient could benefit from lifestyle modification to accomplish medication step-down or cessation in concert with his goals. The recommended behaviors include:

- Weight loss for those who are overweight or obese,
- Moderate physical activity on most days of the week,
- Reduced intake of dietary sodium to < 100 mmol/day (2.4 g/day),
- adopting a diet rich in fruits, vegetables, and low-fat dairy products,
- reducing dietary intake of saturated fat, total fat, and cholesterol,
- moderation of daily alcohol intake to no more than two drinks for men and one for women, and
- smoking cessation.

The evidence is mounting that supports potassium supplementation. Available evidence is less clear regarding calcium and magnesium supplementation, intake of fish oil, and stress management. Table 1 provides a brief summary of the clinical trial findings from normotensive and hypertensive trials of these targeted interventions. Despite high recidivism for lifestyle modifications and few trials examining long-term effects on clinical cardiovascular events, there is some support for sustained risk factor reduction despite recidivism several years postintervention. These data support the importance of systematic attention to lifestyle management in clinical practice.

Multiple studies indicate that even modest adult weight gain may increase the occurrence of hypertension, whereas weight loss substantially decreases this risk. A recent review of lifestyle factors in the treatment of hypertension concludes that the most promising intervention appears to be weight loss for overweight persons. An approximate 10-pound reduction in weight affords a blood pressure reduction of 7.2/5.9 mmHg. Findings from the TONE (Trial of Nonpharmacologic Interventions in the Elderly) study are particularly instructive for the patient in this case. Those assigned to the weight loss intervention lost more weight and a larger percentage remained free of blood pressure elevation >150/90 mmHg, resumption of antihypertensive medication or a blood pressure–related clinical complication up to 30 months after attempted withdrawal of medication.

An overall healthy eating pattern with minimal-to-moderate alcohol intake is important to preventing and controlling hypertension. Results

Table 1.   Impact of Lifestyle Interventions on Blood Pressure in Normotensive and Hypertensive Adults: Results from Aggregate and Meta-analyses of Short Term Trials*

Intervention	Normotensive Trials		Hypertensive Trials	
	Targeted Change (Median or Mean)	Change in SBP/DBP	Targeted Change	Change in SBP/DBP
Sodium reduction (2.4 g/day)	−100 mmol/day	−2.3/−1.4	−100 mmol/day	−5.8/−2.5
Weight loss	−4.5 kg	−2.0/−2.0	−4.5 kg	−7.2/5.9 kg
Alcohol reduction	−2.0 drinks/day	−2.9/−2.6	−2.7 drinks/day	−4.6/−2.3
Exercise	Habitual	−7.0/ −5.8	3 times/week	−10.3/ −7.5
Dietary patterns	DASH diet	−5.5/−3.0	DASH diet	−11.4/−5.5
Potassium increase	+75mmol/day	−1.8/1.0	>3 g/day	−5.5/−3.5
Fish oil	>3 g/day	−1.0/−0.5	>3 g/day	−5.5/−3.5
Calcium increase	−1.0 g/day	−0.5/−0.3	1.0 g/day	−1.7/0.0

*Note that extent of blood pressure change from each intervention should not be compared because the participants, the type and duration of intervention, and the basic design of the trials differed substantially.

Adapted from Miller EG, Erlinger TP, Young DR, et al: Lifestyle changes that reduce blood pressure: Implementation in clinical practice. J Clin Hypertens 1:191–198, 1999; with permission.

SBP = Systolic blood pressure, DBP = diastolic BP, DASH = Dietary Approaches to Stop Hypertension.

of the Dietary Approaches to Stop Hypertension (DASH and DASH sodium) studies support this notion. Persons with hypertension who ate a diet rich in fruits and vegetables and low-fat dairy products, and low in saturated fats over an 8-week study period reduced their systolic blood pressure by 11.4 mmHg and diastolic blood pressure by 5.5 mmHg over the control diet group. Sodium restriction, in combination with the DASH diet resulted in an 11.5 mmHg decline in blood pressure in patients with hypertension and also lowered blood pressure in normotensives. Sodium reduction, especially for salt-sensitive groups, and increased intake of dietary potassium, especially for those with a normal-high sodium intake, may be important public health benefits. Restriction of saturated fat to < 7% of calories and < 200 mg/day of dietary cholesterol are also recommended for elevated lipoprotein levels. In hypertensive persons who are heavy drinkers, a two to three drink/day reduction in alcohol consumption can contribute 4.6/-2.3 mmHg reduction in blood pressure. Medium-to-high intensity dietary counseling interventions are most likely to produce the greatest behavioral change.

Increased physical activity can lower blood pressure. Specific recommendation regarding the quantity and type of physical activity anticipated to bring about positive health effects remains unclear although all frequencies, intensities, and types of activity lower blood pressure. An early estimate from aggregated data analyses indicates that the mean reduction in SBP/DBP among patients with hypertension who engage in such moderate physical activity over most days of the week is 10/7 mmHg. More recent evidence moderates this effect with a still impressive 4/3 reduction even in persons whose mean body mass indices are in the normal range.

Although it is difficult to sort out the individual effects of a given risk factor, recent evidence indicates that smoking approximately doubles the cardiovascular risk resulting from an increased systolic blood pressure. Activation of the sympathetic nervous system is the most likely mechanism, coupled with effects on left ventricular geometry and large artery intima-medial thickness and elasticity. Interestingly, the effects of smoking seem to be reversible and the quantity of smoking does not influence the degree of excess risk among smokers. Despite these potentially positive benefits, health care providers continue to miss many opportunities to counsel on smoking cessation.

Implementing lifestyle modifications in routine health care practice still falls short of the goal. Less than one half of all physicians provide lifestyle advice, despite its recognized benefit in motivating reticent patients to initiate behavioral changes. Most international organizations and individual risk factor guidelines in the United States advocate the assessment of composite cardiac risk as an initial step in the prevention and management of hypertension.

Risk assessment provides a tool for healthcare-provider counseling and intervention with patients who agree to embark on lifestyle therapy. Using a one page in-office questionnaire to assess patient readiness to change with counseling targeted to "stage" of readiness has demonstrated benefit (see Table 2).

Table 2. Patient's Motivational Readiness to Make Lifestyle Changes: Prochaska's "Stages of Change" Model

Level	Definition	Counseling
Precontemplation	Not intending to change	Brief advice on recommended changes
Contemplation	Intending to change, but none made	Brief advice on recommended changes with discussion of barriers/facilitators
Preparation	Making some lifestyle changes, but inconsistently	Detailed education and set specific, measurable goals. Written contract.
Action	Making lifestyle changes and meeting goals for < 6 months	Continued monitoring and revision of written contract to incorporate multiple changes
Maintenance	Have made lifestyle changes and maintained for > 6 months	Continued supportive counseling

Adapted from Prochaska JO, DiClemente CC: Stages and processes of self change in smoking: Towards an integrative model of change. J Consult Clin Psychol 51:390–395, 1983, with permission.

Recognizing the difficulties associated with multiple lifestyle changes, this gentleman and his health care provider identified a staged approach to modifying his treatment regimen based on his readiness to change specific behaviors and his cardiovascular risk estimates. According to the Framingham Risk model, this patient has a 25% 10-year risk for coronary artery disease. Priority was placed on weight loss to reduce his blood pressure and improve his lipid profile. A weight loss goal of 3 pounds/month and an LDL goal of < 100 mg/dl was set. A nutritionist was consulted for sodium and caloric restriction, and the patient initiated a 2.4 sodium DASH diet with total saturated fat < 7 % of calories and cholesterol < 200 mg/day. He and his family negotiated a shared exercise program, identifying several targets and associated rewards for achieving weight loss goals. After three months, he had lost 15 pounds and his LDL level had improved (130 mg/dl). His triglyceride level was now 250 mg/dl and his total cholesterol was 220 mg/dl with a mild increase in HDLs to 42 mg/dl. His blood pressure was now 124/80 mmHg and his dose of antihypertensive was reduced to one pill daily of bisoprolol/hydrochlorothiazide 5/6.25 mg.

Encouraged by his significant progress, he was ready to initiate the next lifestyle modification. He selected reduction in alcohol intake with a goal of no more than two beers per day. Over the next 6 months, he was able to sustain his overall dietary changes, continue with moderate exercise 3–4 days/week, and reduce his binge drinking to six beers on one weekend per month. His blood pressure remained stable and a trial cessation of all antihypertensive medications was initiated. Within another 2 months he stopped smoking. Over the next year, he gradually reduced his alcohol intake to consistently moderate levels. Eighteen months after initiating lifestyle changes, his blood pressure off all antihypertensive medications was 128/82 and his lipids levels were normalized with an LDL of 110. His 10-year cardiovascular risk reassessed at < 10%. His weight remained stable at 185 pounds with a BMI of 25, and his waist circumference measured 36 inches.

Clinical Pearls

1. Risk factor assessment by using a Framingham-based assessment tool is an important component of managing primary hypertension.
2. Lifestyle modification can reduce or eliminate the need for pharmacotherapy in some individuals.
3. Weight loss is the greatest contributor to reducing blood pressure.
4. Primary care providers play an important role in motivating and counseling lifestyle changes.
5. The "Stages of Change" model and written contracts or prescriptions with specific, attainable, realistic, measurable targets can be used to enhance adherence to lifestyle modifications.

REFERENCES

1. Pignone MP, Ammerman A, Fernandez RD, et al: Counseling to promote a healthy diet in adults: A summary of the evidence for the US Preventive Services Task Force. Am J Prev Med 24:75–92, 2003.
2. Blumenthal JA, Sherwood A, Gullett EDC, et al: Biobehavioral approaches to the treatment of essential hypertension. J Consult Clin Psych. 70:569–589, 2002.
3. Khalili P, Nilsson PM, Nilsson JA, Berglund G: Smoking as a modifier of the systolic blood pressure induced risk of cardiovascular events and mortality—a population-based prospective study of middle-aged men. J Hypertens 20:1759–1764, 2002.
4. Whelton SP Chin A, Xin X, He J. Effect of aerobic exercise on blood pressure: A meta-analysis of randomized, controlled trials. Ann Intern Med 136:493–503, 2002.
5. Executive summary of The Third Report of the National Cholesterol Education Program (NCEP) Expert Panel on Detection, Evaluation, and Treatment of High Blood Cholesterol In Adults (Adult Treatment Panel III). JAMA 285:2486–2497, 2001.
6. Sacks FM, Svetkey LP, Vollmer WM, et al: A clinical trial of the effects on blood pressure of reduced dietary sodium and the DASH dietary pattern (the DASH Sodium Trial). N Engl J Med, 344:3–10, 2001.
7. He J, Whelton PK, Apel LH, et al. Long term effects of weight loss and dietary sodium reduction on incidence of hypertension. Hypertension 35:544–549, 2000.
8. Chobanian AV, Bakris GL, Black HR, et al: National Heart, Lung, and Blood Institute Joint National Committee on Prevention, Detection, Evaluation, and Treatment of Blood Pressure; National High Blood Pressure Education: The Seventh Report of the Joint National Committee on Prevention, Detection, Evaluation, and Treatment of Blood Pressure: the JNC VII report, JAMA 289(19):2560–2572, 2003.

PATIENT 14

A 16-year-old boy with hypertension

A 16-year-old boy was found during a school physical to have a blood pressure of 160/100. Subsequent evaluation reveals his sister was diagnosed with hypertension at age 14, his father remains hypertensive despite treatment with four antihypertensive agents, and his paternal grandmother had hypertension and died of a stroke at age 45. He has no significant medical history, and review of systems is negative.

Physical Examination: Temperature 98.2°F, pulse 72, blood pressure 164/102, respiratory rate 16. General: well-developed, well-nourished adolescent appearing his stated age; no apparent distress. Chest: clear. Cardiac: no heave, point of maximum intensity not displaced, normal S_1 and S_2, no S_3 or S_4, no murmurs, no thrill, no jugular venous distension. Abdomen: normal bowel sounds, no organomegaly. Extremities: no edema. Skin: normal facial and axillary hair. Genitourinary: Tanner Stage V.

Laboratory Findings: WBC 8000/μl with normal differential. Hct 52%; sodium 130 mmol/L, chloride 106 mmol/L, bicarbonate 25 mmol/L, potassium 3.1 mmol/L, BUN 12 mg/dl, creatinine 0.9 mg/dl, glucose 100 mg/dl. Upright plasma aldosterone level 1410 pmol/L (normal, 140 to 1110 pmol/L), plasma renin activity decreased.

Question: What pharmaceutical agent would be most likely to lower his blood pressure to normal?

Answer: Dexamethasone

Discussion: Glucocorticoid-remediable aldosteronism (GRA) is a rare, autosomal dominant cause of early-onset hypertension. It is sometimes accompanied by hypokalemia with an inappropriately elevated kaluresis, hyperaldosteronism, and decreased plasma renin levels. Elevated levels of 18-hydroxycortisol and 18-oxocortisol in plasma urine are diagnostic of the condition. It is not known why some family members who carry their family's mutation do not express all the signs of the disorder.

The condition was first described in a father and son who had hypertension, low plasma renin activity, and increased aldosterone secretion that could be reduced by the administration of dexamethasone. Several similar families have subsequently been investigated. Hemorrhagic stroke is particularly common in patients with GRA, often due to rupture of a berry aneurysm. In this case-study family, three generations are affected by early-onset or refractory hypertension, and one affected member had a cerebrovascular accident.

The underlying etiology is a fusion gene product that contains DNA sequences from both the aldosterone synthase gene (*CYP11B2*) and the steroid 11β-hydroxylase gene (*CYP11B1*). These genes are adjacent to each other on the long arm of chromosome 8 with *CYP11B2* lying 5′ to *CYP11B1*, separated by only 30 to 45 kb of DNA. There is about 95% sequence similarity in the coding regions of the two genes, with some differences being found in the 5′ regulatory sequences and other differences in exon 5 being responsible for substrate specificity. Unequal crossing over during meiosis produces a fusion gene that contains the *CYP11B1* sequence at the 5′ end and *CYP11B2* sequence at the 3′ end. The fusion gene product is located between normal copies of *CYP11B2*, located 5′ to the fusion gene, and *CYP11B1*, located 3′ to the fusion gene. All chimeric genes identified so far contain a break point located downstream of exon 2 and upstream of exon 5. *In vivo* expression studies of DNA constructs have confirmed that this region is responsible for substrate specificity.

Expression of the fusion gene product is under the control of adrenocorticotropic hormone (ACTH) and suppressible by glucocorticoids. Once the "gain of function" mutation is established, the chromosome containing the three genes undergoes duplication and division during meiosis as all other chromosomes do, leading to the autosomal dominant transmission pattern seen in affected families. DNA testing for the fusion gene has allowed studies of families with hypertension due to GRA. It is not known why some mutation carriers are normotensive and normokalemic.

CYP11B2 is normally expressed in the zona glomerulosa under the control of angiotensin II, whereas *CYP11B1* is usually expressed in the zona fasciculata. The hybrid cytochrome P450 in GRA is expressed in the zona fasciculata, where it is able to produce aldosterone from corticosterone but is also able to catalyze the production of 18-oxocortisol from cortisol. Aldosterone binds mineralocorticoid receptors in the distal nephron, increasing activity of the epithelial sodium channel (ENaC), which increases net reabsorption of sodium. The resulting increased cardiac output and renal blood flow increases chloride delivery to the juxtaglomerular apparatus. Renin secretion is diminished, with decreased production of angiotensin II. Aldosterone production is not affected substantially because it continues to be produced by the chimeric protein after stimulation by ACTH.

Salt restriction and replacement doses of glucocorticoids are one major treatment for GRA. Suppression of steroidogenesis in the zona fasciculata reduces the mineralocorticoid excess. Dexamethasone has caused hypercortisolism in some patients. Children are difficult to treat because glucocorticoid requirements vary with developmental changes.

Other treatments include spironolactone, a mineralocorticoid antagonist that acts by inhibiting competitively the mineralocorticoid receptor, and amiloride, an antagonist of ENaC. If not treated, prolonged hypertension can lead to a fixed hypertension due to changes in the renal vasculature.

This patient should undergo a trial of treatment with a glucocorticoid for 4 weeks to rule out primary aldosteronism. The diagnosis of GRA can be confirmed by DNA analysis of the affected family members. Consideration should be given to cerebrovascular imaging studies to evaluate possible aneurysms. Due to his age, frequent monitoring for hypercortisolism is needed while he is taking glucocorticoids.

Clinical Pearls

1. A family history of early onset hypertension and refractory hypertension is an important clue to the etiology.
2. Hypokalemia is variable in this condition. Screening relatives for low serum potassium levels to identify those with abnormal mineralocorticoid production may miss some affected members.
3. In addition to salt restriction, treatment should focus on suppressing ACTH or inhibiting the effect of aldosterone on ENaC.
4. DNA testing can identify presymptomatic family members at high risk of developing refractory hypertension.
5. Cerebrovascular disease is particularly common in GRA.
6. Some patients with hyperaldosteronism and a positive dexamethasone suppression test do not have a chimeric *CYP11B2/CYP11B1* mutation.

REFERENCES

1. Fardella CE, Pinto M, Mosso L, et al: Genetic study of patients with dexamethasone-suppressible aldosteronism without the chimeric *CYP11B1/CYP11B2* gene. J Clin Endocrinol Metab 86:4805–4807, 2001.
2. Litchfield WR, Anderson BF, Weiss RJ, et al: Intracranial aneurysm and hemorrhagic stroke in glucocorticoid-remediable aldosteronism. Hypertension 31:445–450, 1998.
3. Gates LJ, MacConnachie AA, Lifton RP, et al: Variation of phenotype in patients with glucocorticoid-remediable aldosteronism. J Med Genet 33:25–28, 1996.
4. Lifton RP, Dluhy RG, Powers M, et al. A chimeric 11-hydroxylase/aldosterone synthase gene causes glucocorticoid-remediable aldosteronism and human hypertension. Nature 355:262–265, 1992.
5. Rich GM, Ulick S, Cook S, et al: Glucocorticoid-remediable hypertension in a large kindred: Clinical spectrum and diagnosis using a characteristic biochemical phenotype. Ann Intern Med 116:813–820, 1992.
6. Lifton RP, Dluhy RG, Powers M, et al: Hereditary hypertension caused by chimeric gene duplications and ectopic expression of aldosterone synthase. Nat Genet 2:66–74, 1992.
7. New MI, Peterson RE. A new form of congenital adrenal hyperplasia. J Clin Endocrinol Metab 27:300–305, 1967.
8. Sutherland DJ, Ruse JL, Laidlaw JC. Hypertension, increased aldosterone secretion, and low plasma renin activity relieved by dexamethasone. CMAJ 95:1109–1119, 1966.

PATIENT 15

A 37-year-old woman with migraine headaches and hypertension

A 37-year-old woman presents to the hypertension clinic for evaluation of migraine headaches and hypertension that she has had for 2–3 months. She was seen 2 weeks prior by a cardiologist who conferred the diagnosis of hypertension. An EKG and an echocardiogram were obtained at that time and reported to be normal. She was prescribed atenolol 50 mg that she has continued to take until the current appointment. She has had migraine headaches for 5 years, which have worsened in severity over the last 2–3 months. Her blood pressure has remained consistently high even during headache-free periods. In addition to atenolol 50 mg, she uses a butalbital and acetaminophen combination-product as needed for headaches and takes Celexa 20 mg daily. Captopril, 6.25 mg twice daily was added to her current regimen. At home, after a single dose of Captopril she began vomiting. She discontinued the medication and returned to clinic 2 days later. Her blood pressure at that time was 190/90 mmHg.

Physical Examination: Pulse 90, blood pressure 170/90, BMI 19. General: thin, appears uncomfortable due to headache. Neck: no bruits or masses. Retina: no papilledema, no arteriolar narrowing. Cardiac: regular rhythm without murmurs. Lungs: clear bilaterally. Abdomen: flat, normal bowel sounds, no palpable masses, no bruits.

Laboratory Findings: CBC: normal. K^+ 4.2 mEq/L, HCO_3^- 24 mEq/L, BUN 13 mg/dl, creatinine 0.8 mg/dl. Urinalysis: no red blood cells, blood, or protein. Thyroid stimulating hormone 2.0. Aldosterone 7 ng/ml (normal 1.3–3.0 ng/dL), plasma renin activity 1.9 ng/ml/hr (normal 1.3-4.0 ng/ml/hr).

Question: What diagnosis should be considered in this woman with severe hypertension?

Diagnosis: Fibromuscular dysplasia with renovascular hypertension

Discussion: Renal artery stenosis (RAS) that leads to renovascular hypertension has a low prevalence in primary care practices. The prevalence increases with severity of hypertension and among patients with hypertension at the extremes of life. For reasons that are not clear, the prevalence of RAS is more common in Caucasians than in African Americans, and is extremely rare in African American men < 40 years of age.

Renovascular hypertension (RVH) is a clinical state that results from unilateral or bilateral renal ischemia. The diagnosis of RVH is made by identification of renal arterial obstruction and evidence of excessive renin production by the affected kidney. RVH must be distinguished from renal vascular disease because the latter may exist without associated hypertension. Because RVH is the most common correctable form of secondary hypertension and failure to correct the vascular abnormality may result in progressive renal failure, it is important to recognize RVH in clinical practice.

The association between constriction of the renal artery and hypertension was first demonstrated by Goldblatt whose work with dogs demonstrated that hypertension related to renal ischemia may be corrected by nephrectomy of the ischemic kidney. RAS, the obstruction of renal blood flow, may result from atherosclerosis, fibromuscular dysplasia, or uncommon causes such as extrinsic compression of the renal artery, thrombosis, or vasculitis. As the renal artery lumen narrows by at least 70–80%, the renin-angiotensin-aldosterone system is activated, leading to increased angiotensin II and aldosterone secretion. The affected kidney is dependent on the vasoconstrictor action of angiotensin II at the afferent and efferent arterioles for maintenance of glomerular filtration. Excessive aldosterone increases sodium absorption and thus increases blood pressure.

Fibromuscular dysplasia, due to hyperplasia of the renal artery branches, occurs most often in young, white women between the ages of 20 and 40 years. Medial fibromuscular dysplasia accounts for 85%, perimedial for 10–15% percent, and intimal hyperplasia for 5% of the cases. On arteriogram, the renal vessels may have a beaded appearance, with stenotic areas most often located in mid-to-distal vessels. Angioplasty is the desired treatment for fibromuscular dysplasia.

Atherosclerotic renovascular disease, most commonly seen in men with a history of smoking, usually causes a sudden increase in blood pressure in previously normotensive or controlled hypertensive patients. Other clinical features that should prompt an investigation for RAS are the presence of severe hypertensive retinopathy, a systolic–diastolic abdominal bruit, evidence of generalized atherosclerosis, or recurrent pulmonary edema. Worsening of renal function following the initiation of angiotensin-converting enzyme (ACE) inhibitors or angiotensin II receptor blockers warrants a search for RAS. These agents may cause acute renal failure when used in patients with bilateral RAS or stenosis of a solitary kidney.

Atherosclerotic plaque in RAS occurs more commonly in the proximal portion of the renal artery. Branch lesions also can occur. Angioplasty with stent placement or surgical bypass is the desired treatment followed by aggressive medical management of hypertension and risk factor modification.

When RAS is considered in the differential diagnosis for secondary hypertension, the decision to proceed with noninvasive testing versus arteriogram must be considered. The selection of diagnostic tests is a subject of much debate and investigation, often requiring collaboration between a hypertension specialist, radiologists, and surgeons. A number of noninvasive tests may provide evidence for further investigation, although there remains concern for false-negative tests, since patients with RAS may be missed. The decision to proceed with an arteriogram is based on results of preliminary tests, index of suspicion, and profile of the patient. Noninvasive test options include:

Renal artery duplex sonography: Renal artery stenosis may be detected by ultrasound imaging of blood flow in the renal arteries. Smaller, more distal vessels may be difficult to visualize, particularly in obese subjects or in association with poor bowel preparation. This screening test has the potential to discriminate between unilateral and bilateral disease but is operator-dependent and time-consuming.

Captopril renal scan: Radioisotope scanning is enhanced with the use of the ACE inhibitor, captopril, prior to the renogram. The use of an ACE inhibitor alters the hemodynamics of renal flow resulting in a decline in glomerular filtration rate (GFR) in a stenotic kidney and increased GFR in a normal kidney. A positive scan is one in which there is delayed or decreased uptake of the radionucleotide tracer in one kidney (the stenotic kidney) relative to the nonstenotic kidney.

Magnetic resonance imaging (MRI): This imaging modality has a sensitivity of 100% and specificity of 70–90% in studies done in specialty centers, when compared to renal arteriography, the gold standard for detection of RAS. This is a particularly useful noninvasive evaluation in patients with impaired renal function in whom arteriography poses additional risk.

Renal arteriography with renal vein renins: A combination of renal arteriography and renal vein renin sampling provides an anatomic and functional evaluation for renovascular disease. A renal-vein renin concentration from the ischemic kidney, which is 1.5 times greater than renin from the contralateral kidney, predicts an improvement of hypertension with correction of the stenosis. A stenosis of < 60% may not result in increased renin production, so correction of the obstruction may not be beneficial.

Arteriography is the "gold standard" test for RAS. The decision to proceed to this invasive procedure is based upon the result of noninvasive tests, the clinical suspicion that RAS is present, and the surgical risk for subsequent revascularization. If a patient is not a candidate for revascularization surgery or angioplasty, he should not be subjected to the risks associated with arteriography which include bleeding, infection, vascular dissection, and emergent surgery.

Among the noninvasive tests that are no longer considered useful are intravenous pyelograms, split renal function tests, and plain abdominal radiographs. These have been shown to lack sensitivity and specificity, whereas other tools have proven to be more useful in the detection of RAS.

Randomized, controlled clinical trials are needed to determine an algorithmic approach to the diagnosis of RVH. In general, the current recommendation for choosing diagnostic tests is based upon the "clinical suspicion" that a patient has RVH. In a patient with mild or moderate hypertension and no clinical clues of underlying renovascular disease, further evaluation is not indicated. A moderate-risk patient may have refractory hypertension, sudden onset of poorly controlled hypertension, presence of abdominal bruits or evidence for peripheral vascular disease, or other clinical clues suggestive of RVD. Noninvasive testing is recommended for such patients. The choice of test is based upon factors such as availability of imaging techniques, operator expertise, and the patient profile. The high-risk patient is one that may forego noninvasive testing altogether and proceed directly to arteriography. These patients include those with a diastolic blood pressure > 120 mmHg and clinical evidence of vascular disease, evidence of renal insufficiency, or an increase in creatinine following initiation of ACE inhibitor or angiotensin II receptor antagonists. For such patients, direct referral for renal arteriography may be considered. If reliable testing is not available, the patient should be referred to specialist centers.

Medical therapy alone does not correct the underlying ischemia in RVD. Revascularization with surgical bypass or angioplasty with stent placement are the favored treatment. Medical management for RVH may be appropriate for individuals who cannot proceed with revascularization. ACE inhibitor or angiotensin receptor antagonists should be used with great caution in patients with RVD. In patients with bilateral RAS or in the patient with a solitary kidney, the use of such agents may precipitate acute renal failure as a result of reduced glomerular filtration and renal hypoxia. In the patient with unilateral disease, however, the use of these agents may be required to maintain blood pressure control, given the underlying pathophysiology of RVH. The majority of patients with RVD have underlying primary hypertension or renal insufficiency. Even with an optimal result from revascularization, most patients require continued antihypertensive medications.

This young woman with severe headaches and hypertension was referred directly for renal arteriography (see Figure). A distal stenosis on one kidney was found to be critical. Successful angioplasty was performed resulting in sustained blood pressure reduction. She is no longer on antihypertensive therapy and seldom has a migraine headache.

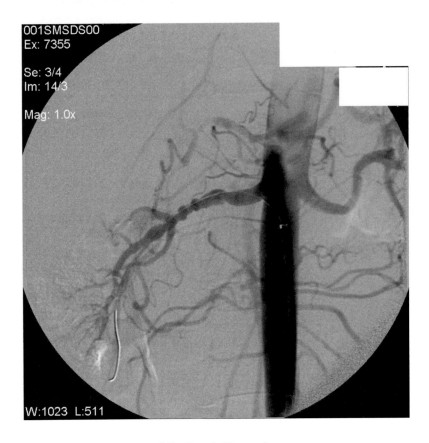

001SMSDS00
Ex: 7355

Se: 3/4
Im: 14/3

Mag: 1.0x

W:1023 L:511

Clinical Pearls

1. Fibromuscular dysplasia should be considered in a young woman with new-onset hypertension.
2. The diagnostic approach for the evaluation of RAS depends on the clinical presentation and a clinical suspicion for its occurrence.
3. Renal arteriography is the "gold standard" for diagnosing RAS.
4. The choice of a noninvasive test for the detection of RAS is based upon factors such as availability of imaging techniques, operator expertise, and the patient profile.
5. The treatment for fibromuscular dysplasia is angioplasty.
6. Angiotensin II receptor antagonists and ACE inhibitors should be used with caution in patients suspected of having RAS. An increase of serum creatinine or an extreme blood pressure reduction after initiation of these drugs should heighten concern for RAS.

REFERENCES

1. Safian RD, Textor SC: Medical progress: Renal-artery stenosis. N Engl J Med 344(6):431–442, 2001.
2. Canzanello VJ, Textor SC: Noninvasive diagnosis of renovascular disease. Mayo Clin Proc 69:1172–1181, 1994.
3. Wilcox CS: Use of angiotensin-converting enzyme inhibitors for diagnosing renovascular hypertension. Kidney Int 44:1379–1390, 1993.
4. Mann SJ, Pickering TG: Detection of renovascular hypertension: State of the art. Ann Intern Med 117:845–853, 1992.
5. Working Group on Renovascular Hypertension: Detection, evaluation, and treatment of renovascular hypertension. Arch Intern Med 147:820–829, 1987.
6. Harrison EG Jr, McCormack LJ: Pathologic classification of renal arterial disease in renovascular hypertension. Mayo Clin Proc 46:161–167, 1971.
7. Goldblatt H, Lynch J, Hanzal RF, Summerville WW. Studies on experimental hypertension. I. The production of persistent elevation of systolic blood pressure by means of renal ischemia. J Exp Med 1934:59:347–378.

PATIENT 16

A patient with von Recklinghausen's neurofibromatosis
and hypertension

A 64-year-old woman with von Recklinghausen's neurofibromatosis presents to the hypertension clinic upon referral from her primary care provider. The patient has longstanding hypertension, which has been controlled with a regimen consisting of lisinopril and hydrochlorothiazide. Over the last year her blood pressure has become increasingly difficult to control, despite adherence to her current regimen with addition of a calcium channel blocker, dietary salt restriction, and weight maintenance. The patient has no complaints of palpitations, headaches, diarrhea, constipation, or weight loss.

Physical Examination: Blood pressure 160/110, pulse 100. General: thin; multiple neurofibromas on total body and freckling in the axilla and back.

Laboratory Findings: 24-hour urinary total metanephrines 28 μmol/d (upper reference limit = 6), plasma free metanephrines 13 nmol/L (upper reference limit = 0.3). Hematocrit 48%. BUN 25 mg/dl, creatinine 1.5 mg/dl. Abdominal MRI: 3.5-cm left adrenal mass.

Question: What etiology should be considered in the medical management of hypertension in this patient?

Diagnosis: Pheochromocytoma

Discussion: Patients with pheochromocytoma should be operated upon once medical management has been initiated. The surgical manipulation and removal of this tumor may result in cardiovascular and hemodynamic disasters. An experienced team of internists, surgeons, and anesthesiologists is required. An understanding of the role of excess catecholamines is critical in the management of patients with pheochromocytoma, as perioperative morbidity and mortality is very high.

The use of adrenergic blockade has resulted in reduction in the mortality related to resection of pheochromocytomas. Patients who are hemodynamically stable but who require resection of a catecholamine-secreting tumor may be managed with the use of medications given orally. In general, it is recommended that preoperative alpha-blockade with phenoxybenzamine 10 mg by mouth once daily be given. Doses are increased to achieve blood pressure control. Prazosin 1–2 mg orally three times daily may also be used. The use of alpha-blockade may reverse hypovolemia, decrease complications with anesthesia, and control blood pressure during the preoperative period. Treatment with alpha-blockade is recommended for 2–3 weeks before surgery.

Beta-blockade may be needed to control the tachycardia associated with catecholamine excess. Initiation of beta-blocker therapy should always follow alpha-blocker therapy. The use of beta-blockers before alpha-blockade in patients with catecholamine excess may result in unopposed alpha-receptor stimulation leading to peripheral vasoconstriction and an increase in blood pressure. This is more likely to occur with the use of non-selective beta-blockers (propranolol or nadolol) which inhibit the vasodilator effect of epinephrine. For this reason, cardioselective beta-blockers such as metoprolol or atenolol should be used in the management of hypertension in patients with pheochromocytomas.

Metyrosine, an inhibitor of tyrosine hydroxylase, blocks the conversion of tyrosine to dihydroxyphenylalanine (DOPA) and, therefore, the synthesis of catecholamines. Metyrosine may be used with phenoxybenzamine or prazosin in the preoperative period to decrease the catecholamine content of the pheochromocytoma. An acute hypertensive crisis may be treated with phentolamine, a short-acting alpha-adrenergic blocker. A continuous infusion of nitroprusside may also be used in the perioperative period for hypertensive crises. Intravenous fluids should be used preoperatively to avoid postoperative hypotension, a common complication of surgery.

This patient was managed with the prazosin for 2 weeks, followed by the addition of atenolol for blood pressure control. One month after identification of the pheochromocytoma, she was admitted for hydration prior to a successful surgical resection.

Clinical Pearls

1. Alpha-blockers such as phenoxybenzamine or prazosin should be the initial drug used for the control of hypertension in patients with a pheochromocytoma.
2. Beta-blockers should never be used before alpha-blockers in patients with suspected pheochromocytoma. The use of beta-blockers may result in a dramatic increase in blood pressure.
3. Surgical removal of pheochromocytomas should be managed be experienced anesthesiologists and surgeons. Patients are at high risk for hypertensive crises, arrhythmias, and stroke.

REFERENCES
1. Pacak K, Linehan WM, Eisenhofer G, et al. Recent advances in genetics, diagnosis, localization, and treatment of pheochromocytoma. Ann Intern Med 134:315, 2001.
2. Bravo EL. Evolving concepts in the pathophysiology, diagnosis, and treatment of pheochromocytoma. Endocr Rev 15:356, 1994.

Thomas Kristopher Harrell, PharmD
Honey East Holman, MD

PATIENT 17

A 44-year-old man with elevated total cholesterol

A 44-year old man comes to your office after he was told that he had an abnormal cholesterol reading during a health fair. He has no known significant previous medical history, and system review is negative. He does not smoke cigarettes. He takes no medications. His family history is negative for premature coronary artery disease.

Physical Examination: Pulse 88, blood pressure 162/92, respiration 16, BMI 32. General: moderate obesity; well-developed; appears stated age: Funduscopic: A-V nicking noted. Skin: normal. Abdomen: obese, no masses or bruits. Extremities: normal strength. Cardiac: normal. Lungs: normal.

Laboratory Findings: Fasting lipid panel: total cholesterol 253, triglycerides 148, HDL-C 41, LDL-C 182. Electrolytes: glucose 105 mg/dl, BUN and creatinine normal. Liver enzymes: AST 23, ALT 29. Thyroid-stimulating hormone 1.0

Question: What do the laboratory findings suggest as a diagnosis?

Diagnosis: Dyslipidemia (specifically, elevated LDL level)

Discussion: A large percentage of patients have both hypertension and dyslipidemia, which are two of the primary risk factors for cardiovascular disease. Elevated cholesterol levels have been observed in as many as 40% of the hypertensive population.

Numerous observational studies have demonstrated that elevated cholesterol levels correlate with the mechanisms responsible for blood pressure increases and peripheral vascular resistance. Thus, it has been postulated that reduction of plasma cholesterol may also result in a decrease in blood pressure and reduction of cardiovascular disease risk. Furthermore, studies have suggested that patients with both hypertension and dyslipidemia should be treated aggressively for both risk factors in order to achieve a substantial reduction in morbidity and mortality associated with cardiovascular disease.

The most common class of drugs used to treat dyslipidemia include the statins or HMG-CoA reductase inhibitors. These agents are also the most potent agents available to treat abnormal cholesterol levels. Statins have been shown to decrease morbidity and mortality in both primary and secondary prevention of cardiovascular disease. Statins have also been suggested to have effects beyond cholesterol lowering, including improvement of endothelial function and improved blood pressure control. The direct mechanism for these additional benefits is unknown, but may involve the ability to prevent renal vascular hypertrophy and improvement of the pressure-natriuresis relationship. Statins may have a vasodilatory effect by up-regulating nitric oxide synthase, which results in improved arterial compliance (especially of the larger arteries). Others theorize that statins may decrease the vasoconstriction and pressor response of angiotensin II or norepinephrine. This theory would suggest statins would work synergistically with drugs such as angioteasin-converting enzyme (ACE) inhibitors, calcium channel blockers, and angiotensin II receptor blockers in lowering both cholesterol level and blood pressure. Studies are currently ongoing to evaluate the effectiveness of fixed combinations of statins and certain classes of antihypertensive medications for the treatment of patients with both hypertension and dyslipidemia.

Treatment of dyslipidemia is usually based on guidelines from the National Cholesterol Education Program Adult Treatment Panel III (NCEP ATP III). These guidelines were published in May 2001, an update of previous guidelines. These guidelines establish cardiac risk factors (other than LDL cholesterol) as HDL < 40 mg/dl; blood pressure > 140/90 or taking antihypertensive medications; age (men > 45 years, women > 55 years); family history of early coronary artery disease (first-degree relative: female < 65 or male < 55); and tobacco use.

Patients are evaluated for the number of cardiac risk factors, and treatment decisions are based on risk assessment. As we look at our case, we see that our patient has two risk factors—a low HDL and high blood pressure. The combination causes his risk to escalate. If he had only one or the other, then his 10-year risk of having an event would be less than 10%. Because he has both risk factors, a Framingham calculation should be performed (see tables).

Because our patient is male, we use the Framingham risk assessment for men. He gets 0 points for his age, 8 points for his total cholesterol, 0 points because he does not smoke, 2 points for his HDL, and 2 points for his blood pressure. His Framingham risk calculates to be 10%. If his blood pressure were 128/88 then his risk would be 6%. This difference would change his goal LDL level, and would make the difference in medication versus no medication. With a < 10% risk, drug therapy would be indicated for LDL levels greater than or equal to 160. His blood pressure elevates his risk level, and medication would be indicated for LDL levels greater than or equal to 130.

Treatment of his hypertension is determined based on guidelines from Seventh Report of the Joint National Committee on Prevention, Detection, Evaluation, and Treatment of High Blood Pressure (JNC VII). According to the JNC VI, the patient's blood pressure goal should be < 140/90. Because the patient has both dyslipidemia and hypertension, both conditions warrant aggressive management. Lifestyle modifications are important factors in both disease states, so a strong emphasis should be placed on losing weight, reducing saturated fats and sodium intake, while increasing physical activity. Modest weight loss may cause significant lowering of blood pressure; however, lifestyle modifications will only maximally lower cholesterol by 10–15%. Commonly, medications will be required in combination with the therapeutic lifestyle changes for a patient to reach lipid goals.

Medications used to treat hypertension can significantly alter lipid parameters, and this is important to keep in mind when treatment is initiated. For instance, thiazide and loop diuretics, may at least transiently increase total cholesterol, triglycerides, and LDL levels. Likewise,

Framingham Point Scores—Estimate of 10-Year Risk for Men

By Age Group and Total Cholesterol

Total Cholesterol	Age 20-39	Age 40-49	Age 50-59	Age 60-69	Age 70-79
<160	0	0	0	0	0
160-199	4	3	2	1	0
200-239	7	5	3	1	0
240-279	9	6	4	2	1
280+	11	8	5	3	1

By Age and Smoking Status

	Age 20-39	Age 40-49	Age 50-59	Age 60-69	Age 70-79
Nonsmoker	0	0	0	0	0
Smoker	8	5	3	1	1

By Age

Age	Points
20-34	−9
35-39	−4
40-44	0
45-49	3
50-54	6
55-59	8
60-64	10
65-69	11
70-74	12
75-79	13

By HDL Level

HDL	Points
60+	−1
50-59	0
40-49	1
<40	2

By Systolic Blood Pressure and Treatment Status

Systolic BP	If Untreated	If Treated
<120	0	0
120-129	0	1
130-139	1	2
140-159	1	2
160+	2	3

10-Year Risk by Total Framingham Point Scores

Point Total	10-Year Risk
<0	<1%
0	1%
1	1%
2	1%
3	1%
4	1%
5	2%
6	2%
7	3%
8	4%
9	5%
10	6%
11	8%
12	10%
13	12%
14	16%
15	20%
16	25%
17 or more	30%

Framingham Point Scores—Estimate of 10-Year Risk for Women

By Age Group and Total Cholesterol

TOTAL CHOLESTEROL	AGE 20-39 YR	AGE 40-49 YR	AGE 50-59 YR	AGE 60-69 YR	AGE 70-79 YR
<160	0	0	0	0	0
160-199	4	3	2	1	1
200-239	8	6	4	2	1
240-279	11	8	5	3	2
280+	13	10	7	4	2

By Age and Smoking Status

STATUS	AGE 20-39 YR	AGE 40-49 YR	AGE 50-59 YR	AGE 60-69 YR	AGE 70-79 YR
Nonsmoker	0	0	0	0	0
Smoker	9	7	4	2	1

By Age Group

AGE	POINTS
20-34	−7
35-39	−3
40-44	0
45-49	3
50-54	6
55-59	8
60-64	10
65-69	12
70-74	14
75-79	16

By HDL Level

HDL	POINTS
60+	−1
50-59	0
40-49	1
<40	2

By Systolic Blood Pressure and Treatment Status

SYSTOLIC BP (MMHG)	IF UNTREATED	IF TREATED
<120	0	0
120-129	1	3
130-139	2	4
140-159	3	5
160+	4	6

10-Year Risk by Total Framingham Point Scores

POINT TOTAL	10-YEAR RISK
<9	<1%
9	1%
10	1%
11	1%
12	1%
13	2%
14	2%
15	3%
16	4%
17	5%
18	6%
19	8%
20	11%
21	14%
22	17%
23	22%
24	27%
25 or more	30%

beta-blockers may increase triglycerides and decrease HDL levels. The exact mechanism and significance of these effects are unknown. Nevertheless, both diuretics and beta-blockers have both been shown to reduce the rate of cardiovascular events despite these fluctuations in lipids. Alpha-antagonists have been shown to modestly lower total cholesterol and raise HDL levels, but are not recommended as first-line antihypertensive agents even if a patient has both dyslipidemia and hypertension. ACE inhibitors, angiotensin receptor blockers (ARBs), and central adrenergic agonists have no effects on lipids.

The present patient is an obese man with both hypertension and dyslipidemia, previously undiagnosed. His blood pressure goal is < 140/90.

His LDL goal is < 130. For both conditions, the patient is advised to begin therapeutic lifestyle changes, which include a low-fat, low-sodium diet, as well as increased physical activity and weight reduction. Drug therapy was initiated for both his hypertension and dyslipidemia, which included hydrochlorothiazide 12.5 mg daily and simvastatin 20 mg each evening. The baseline chemistry and liver panels were verified to ensure adequate renal and hepatic function. Additional laboratory tests to monitor for therapeutic and adverse effects will be obtained when the patient returns to the clinic in 6 weeks. Blood pressure checks will be done periodically via home monitoring until the patient returns for his next visit.

Clinical Pearls

1. Hypertension and dyslipidemia are two of the most important risk factors for cardiovascular disease that occur concomitantly in a large proportion of patients.
2. High cholesterol levels can cause an increase in peripheral vascular resistance and impaired renal perfusion and thus cause indirect and direct increases in blood pressure.
3. In patients with both hypertension and dyslipidemia, both risk factors should be treated aggressively to reduce risk for cardiovascular disease.
4. Statins are the most potent agents used to treat dyslipidemia, which may offer additional benefits other than cholesterol-lowering effects, including improvement in endothelial function, direct vasodilation, and inhibition of the pressor response.

REFERENCES

1. Chobanian AV, Bakris GL, Black HR, et al: National Heart, Lung, and Blood Institute Joint National Committee on Prevention, Detection, Evaluation, and Treatment of Blood Pressure; National High Blood Pressure Education: The Seventh Report of the Joint National Committee on Prevention, Detection, Evaluation, and Treatment of High Blood Pressure: the JNC VII report, JAMA 289(19):2560–2572, 2003.
2. Borghi CB, Dormi A, Veronesi M, et al. Use of Lipid-Lowering Drugs and Blood Pressure Control in Patients with Arterial Hypertension. J Clin Hypertens 4:277–285, 2002.
3. Expert Panel on Detection, Evaluation, and Treatment of High Blood Cholesterol in Adults (Adult Treatment Panel III). Executive Summary of the Third Report of the National Cholesterol Education Program (NCEP). JAMA. 285:2486–2497, 2001.
4. Glorioso N, Troffa C, Filigheddu F, et al. Effect of the HMG-CoA reductase inhibitors on blood pressure in patients with essential hypertension and primary hypercholesterolemia. Hypertension 34:1281–1286, 1999.

George E. Habeeb, Jr., MD
Kimberly G. Harkins, MD

PATIENT 18

A 62-year-old woman with uncontrolled hypertension

A 62-year-old woman presents to her primary care physician for evaluation of uncontrolled hypertension. She has known type 2 diabetes mellitus of a 10-year duration treated in the past with oral hypoglycemic agents. Recently hyperglycemia has required conversion to insulin injections. She has occasional dyspnea on exertion, but no chest pain. She is followed by ophthalmology for diabetic retinopathy. Her current medications include insulin injections and hydrochlorothiazide 12.5 mg daily.

Physical Examination: Blood pressure 165/90, pulse 90, BMI 42. General: obese, no distress. Funduscopic: nonproliferative retinopathy. Neck: no bruits, no mass, normal jugular venous pressure. Extremities: pitting bilateral edema of ankles and feet. Neurological: mild decreased sensation of both feet.

Laboratory Findings: CBC normal. Na 140 mEq/L, K^+ 3.9 mEq/L, Cl^- 123 mmol/L, CO_2 29 mmol/L, glucose 263 mg/dl, BUN 16 mg/dl, creatinine 1.6 mg/dl. Spot urinalysis: protein 100 mg/dl. EKG: sinus mechanism with left ventricular hypertrophy (LVH).

Question: What co-morbid condition contributes to uncontrolled blood pressure?

Diagnosis: Diabetic nephropathy

Discussion: Diabetes mellitus is the most common cause of end-stage renal disease in the United States. The incidence of type 2 diabetes mellitus is projected to double by 2010. Certain variants of the angiotensin-converting enzyme (ACE) genotypic alleles predispose to the onset and progression of diabetic nephropathy in type 2 diabetes mellitus with insulin resistance.

Hyperglycemia and insulin resistance are significant predictors for diabetic nephropathy. Hyperglycemia has pathologic effects on the nephron and the renal interstitium. High extracellular glucose can activate cytokines that are prosclerotic and lead to evolving glomerular and tubular interstitial fibrosis. Activation of the renin-angiotensin-aldosterone system (RAAS) contributes to increased glomerular capillary pressure and cellular hypertrophy with more extracellular matrix deposition. The results may be proteinuria and decline in renal function.

It is hypothesized that the systemic RAAS is suppressed in diabetics, whereas intrarenal RAAS is active, producing local angiotensin II and inhibiting systemic renin release. The local angiotensin II then binds to AT1 receptors to increase vascular resistance, reduce renal blood flow, and to promote increased matrix of glomerular mesangium and tubular interstitium. Blockade of AT1 receptors increases intrarenal nitric oxide production, stimulates natriuresis, and inhibits proliferation of abnormal cell growth and matrix deposition. ACE inhibition may exert similar benefits.

In the United Kingdom Prospective Diabetes Study, tight blood pressure and glucose control lowered relative risk of cardiovascular events, cerebrovascular events, microvascular complications, diabetic endpoints, and diabetic deaths.

The goal blood pressure for diabetics is < 130/80 mmHg. It is currently recommended that ACE inhibitors or angiotensin receptor blockers be included in the treatment regimen of diabetics with proteinuria. Clinical trials are in progress to determine if there is additional benefit from the combination of these two medication classes in patients with proteinuria.

A number of landmark clinical trials have shown benefits from ACE inhibitors and angiotensin receptor blockers on insulin resistance and diabetic nephropathy. The Heart Outcomes Prevention Evaluation (HOPE) substudy revealed that ramipril was associated with lower rates of new-onset type 2 diabetes mellitus. The Irbesartan in Patients with Type II Diabetes and Microalbuminuria Study II (IRMA II) showed that irbesartan was renoprotective and prevented development of type 2 diabetic nephropathy in diabetic hypertensives with microalbuminuria. A similar trial, Irbesartan Diabetic Nephropathy Trial (IDNT), demonstrated that irbesartan decreased progression of type 2 diabetic nephropathy independent of blood pressure lowering. The Reduction of End-Points in Non-Insulin Dependent Diabetes Mellitus with Angiotensin II Antagonist Losartan (RENAAL) Trial showed that losartan preserved renal function in patients with type 2 diabetes and nephropathy and reduced first hospitalizations for heart failure.

This patient presented with uncontrolled diabetes mellitus, hypertension, diabetic retinopathy, LVH, edema, and proteinuria. She is obese, a condition which makes glycemic and blood pressure control more challenging. She will need regular follow-up with ophthalmology. The level of proteinuria falls within the category of microalbuminuria, predicting increased risk of cardiovascular morbidity and mortality. There is direct correlation with the level of proteinuria and the incidence for stroke and cardiac events. This patient will need an echocardiogram for further evaluation of LVH, an independent marker for cardiovascular risk. Overall, this patient needs both aggressive blood pressure and glucose or glycemic control. An ACE inhibitor or angiotensin receptor blocker should be added to her current therapy.

Clinical Pearls

1. Tight glucose and blood pressure control can lower morbidity and mortality in diabetes mellitus.
2. Proteinuria is an independent risk factor for mortality in type 2 diabetes mellitus.
2. ACE inhibitors or angiotensin receptor blockers should be used for treatment of diabetic nephropathy.
3. The blood pressure goal for diabetics is < 130/80 mmHg.

REFERENCES

1. Yusuf S, Gerstein H, Hoogwerf B, et al: Heart outcomes prevention evaluation substudy: Ramipril and the development of diabetes. JAMA 286:1882–1885, 2001.
2. Parving H-H, Lehnert H, Brochner-Mortensen J, et al: Irbesartan in patients with type II diabetes and microalbuminin study II. N Engl J Med 345:870–878, 2001.
3. Lewis EJ, Hunsicker LG, Clark WR, et al: Irbesartan diabetic nephropathy trial. N Engl J Med 345:851–860, 2001.
4. Brenner BM, Cooper, ME, de Zeeuw D, et al: Reduction of end points in non-insulin dependent diabetes mellitus with angiotensin II antagonist losartan. N Engl J Med 345:861–869, 2001.
5. Burns KD: Angiotensin II and its receptors in the diabetic kidney. Am J Kidney Dis 36:449–467, 2000.
6. Kuramoto N: Effect of ACE gene on diabetic nephropathy in NIDDM patients with insulin resistance. Am J Kidney Dis 33:276–282, 1999.
7. UKPDS Group: United Kingdom Prospective Diabetes Study 38. BMJ 317:703–713, 1998.

PATIENT 19

A 63-year-old man with right-sided weakness and slurred speech

A 63-year-old man presents to the emergency department after he was discovered by his coworkers at 4:45 P.M. sitting with his head down on his desk. He was noted to have slurred speech and difficulty moving his right arm and leg. He does not remember when the symptoms began, but a coworker reported that he seemed fine when they ate lunch together from 12:00 to 12:30 P.M. He denies headache, stiff neck, and visual changes. He has been receiving warfarin to treat a deep vein thrombosis he sustained following a long airplane flight and atorvastatin for hyperlipidemia. There is a family history of stroke and myocardial infarction.

Physical Examination: Temperature 99.1°F, pulse 110, respiratory rate 20, blood pressure 160/95. General: anxious, awake, alert. HEENT: decreased nasolabial fold on right, fundus without hemorhages, papilledema, or exudates. Neck: no bruits. Chest: clear to auscultation and percussion. Cardiac: no murmurs, rubs, or gallops. Extremities: left calf circumference greater than right. Neurological: decreased sensitivity to pin prick, light touch, and temperature on the right throughout.

Laboratory Findings: WBC 8500/μl, with normal differential. Hct 42%, Hgb 13.6, platelets 250,000/μl. Prothrombin time 26.5 seconds, natural ratio 2.2, activated partial thromboplastin time 30 seconds. Electrolytes, glucose, BUN, creatinine: normal. Oxygen saturation 98%. EKG: normal rhythm, tachycardic to 110. Chest radiograph: unremarkable. Head CT scan: normal, without evidence of hemorrhage.

Question: What is the cause of the neurologic deficits in this patient?

Diagnosis: Acute ischemic stroke

Discussion: Elevated blood pressures are commonly seen following an acute ischemic stroke, even in patients who were previously normotensive. There is evidence that elevated blood pressure following stroke is associated with poorer outcomes. Less clear is whether reducing the patient's blood pressure acutely following an ischemic stroke is of benefit.

Causes of "new-onset" hypertension in ischemic stroke patients include fear or pain, elevations in intracranial pressure (the Cushing reflex), and disruption of cerebral blood flow autoregulation. The "shift to the right" of the cerebral blood flow autoregulation curve puts the patient at risk of hypoperfusion if the mean arterial pressure (MAP) is lowered pharmacologically. In addition, blood flow to the ischemic area of the brain from collateral vessels is dependent upon arterial blood pressure. Lowering the blood pressure may reduce blood flow to at-risk neurons that might otherwise have survived. The dilemma is that *elevated* blood pressure is associated with an increased risk of hemorrhagic transformation and cerebral edema.

The question of what blood pressure is too high remains unsettled. Most recommendations agree that pressures that put the patient at risk for hypertensive encephalopathy (systolic > 220 mmHg, diastolic > 110–130 mmHg or MAP > 130 mmHg) should be treated. In the International Stroke Trial, the risk of early death increased by 3.8% for every 10 mmHg increase in systolic blood pressure over 150 mmHg. However, the trial did not provide evidence that lowering systolic pressures in the 150–220 mmHg range improved patient outcome.

Acutely, patients should be assessed for evidence of end-organ damage or a concurrent condition that would require blood pressure modification. These would include aortic dissection, acute renal failure, heart failure, myocardial infarction, hypertensive encephalopathy, or evidence of hemorrhagic transformation. In this patient, there was no evidence of end-organ damage.

In the absence of such complications, the next factor to consider is whether the patient is a candidate for treatment with a thrombolytic agent. Pressures > 185 mmHg systolic or < 110 mmHg diastolic are contraindications to the use of alteplase. A moderate blood pressure reduction with nitroprusside or labetalol may be initiated, and pressures should remain below 185/110 mm Hg for 24 hours post-treatment. However, one should not extrapolate that these guidelines are appropriate for patients not receiving thrombolytics.

Because this patient was receiving warfarin and it was unclear if his stroke was within 3 hours, thrombolytic therapy was not offered. How to manage his blood pressure is now much less clear.

Trials with beta receptor antagonists and some calcium channel blockers suggest these agents may worsen outcomes. A trial of nimodipine given within 6 hours of stroke onset found a borderline significant poorer outcome at 3 months in the treatment group even though no significant difference in blood pressure at 24 hours was noted. Small trials with angiotensin-converting enzyme (ACE) inhibitors suggest they may lower blood pressure without significantly impairing cerebral blood flow. A trial of candesartan administered within 72 hours of the onset of cerebral ischemia was halted after a significant decrease in morbidity and mortality at 3 months was noted in the treatment group.

If this patient were on antihypertensives at home, should they be continued in the hospital? A survey of physicians with an interest in stroke found that more would tend to continue the medications than not, but over half indicated that they were not sure what to do. The Efficacy of Nitric Oxide in Stroke Trial (ENOS) will randomize patients to either continue or stop prior antihypertensive therapy in the hours following a stroke. Further, this trial will assess the risk and benefit of lowering blood pressure within 48 hours with a nitroglycerin patch.

The blood pressure of most patients returns to their prestroke baseline within 4–7 days, regardless of whether antihypertensives are given. At 1–2 weeks poststroke, the patient's blood pressure should be reassessed and, if appropriate, a regimen of maintenance antihypertensive medications may be initiated.

The present patient was admitted to the intensive care unit where his blood pressure was closely monitored. Four hours after he was admitted, his pressure increased to 200/105 mmHg and he was given intravenous enalapril at 1.25 mg. His pressure fell to 180/90 within 30 minutes. The following morning his pressure was 150/85 and by the next day it was 130/80. He continued to have right-sided weakness and difficulty speaking. His pressure remained normal for the remainder of his hospital stay and he was transferred to a rehabilitation facility without antihypertensive medications.

Clinical Pearls

1. Patients presenting with ischemic stroke often have elevated blood pressures, even if they were previously normotensive.
2. After an ischemic stroke, blood pressure usually spontaneously declines, to the patient's prestroke level within 4–7 days even without antihypertensive treatment.
3. Low blood pressure is a predictor of poor outcome as well. In the International Stroke Trial, patients with an a systolic blood pressure of < 150 mmHg had, for every 10 mmHg fall in blood pressure, an increased risk of early death of 17.9%.

REFERENCES

1. Johnston SG, Higashida RT, Barrow DL, et al. Major ongoing stroke trials. Stroke 33:2525–2535, 2002.
2. Leonardi-Bee J, Bath PMW, Phillips SJ, et al: Blood pressure and clinical outcomes in the International Stroke Trial. Stroke 33:1315–1320, 2002.
3. Shrader J, Lüders S, Kulschewski A, et al: ACCESS Study: Acute candesartan cilexetil evaluation in stroke survivors. Am J Hypertens 15:17A, 2002.
4. Blood Pressure in Acute Stroke Collaboration (BASC): Interventions for deliberately altering blood pressure in acute stroke. Cochrane Database Syst Rev Issue 4, 2002.
5. Blood Pressure in Acute Stroke Collaboration: Vasoactive drugs for acute stroke. Cochrane Database Syst Rev Issue 4, 2002.
6. Bath PM: Efficacy of Nitric Oxide in Stroke (ENOS) Trial. Stroke 32:2450–2451, 2001.
7. Horn J, de Haan RJ, Vermeulen M, et al: Very Early Nimodipine Use in Stroke (VENUS): a randomized, double-blind, placebo-controlled trial. Stroke 32:461–465, 2001.
8. Adams HP Jr, Brot TG, Crowell RM, et al: Guidelines for the management of patients with acute ischemic stroke. A statement for healthcare professionals from a special writing group of the Stroke Council, American Heart Association. Stroke 25:1901–1914, 1994.
9. Brott T, Lu M, Kothari R, et al: Hypertension and its treatment in the NINDS rt-PA stroke trial. Stroke 29:1504–1509, 1988.

PATIENT 20

A 40-year-old man with hypertension, morning headaches, and hypersomnolence

A 40-year-old obese man presents to a follow-up outpatient clinic visit with complaints of headaches, fatigue, and excessive daytime sleepiness over the past year. During this time he admits to a weight gain of about 30 pounds. His headaches occur mostly in the morning after awakening. He usually takes ibuprofen at breakfast with relief shortly before lunch. He has also noticed that he gets tired easily during the day. Recently he had a car accident in which he fell asleep at the wheel, prompting this clinic visit. His past medical history is significant for hypertension that is poorly controlled on hydrochlorothiazide and metoprolol. He takes no other medicines. He has also recently been seen in the emergency department with chest pain, but was sent home after a negative exercise stress test.

Physical Examination: Temperature 98.7°F, pulse 82, respiratory rate 17, blood pressure 160/100, weight 257 pounds, BMI 38. General: tired-looking, obese, no distress. Chest: clear to auscultation in all lung fields. Cardiovascular: regular rate and rhythm with a normal S_1, loud S_2, and an audible S_3. Mildly elevated jugulovenous pressure. Radial and dorsalis pedis pulses present. Extremities: mild lower extremity edema.

Laboratory Findings: WBC 7500 μl with normal differential. Hgb 15, Hct 48%. Serum electrolytes, glucose, BUN, creatinine: normal. Routine urinalysis: no protein or sediment. EKG: normal sinus rhythm with criteria met for right ventricular hypertroply. Chest x-ray: prominent vasculature with no evidence of infiltrates or edema.

Question: Considering this man's symptoms, physical examination, and laboratory findings, what is the most likely diagnosis?

Diagnosis: Obstructive sleep apnea

Discussion: In this case, the patient most likely has obstructive sleep apnea (OSA). It is estimated that nearly 3 million men and 1.5 million women have OSA in the United States. OSA is an often overlooked risk factor for life-threatening diseases such as hypertension. In fact, this substantial group of patients may make up a majority of patients previously labeled with essential hypertension. The link between OSA and hypertension is a source of intense debate. This debate centers on whether OSA is an independent risk factor for hypertension or whether confounding factors common to both (obesity, alcohol consumption, or smoking) are truly to blame.

Sleep-disordered breathing is a broad category that encompasses conditions characterized by repeated episodes of apnea and hypopnea that occur during sleep. The problem arises because of a temporary obstruction of the upper airway. Hypopnea describes only a temporary decrease in airflow and is often the result of a partial airway obstruction. Apnea, however, is defined as the temporary cessation of airflow during sleep. The airway obstruction is most often at the level of the pharynx. As opposed to central sleep apnea, the ventilatory drive in obstructive apnea is present during the apneic episode. Most problems arise because the pharynx is too small due either to enlarged surrounding structures or abnormal collapsibility of the airway. Studies show that sleep is associated with pharyngeal narrowing and simultaneous increase in respiratory resistance. Pharyngeal narrowing is often excessive in obese patients, with a larger amount of soft tissue surrounding the airway.

The most common manifestations of OSA are snoring and daytime somnolence. The patient may be unaware of snoring. It is imperative to have a bed partner present during the interview to obtain a reliable description of sleep patterns. On the other hand, the daytime somnolence is quite bothersome and the patient often will fall asleep during the interview. Other common manifestations include repetitive night-time arousals causing restless sleep, morning headaches and confusion, daytime cognitive impairment, personality changes, and impotence. On physical examination, the patient is often an obese, middle-aged man with a very large neck that crowds the upper airway. There may be tonsillar or uvular enlargement compounding the obstruction. Uncontrolled hypertension or isolated diastolic hypertension is often present, despite a multidrug regimen. There also may be signs of right-sided heart failure, such as elevated jugular venous pressure and peripheral edema with clear lung fields.

Even though these symptoms may make the diagnosis obvious, the true diagnosis of OSA must be made by examining the patient during sleep. This is often done in a sleep lab by using **polysomnography** or a "**sleep study**." A complete study includes electroencephalography, electromyography, electrooculography, electrocardiography, oximetry, and measurement of respiratory effort and airflow. Polysomnography remains the gold standard for the diagnosis of sleep apnea. The number of apneas and hypopneas per hour of sleep witnessed during these studies are combined to form the apnea-hypopnea index (AHI). This index establishes the severity of the sleep disturbance and offers a definition for diagnosing true sleep apnea. Most testing facilities define obstructive sleep apnea as an AHI > 5 per hour of sleep, each lasting >10 seconds, but treatment is often recommended in patients with AHI > 15.

The most widely accepted method of treatment for obstructive sleep apnea is continuous positive airway pressure (CPAP). CPAP works by providing pressurized air during each spontaneous breath, thereby improving the patency of the upper airway. An alternative to CPAP for those who cannot tolerate it or in whom CPAP is not effective, is surgery. The upper airway is reconfigured by procedures such as uvulopalatopharyngoplasty. Unfortunately, this procedure has only a 50% success rate in alleviating OSA symptoms.

Interest in OSA is increasing because of the growing knowledge of the morbidity that it incurs. There is a very high association between OSA and hypertension. Studies show that in OSA, patients do not exhibit normal nightly falls in blood pressure, thus they are described as "nondippers" (see figure) It is hypothesized that hypoxia leads to stimulation of peripheral chemoreceptors, increasing sympathetic outflow. This increased sympathetic outflow contributes to chronically elevated blood pressure in those with intermittent hypoxia. With increasing severity of apnea, there is an increased correlation with nondipping. Patients with mild sleep apnea are twice as likely to have hypertension and those with moderate-to-severe disease are more than three times more likely to have hypertension. OSA is often overlooked and nearly 80–90% of people are undiagnosed. Several studies have shown that CPAP does improve blood pressure. The improvement in blood pressure from CPAP in patients with sleep apnea is similar to the effect of conventional antihypertensive therapy in non-sleep–apnea patients on preventing strokes and coronary disease. Because of this, sleep apnea should be included as a differential diagnosis in those presenting as this patient did.

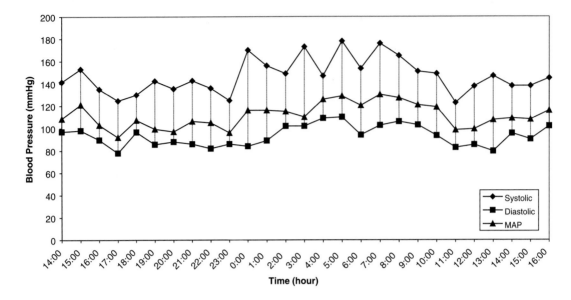

This patient was referred for polysomnography and was found to have an AHI of 43. He was fitted for CPAP and experienced an immediate relief of his symptoms. His blood pressure is now well-controlled with two medications, and he has lost 5 pounds.

Clinical Pearls

1. OSA should be considered in any patient with excessive snoring, daytime sleepiness, repetitive night time arousals causing restless sleep, morning headaches, daytime cognitive impairment, personality changes, and impotence.
2. The gold standard for diagnosing OSA is the sleep study or polysomnography. An apnea-hypopnea index > 5 per hour of sleep is usually used to diagnose OSA.
3. Treatment is usually initiated with AHI >15. CPAP is the treatment of choice, but surgery is an option if CPAP fails to improve symptoms.
4. OSA is an independent risk factor for hypertension. When OSA is treated appropriately, high blood pressure usually improves.

REFERENCES

1. Cuspidi C, Macca G, Sampieri L, et al: Target organ damage and non-dipping pattern defined by two sessions of ambulatory blood pressure monitoring in recently diagnosed essential hypertensive patients. J Hypertens 19: 1539–1545, 2001.
2. Fletcher EC: Invited review. Physiological consequences of intermittent hypoxia: systemic blood pressure. J Appl Physiol 90(4): 1600–1605, 2001.
3. Garcia-Rio F, Racionero MA, Pino JM, et al. Sleep apnea and hypertension. Chest 117(5): 1417–1425, 2000.
4. Nieto FJ, Young TB, Lind BK, et al. Association of sleep-disordered breathing, sleep apnea, and hypertension in a large community-based study. Sleep Heart Health Study. JAMA 283(14): 1829–1836, 2000.
5. Peppard PE, Young T, Palta M, et al. Prospective study of the association between sleep-disordered breathing and hypertension. N Engl J Med 342(19): 1378–1384, 2000.
6. Portaluppi F, Provini F, Cortelli P, et al. Undiagnosed sleep-disordered breathing among male nondippers with essential hypertension. J Hypertens 15(11): 1227–1233, 1997.

PATIENT 21

A 28-year-old pregnant woman with hypertension and proteinuria

A 28-year-old pregnant woman presents to the emergency department with complaints of nausea, vomiting, and headache. The patient states the symptoms have become progressively worse over the past few days. According to the patient, an obstetrician had followed her early during her pregnancy. However, she since lost insurance coverage secondary to becoming unemployed, and she has not returned for follow-up appointments. The patient is currently at 36 weeks of gestation, and states she was at 16 weeks of gestation at her last obstetrician visit. Her only medication is prenatal vitamins.

Physical Examination: Temperature 98.9°F, pulse 79, respiratory rate 18, blood pressure 173/119. General: anxious, appears fatigued. Funduscopic: normal. Cardiac: regular rhythm, no murmurs. Abdomen: normal size for gestational age, nontender, no bruits. Neurological: hyperreflexia. Extremities: 2^+ pitting edema.

Laboratory Findings: Hemogram: WBC normal, Hct 36%, platelets 98,000/μl. Chemistries: electrolytes, glucose, BUN, creatinine normal. Spot urinalysis: 2^+ proteinuria. AST, ALT normal.

Question: What diagnosis best describes the symptom complex?

Diagnosis: Preeclampsia

Discussion: Preeclampsia is a complex systemic syndrome specific to pregnancy that is characterized by blood pressure elevation and proteinuria. It can occur during any pregnancy, and usually appears after 20 weeks of gestation. If preeclampsia occurs in a woman with chronic hypertension, it is referred to as superimposed preeclampsia, which results in a worse prognosis for both the mother and fetus.

Although the etiology of preeclampsia is unknown, many consider the placenta the initiating factor. Placental hypoperfusion is believed to stimulate a maternal response that is characterized by the clinical syndrome. Other etiological theories may also be implicated including genetic susceptibility and possible immunologic mechanisms. The difficulty in identifying a specific etiology is likely attributable to a complex interaction between multiple mechanisms in the overall pathogenesis of preeclampsia.

During a normal pregnancy, necessary cardiovascular, renal, and hormonal accommodations are made to meet the needs of the fetus. These physiologic changes include vasodilation and decreased peripheral vascular resistance, followed by increased total fluid volume and cardiac output. Renal blood flow also increases. With preeclampsia, these normal hemodynamic and renal adjustments are altered: hypertension and increased peripheral vascular resistance occur secondary to vasoconstriction, resulting in decreased intravascular volume, as well as reduced renal blood flow.

The clinical syndrome may be classified as mild to severe and may progress rapidly from one classification to the next. The presenting clinical signs are highly nonspecific, and, consequently, diagnosis may be challenging. The syndrome usually presents after 20 weeks of gestation, and is characterized by new-onset hypertension ($\geq$ 140/90 mmHg) and proteinuria ($\geq$ 300 mg/dl). In patients with chronic hypertension, superimposed preeclampsia should be suspected when proteinuria develops or worsens, or when sudden increases in blood pressure occur. Hyperreflexia is a common neurologic finding in patients with preeclampsia. Previously, edema has been considered a marker for preeclampsia. However, because edema commonly occurs during normal pregnancy, its usefulness as a diagnostic tool is questionable. Other findings increase the certainty of diagnosis and possibly indicate a more severe course, including the following: a blood pressure > 160/110 mmHg, proteinuria > 2 g/day, persistent headache, visual disturbances, epigas-

tric pain, nausea, or vomiting. Laboratory testing may reveal thrombocytopenia, or hepatic or renal dysfunction. High-risk populations should be closely monitored for the development of preeclampsia; these include women with chronic hypertension, renal disease, a positive personal or family history of preeclampsia, or more than one fetus for the given pregnancy.

The management of preeclampsia is dependent upon disease severity. It may be possible to delay delivery in patients with mild preeclampsia, allowing for continued fetal development. Intensive maternal and fetal evaluation for the development of fetal demise, end-organ damage, or eclampsia is warranted in patients with severe preeclampsia. Eclampsia is defined as the development of seizures in a woman with preeclampsia, which cannot be attributed to other causes. Delivery should be considered if maternal symptoms worsen, end-organ damage becomes apparent, or fetal deterioration occurs.

Although therapeutic intervention does not alter the underlying pathophysiologic mechanism, it may slow the progression of the syndrome, thereby allowing for postponed delivery and continued fetal development. The use of antihypertensive agents for the treatment of preeclampsia is controversial. Concern arises over the possibility of excessive blood pressure reduction resulting in diminished placental blood flow. In addition, there is disagreement over the level at which hypertension should be treated. Although therapy is generally indicated in cases with sudden or extreme blood pressure elevations, mild hypertension may not necessitate the use of antihypertensives. The decision to treat pharmacologically should be made on an individual basis. Hydralazine, a direct vasodilator, and labetalol, an alpha- and beta-blocker, are commonly used. Both agents have been shown to be effective in lowering blood pressure in patients with preeclampsia. The short-acting calcium channel blocker, nifedipine, may also be used. However, this agent should be used cautiously, as nifedipine may lead to a significant decrease in blood pressure and result in fetal distress.

A significant complication of preeclampsia is the development of eclampsia. Parenteral magnesium sulfate may reduce the risk of progression from preeclampsia to eclampsia. Patients with severe preeclampsia may obtain a greater benefit, whereas benefit in patients with mild preeclampsia remains unclear. Magnesium sulfate has been shown to be more effective in preventing eclampsia than the anticonvulsant phenytoin. Post delivery, maternal symptoms generally begin to resolve within 24 to 72 hours.

Another complication that may arise from preeclampsia is the HELLP syndrome, which is associated with hemolysis, elevated liver enzymes, and low platelet count. The HELLP syndrome affects pregnant patients at or beyond 20 weeks of gestation and consists of the triad of hypertension, elevated liver enzymes, and low platelets. Acute fatty liver of pregnancy (AFLP) is a rare, but a severe complication with a near 50% mortality rate for both mother and fetus. AFLP quite often presents as preeclampsia with jaundice and significant hepatic and renal dysfunction that requires liver biopsy for diagnosis. Some authorities view these entities as progression of the same disease along a spectrum, whereas others consider them to be separate disease processes. Treatment of HELLP syndrome and AFLP is prompt delivery of the fetus and supportive care.

This patient has signs and symptoms suggestive of preeclampsia: hypertension, headache, nausea, and vomiting. Laboratory results revealed proteinuria and thrombocytopenia, which further support the diagnosis of preeclampsia. She was treated with parenteral hydralazine and magnesium sulfate. After delivering a healthy infant, her blood pressure and proteinuria normalized and her symptoms abated.

Clinical Pearls

1. Preeclampsia is a multisystem disorder of unknown etiology, which affects various organ systems, including the kidneys, brain, liver, and vasculature.
2. Nonspecific signs, such as hypertension, proteinuria, headache, visual disturbances, edema, nausea, vomiting, and epigastric pain, characterize the clinical syndrome.
3. The medical management of preeclampsia varies according to disease severity, and may include delivery or pharmacologic therapy to lower blood pressure and to prevent eclampsia.
4. The ultimate goal of managing preeclampsia is the delivery of a healthy infant without compromising maternal well being.

REFERENCES
1. Kaplan NM: Hypertension with pregnancy and the pill. In Neal W (ed): Kaplan's Clinical Hyptertension, 8th ed. Philadelphia, Lippincott Williams & Wilkins, 2002.
2. Lenfant D, National Education Program Working Group on High Blood Pressure in Pregnancy: Report on high blood pressure in pregnancy. Am J Obstet Gynecol 183(1):S1–S22, 2000.
3. Seely EW, Lindheimer MD: Pathophysiology of preeclampsia: In Izzo JL Jr, Black HR (eds): Hypertension Primer: The Essentials of High Blood Pressure, 2nd ed. Baltimore, Lippincott Williams & Wilkins, 1999.
4. August P: Management of pregnant hypertensive patients. In Izzo JL Jr, Black HR (eds): Hypertension Primer: The Essentials of High Blood Pressure, 2nd ed. Baltimore, Lippincott Williams & Wilkins, 1999.

Michael Mohundro, PharmD
Marion R. Wofford, MD, MPH

PATIENT 22

A 78-year-old woman with a wide pulse pressure

A 78-year-old woman presents to the family medicine clinic for her annual physical. The patient has no complaints and appears healthy. Her review of systems is noncontributory and the family history is unremarkable. Currently, her medication includes Fosamax 70 mg once a week for previously diagnosed osteoporosis, a multivitamin once a day, and a baby aspirin once a day.

Physical Examination: Temperature 98.8°F, pulse 85, respirations 17, blood pressure 180/80 (sitting), 175/78 (standing). General: thin, no apparent distress. Skin: color and turgor normal. HEENT: normal. Cardiac: regular rate and rhythm, no murmurs. Neurological: deep tendon reflexes normal. Extremities: pulses 2 +/= in all, no edema.

Laboratory Findings: Chemistries and complete blood count, normal. TSH normal. Urinalysis no protein.

Question: What is the classification of this patient's blood pressure?

Diagnosis: Isolated systolic hypertension

Discussion: Isolated systolic hypertension (ISH), defined as a systolic blood pressure (SBP) ≥ 140 mmHg and a diastolic blood pressure ≤ 90 mmHg, is the most common form of hypertension in patients > 60 years of age. Systolic blood pressure continues to increase with age, whereas DBP declines after the age of 50 resulting in an increased pulse pressure, the difference between SBP and DBP (see figure). Risks to patients with an elevated SBP and a DBP < 90 mmHg have been clearly demonstrated and include stroke and other cardiovascular events. Pulse pressure is useful in assessing risk in this population, however treatment is based upon reduction of systolic and diastolic blood pressures.

ISH with a wide pulse pressure is most likely the result of the progressive loss of arterial elasticity or compliance. A loss in elasticity in large capacitance arteries leads to increased pressure and the summation of both the initial and reflected pulse waves upon the vessel wall. This is reflected as an exaggerated elevation in the systolic pressure when compared to the diastolic pressure.

The benefits of treatment have also been shown in the a number of clinical trials including the Systolic Hypertension in the Elderly Program (SHEP) and the Systolic Hypertension in Europe Trial (Syst-Eur). The Joint National Committee (JNC) recommends an initial blood pressure reduction to > 160 mmHg for patients with a SBP > 180 mmHg and a reduction of 20 mmHg for those whose SBP is between 160 and 179 mmHg. The long-term treatment goals for patients with ISH are the same as for all patients with hypertension: ≤ 140/90 mmHg.

It is important to consider secondary and "white-coat" hypertension in elderly patients with newly diagnosed hypertension. A careful history, physical examination, and appropriate laboratory values are used to evaluate for secondary causes. Given that the chemistries, renal function and thyroid tests, and the review of systems were normal in this 78-year-old woman, other etiologies need not be considered at this point. The elderly patient often has elevated office blood pressures or "white-coat" hypertension. Reliable ambulatory or home blood pressure readings should be obtained when possible. Another complicating factor is the potential for misdiagnosis due to pseudohypertension. Psuedohypertension results from the same atherosclerotic process that causes isolated systolic hypertension. Stiffness in the brachial artery leads to difficulty in compression and falsely elevated readings of the true intraluminal pressure.

When starting therapy, education regarding lifestyle modifications should be provided as for all patients with hypertension. Smoking cessation, dietary sodium limitation to < 2.4 g/day and adequate dietary intake of calcium, magnesium,

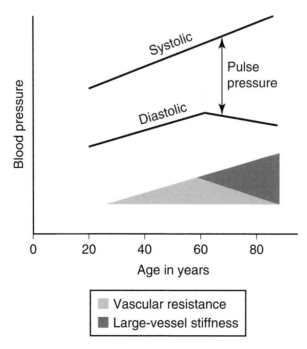

EFFECT OF AGING ON VASCULAR RESISTANCE, LARGE-VESSEL STIFFNESS, AND BLOOD PRESSURE

and potassium should be maintained. Sodium restriction in the elderly may pose a problem due to decreased taste sensation and increased reliance on processed food. Alcohol intake should also be limited and kept to less than one ounce per day. Patients who are obese should be instructed to increase their aerobic activity and to attempt weight loss. Once all nondrug measures have been tried for a sufficient period, drug therapy should be initiated cautiously.

Treatment choices for ISH include low-dose thiazide diuretics or dihydropyridine calcium channel blockers, according to the results of the SHEP and Syst-Eur trials, respectively. The HOPE trial, although not a hypertension trial, also demonstrated significant risk for cardiovascular disease in the elderly with ISH who were treated with angiotensin-converting enzyme inhibitors (ACEIs). Beta-blockers should generally not be chosen as a first-line agent because of increased risk of orthostatic hypotension.

The elderly population has many challenges to treatment and must be monitored carefully. An important point when starting drug therapy is to start with a low dose and titrate up slowly. One of the complications that can occur in this population is orthostatic hypotension, which is due to diminished baroreceptor activity. Orthostatic hypotension can also occur as a result of decreased intravascular volume as well as venous pooling in the legs. Elderly patients should also be checked for postprandial hypotension due to splanchnic pooling. Drug accumulation may be a problem because of the diminished renal and hepatic function associated with aging. Caution should be used in those patients with initially low diastolic blood pressures because the elderly have impaired cerebral autoregulation and cerebral ischemia may occur. Patients should be monitored for subtle signs such as dizziness, confusion, weakness, depression, and unexplained falls, which may indicate one of these problems. In addition, a standing blood pressure is also useful in identifying patients who are at risk or currently have orthostatic hypotension.

The initial treatment goal for this patient with ISH is a systolic blood pressure of < 160 mmHg. She was prescribed 12.5 mg once daily of hydrochlorothiazide, which was titrated to 25 mg once daily over a period of 3 months. Lifestyle changes included a decreased dietary intake of salt and an increase in daily exercise. This treatment resulted in home and office blood pressure reading in the range of 150–168/70–80 mmHg. A low dose of amlodipine was added to the treatment regimen.

Clinical Pearls

1. Isolated systolic hypertension (ISH) has been identified as a risk factor for stroke and cardiovascular events.
2. ISH is a result of loss of arterial wall compliance and the atherosclerotic process.
3. Elderly patients are more prone to "white coat" hypertension than the general population; therefore, accurate home blood pressure measurements should be obtained when possible.
4. The elderly are at risk for orthostatic hypotension. Standing and seated blood pressure measurements should be obtained when evaluating the elderly and before titrating medications.
5. The initial recommendation for therapy in ISH is thiazide diuretic or dihydropyridine calcium channel blockers. ACEIs are also recommended based upon the reduction of cardiovascular events in the high-risk elderly patients. Beta-blockers should be avoided unless there is a comordid disease for which they are indicated.

REFERENCES
1. Izzo JL, Jr, Levy D, Black HR: Importance of systolic blood pressure in older Americans. Hypertension 35:1021–1024, 2000.
2. Savage PJ, Pressel SL, Curb JD, et al: Influence of long-term, low-dose, diuretic-based, antihypertensive therapy on glucose, lipid, uric acid, and potassium levels in older men and women with isolated systolic hypertension: The Systolic Hypertension in the Elderly Program. SHEP Cooperative Research Group. Arch Intern Med 158:741–751, 1998.
3. Staessen JA, Fagard R, Thijs L, et al: Randomized double-blind comparison of placebo and active treatment for older patients with isolated systolic hypertension. Lancet 350:757–764, 1997.
4. Franklin SS, Sutton-Tyrell K, Belle SH, et al: The importance of pulsatile components of hypertension in predicting carotid stenosis in older adults. J Hypertens 15:1143–1150, 1997.
5. Applegate WB, Davis BR, Black HR, et al: Prevalence of postural hypotension at baseline in the Systolic Hypertension in the Elderly Program (SHEP) cohort. J Am Geriatr Soc 39:1057–1064, 1991.
6. Abernethy J, Borhani NO, Hawkins CM, et al: Systolic blood pressure as an independent predictor of mortality in the Hypertension Detection and Follow-up Program. Am J Prev Med 2:123–132, 1986.

PATIENT 23

A 59-year-old woman with weakness and weight gain

A 59-year-old woman presents to the emergency department with complaints of weakness and weight gain. Her family reports that for the last 2 months her blood pressure has been difficult to control and she seems much more anxious and emotional than usual. She attributes a 15-pound weight gain to eating more because of depression. She has been living alone but is requiring more assistance because she is too weak to maintain the house and is having difficulty climbing the stairs to her bedroom. Her past medical history is significant for hypertension for which she has been taking lisinopril/20/12.5 mg and amlodipine 5 mg daily for at least one year. A total hysterectomy was performed at the age of 40 due to uterine fibroids.

Physical Examination: Blood pressure 164/88, pulse 90, weight 185 pounds, BMI 33. General: anxious, truncal obesity, small posterior cervical fat pad, plethora of face. Skin: very thin, bruises on arms, purple striae on the abdomen. Chest: clear. Cardiac: normal rate and rhythm, no murmurs. Abdomen: no palpable masses. Extremities: thin arms and legs, no edema or cyanosis. Neurological: cranial nerves and visual fields are intact, proximal muscle weakness, normal reflexes.

Laboratory Findings: CBC: normal. Na^+ 138 mEq/L, K^+ 3.0 mEq/L, HCO_3^- 27 mEq/L, BUN 13 mg/dl, creatinine 1.1 mg/dl. Fasting glucose 144 mg/dl. Urinalysis: no red blood cells, blood, or protein. A 1-mg overnight dexamethasone suppression test resulted in an 8 AM serum cortisol 9.7 g/dl (normal < 5 g/dl).

Question: What diagnosis does this clinical presentation suggest?

Diagnosis: Cushing's syndrome

Discussion: The diagnosis of Cushing's syndrome, a syndrome due to hypercortisolism, should be considered in this patient. The presentation of this syndrome is variable but includes many features demonstrated in this patient. Some of the features of Cushing's syndrome are nonspecific so the diagnosis may be missed. General features include truncal obesity, hypertension, and psychiatric disorders. Abnormalities of the skin include purple striae, ecchymoses, plethoric facies, hyperpigmentation, hirsutism, and acne. Proximal muscle weakness may be suggested in the review of systems and confirmed by careful physical examination. A number of common metabolic abnormalities are associated with Cushing's syndrome. These include hypokalemic metabolic alkalosis, osteopenia, menstrual disorders, glucose intolerance, diabetes mellitus, kidney stones, and polyuria.

Weight gain in the face, supraclavicular and posterior cervical regions, and abdomen is common in Cushing's syndrome. Chronic hypercortisolism alters the normal inverse relationship between leptin and cortisol, which may contribute to the weight gain in this syndrome.

The skin changes that are seen in this patient such as thin skin, ecchymosis, and striae, are due to the catabolic effects of glucocorticoid. Loss of subcutaneous connective tissue results in easy bruising and striae. These striae appear purple with loss of subcutaneous fat that normally protects superficial capillary beds. Androgen excess is common in women with Cushing's syndrome and results in mild-to-severe hirsutism and acne.

This patient's inability to climb stairs or stand from a sitting position suggests proximal muscle weakness. A decrease in physical activity accentuates the catabolic effect of excess glucocorticoid on skeletal muscle.

The pathogenesis of hypertension in Cushing's syndrome is due to several mechanisms related to coritsol excess. High serum cortisol concentrations overwhelm the ability of the kidneys to convert cortisol to cortisone, resulting in activation of mineralocorticoid receptors. There may be hypersecretion of adrenal mineralocorticoids such as deoxycorticosterone and corticosterone. Increased hepatic synthesis of renin with activation of the renin-angiotensin system also contributes to hypertension in this syndrome. Blocking mineralocorticoid activity with spironolactone may be particularly effective in patients with very high serum cortisol concentrations, especially those with hypokalemia. Treatment of the primary cause of Cushing's syndrome leads to improved blood pressure control.

Glucose intolerance is common in Cushing's syndrome. Chronic excess cortisol results in inappropriate stimulation of gluconeogenesis. Peripheral insulin resistance caused by obesity and direct suppression of insulin release may also contribute to the development of glucose intolerance and diabetes. Of note, the patient presented in this case has not had a prior diagnosis of diabetes but the laboratory results suggest this possibility.

An overnight dexamethasone suppression test is used as a screening tool for Cushing's syndrome. A 1-mg dose of dexamethasone is given between 11 PM and midnight; between 8 and 9 AM on the following morning, a serum coritsol is measured. Normally the cortisol level will suppress to < 5 g/dl, although this screening test has a high false-positive result. An 8 AM serum coritsol of 9.7 g/dl in this patient suggests the need for further testing. A 24-hour urine free cortisol is the single best test for making the diagnosis of Cushing's syndrome.

When clinical and biochemical evidence indicates the possibility of Cushing's syndrome, an experienced endocrinologist should be consulted. Determining the source of excess endogenous cortisol is often a challenge. The first step is to determine whether there is an adrenocorticotropic hormone (ACTH)-dependent or ACTH-independent source of cortisol. Most patients have pituitary tumors, although ectopic ACTH production and adrenal tumors are also included in the differential diagnosis. The proper location of tumors causing Cushing's syndrome requires biochemical and imaging techniques that are best determined by specialized referral centers.

The patient presented here was referred to an endocrinologist. Results of 24-hour urine collections confirmed hypercortisolism with low ACTH secretion. These results indicate an ACTH-independent cause of excess cortisol. Computed tomographic imaging of the adrenal glands revealed a 2.0-cm mass. Following resection of the mass, the electrolyte abnormalities, and hyperglycemia resolved. Her symptoms of muscle weakness slowly improved, and blood pressure became normal.

Clinical Pearls

1. Patients with Cushing's syndrome may present with common findings including diabetes, hypertension, and truncal obesity.
2. Hypertensive patients with ecchymoses, purple striae, and other features related to Cushing's syndrome should be screened for this disorder.
3. Hypokalemia and hypertension may be caused by excess mineralocorticoids, such as cortisol in Cushing's syndrome.
4. High morning cortisol levels after the 1-mg overnight dexamethasone suppression test is a positive screening test for Cushing's syndrome. Further studies are needed to confirm and localize the source of excess endogenous cortisol production.
5. A 24-hour urine free cortisol is the single best test for making the diagnosis of Cushing's syndrome.

REFERENCES

1. Meier CA, Biller BM: Clinical and biochemical evaluation of Cushing's syndrome. Endocrinol Metab Clin North Am 26:741–762, 1997.
2. Ulick S, Wang JZ, Blumenfeld JD, Pickering TG: Cortisol inactivation overload: A mechanism of mineralocorticoid hypertension in the ectopic adrenocorticotropin syndrome. J Clin Endocrinol Metab 74:963, 1992.
3. Kaye TB, Crapo L: The Cushing's syndrome: An update on diagnostic test. Ann Intern Med 112:434–436, 1990.
4. Howlett TA, Rees LH, Besser GM. Cushing's syndrome. Clin Endocrinol Metab 14:911, 1985.

Caryl Sumrall, RN, CFNP, MSN
Brenda M. Davy, PhD, RD, LD

PATIENT 24

A 53-year-old woman with hypertension, dyslipidemia, and hyperinsulinemia

A 53-year-old woman presents to the clinic to establish care. She has a 10-year history of hypertension and is currently taking hydrochlorothiazide 25 mg daily and a calcium channel blocker. She states that she had previously taken an angiotensin-converting enzyme (ACE) inhibitor, but had to discontinue it secondary to a nonproductive cough. She reports no chest pain or tightness and no dyspnea on exertion (DOE). She does report some polyuria, polydipsia, and fatigue that is not worsened with exertion. She does not smoke or drink alcohol, but neither does she exercise on a regular basis. She does not remember the last time her cholesterol was checked. Her last eye examination was 3 years ago and was negative for retinopathy.

Physical Examination: Blood pressure 156/90, otherwise normal. General: moderately obese. Chest: clear to auscultation bilaterally. Cardiac: regular rate and rhythm without murmurs. Abdomen: nontender, no HSM (difficult to tell secondary to obesity). Neck: no thyromegaly. HEENT: tympanic membranes clear, pharynx pink without exudate. Neurologic: deep tendon reflexes 2^+ bilaterally, decreased sensation in bilateral feet. Vascular: 2^+ pedal pulses bilaterally. Eyes: no arteriovenous nicking. Height: 5 foot 5 inches, weight: 190 pounds. BMI: 32 kg/m². Waist circumference: 95 cm (37 inches).

Laboratory Findings: Glucose 123 mg/dl, K$^+$ 4.1 mEq/L, creatinine 1.0 mg/dl, BUN 28 mg/dl, HgbA1c 8.0% (normal < 7.0%). Fasting insulin: 35 μIU/ml (normal 1.9–23 μIU/ml). Total cholesterol: 225 mg/dl (normal < 200 mg/dl), HDL-C: 35 mg/dl (normal 35–59 mg/dl), LDL-C: 151 mg/dl (normal < 130 mg/dl), fasting triglycerides: 195 mg/dl. Urinalysis: trace glucose, trace protein, negative ketones, urine microalbumin 4.55 mg/dl (normal 0.0–2.3 mg/dl), urine creatinine 98.9 mg/dl (normal 60–200 mg/dl), albumin/creatinine ratio 46.0 mg/g (normal 0.0–20.0 mg/g).

Question: What are the treatment options for this patient's metabolic syndrome?

Answer: Lifestyle modification

Discussion: This patient has all of the specified risk determinants (abdominal obesity, triglycerides ≥ 150 mg/dl, HDLs < 50 mg/dl, blood pressure ≥ 130/≥ 85, fasting glucose ≥ 110 mg/dl) for clinical identification of the metabolic syndrome (see table). According to current guidelines, management of the metabolic syndrome has two objectives: to reduce underlying causes of the syndrome (i.e., obesity and physical inactivity) and to treat the lipid and nonlipid abnormalities of the syndrome.

Hypertension, dyslipidemia, and insulin resistance often coexist in individuals with increased abdominal adipose tissue (i.e., visceral obesity). The coexistence of these abnormalities in an individual has been referred to as the metabolic syndrome, syndrome X, and the insulin resistance syndrome. Other abnormalities associated with this syndrome include polycystic ovary syndrome, hyperuricemia, endothelial dysfunction, elevated C-reactive protein concentration, and impaired fibrinolysis. Patients with the metabolic syndrome are at increased risk for atherosclerosis, arterial stiffness, left ventricular hypertrophy, and diastolic dysfunction due to accelerated vascular and cardiac abnormalities. The prevalence of this syndrome has been estimated to be approximately 23% among U.S. adults, with a similar overall prevalence in men and women. Among obese individuals, the prevalence increases to around 60%. Other factors associated with increased risk of the metabolic syndrome include older age, postmenopausal status, Mexican-American ethnicity, smoking, and physical inactivity.

The link between hyperinsulinemia (or insulin resistance) and hypertension is one that has warranted much study and controversy. Insulin resistance results from a defect in the ability of insulin to promote glucose disposal in peripheral tissues. In the initial phase of development of this syndrome, pancreatic beta cells are able to maintain normal blood sugar control by increasing insulin production (i.e., compensatory hyperinsulinemia). Hyperinsulinemia may increase renal sodium and water reabsorption, leading to extracellular volume expansion, which in turn may increase blood pressure. In addition, insulin mediates sympathetic nervous system activity, which may produce increases in heart rate, cardiac output, vascular resistance, and blood pressure. Sympathetic nervous system activity is increased in the postprandial state, as well as in persons with hyperinsulinemia. However, despite these potential mechanistic links, it has also been suggested that insulin resistance and hypertension are parallel consequences of the metabolic syndrome. For example, risk of both disorders increases with obesity, physical inactivity, and advancing age. Thus, the role of insulin resistance in the development of essential hypertension remains controversial, and further study is warranted.

The dyslipidemia associated with the metabolic syndrome is characterized by elevated blood triglyceride and low HDL-C concentrations. Insulin resistance results in a failure of insulin to suppress lipolysis, which increases nonesterified fatty-acid flux to the liver. Very low density lipoprotein (VLDL)/triglyceride concentrations are elevated due to increased hepatic very low density lipoprotein/triglyceride production and release, whereas clearance is decreased.

Patients who have insulin resistance share the same risk factors as those with type 2 diabetes mellitus and are predisposed to earlier onset of cardiovascular disease. Both type 2 diabetes and hypertension are diseases that independently predispose a patient to cardiovascular complications; the presence of both in a patient significantly increases the risk of these complications. Effective blood pressure and glycemic control, in addition to treatment of other cardiovascular risk

Clinical Identification of the Metabolic Syndrome*

Risk Factor	Defining Level
• Abdominal obesity (waist circumference)	
Men	> 102 cm (> 40 in)
Women	> 88 cm (> 35 in)
• Triglycerides	≥ 150 mg/dl
• High-density lipoprotein cholesterol	
Men	< 40 mg/dl
Women	< 50 mg/dl
• Blood pressure	≥ 130/≥85 mmHg
• Fasting glucose	≥ 110 mg/dl

*The diagnosis of the metabolic syndrome is made when three or more of the risk determinants shown are present.
Table modified from reference 3 (NCEP-ATP III guidelines).

factors, decreases the development of macrovascular and microvascular complications, resulting in decreased morbidity and mortality.

All of the abnormalities associated with the metabolic syndrome should be first addressed with weight reduction and increased physical activity. In addition to facilitating weight reduction, regular physical activity will favorably modify blood triglyceride and HDL-C concentrations, blood pressure, and insulin sensitivity. Current recommendations suggest a minimum daily caloric expenditure of 200 kcal/day in moderate physical activity. For example, this recommendation could be achieved by briskly walking 2 miles per day.

Dietary modification is also a critical component of treatment. As with increased physical activity, dietary modification may facilitate weight reduction as well as help to normalize lipids and blood pressure. However, there has been considerable debate as to the optimal dietary approach for the treatment of the metabolic syndrome. In some individuals, the adoption of a high-carbohydrate, low-fat diet may increase blood triglyceride concentrations. For this reason, a moderate fat intake emphasizing monounsaturated fatty acids may be considered. Conversely, a higher intake of fat may promote "passive overconsumption," which would be counterproductive to weight-control efforts. The NCEP ATP III guidelines consider both of these issues and advocate a fat intake between 25 and 35% of total calories (up to 20% from monounsaturated fats), a carbohydrate intake of 50–60% of total calories, and a fiber intake of 20–30 g/day. The dietary pattern used in the DASH trials is an ideal option for patients with the metabolic syndrome.

Treatment of essential hypertension in those with type 2 diabetes or insulin resistance, centers on lowering blood pressure readings to a goal of 135/80 mmHg or less. Studies of hypertension control in patients with type II diabetes show dramatic benefits in reducing risk for cardiovascular events and mortality. Patients with both type 2 diabetes and hypertension may require several antihypertensive medications for optimal blood pressure control. Much study has focused on the role of ACE inhibitors, and, more recently, angiotensin II receptor blockers in patients with both type 2 diabetes and hypertension. Angiotensin II is thought to play a part in the development of insulin resistance, potentially inhibiting insulin signaling pathways at several levels in vascular smooth muscle cells. Subsequently, ACE inhibitors and angiotensin II receptor blockers may prevent the development of type II diabetes that results from the postulated effects on insulin resistance at the cellular level, including inhibition of angiotension II mediated effects on insulin signaling. For hypertension management, the weight of current evidence suggests that thiazide diuretics, angiotensin II receptor blockers, and ACE inhibitors are reasonable first-choice agents, although the majority of patients will require more than one medication.

This patient has multiple conditions that predispose her to both macrovascular and microvascular disease. Furthermore, her urine studies indicated the presence of early nephropathy. More aggressive blood pressure control will help prevent cardiovascular disease. In the past, she experienced side effects with an ACE inhibitor. An angiotensin II receptor blocker was added to her antihypertensive regimen with subsequent improvement in her blood pressure. An insulin sensitizer was added with some improvement in her blood glucose concentrations; she was also referred to a registered dietitian for counseling on a diet and exercise regimen to facilitate weight reduction. She was referred to an ophthalmologist for retinopathy screening. She returned to the clinic after 3 months, reporting a decrease in her symptoms of fatigue, polyuria, and polydipsia, and she had succeeded in losing 8 pounds.

Clinical Pearls

1. The metabolic syndrome is a common condition, with an estimated overall prevalence rate of 23% in the U.S. population. The presence of this condition substantially increases risk for coronary heart disease.
2. Clinical identification of the metabolic syndrome should routinely include assessment of BMI as well as waist circumference, blood pressure, and fasting blood glucose and lipid concentrations.
3. The metabolic syndrome is associated with several modifiable lifestyle factors including obesity, physical inactivity, and smoking. Lifestyle modification and weight reduction, through intensive diet and exercise counseling, should be a substantial component of treatment in patients with this syndrome.
4. Aggressive risk-factor control shows clear and consistent reductions in risk for cardiovascular events and death.

REFERENCES

1. Snow V, Weiss KB, Mottur-Pilson C: The evidence base for tight blood pressure control in the management of type 2 diabetes mellitus. Ann Intern Med 138:587–592, 2003.
2. Park YW, Zhu S, Palaniappan L, et al: The metabolic syndrome. Prevalence and associated risk factor findings in the US population from the Third National Health and Nutrition Examination Survey, 1988–1994. Arch Intern Med 163:427–436, 2003.
3. Expert Panel on Detection, Evaluation, and Treatment of High Blood Cholesterol in Adults: Executive summary of the third report of the National Cholesterol Education Program (NCEP) Expert Panel on Detection, Evaluation, and Treatment of High Blood Cholesterol in Adults (Adult Treatment Panel III). JAMA 285(19):2486–2497, 2001.
4. Ferrannini E: Insulin resistance and blood pressure. In Reaven G, Laws A (eds): Insulin resistance: The metabolic syndrome X. Towtowa, NJ, Humana Press, 1999.
5. Blundell JE, Macdiarmid JI: Fat as a risk factor for overconsumption: Satiation, satiety, and patterns of eating. J Am Diet Assoc 97(suppl):S63–69, 1997.

George E. Habeeb, Jr., MD
Kimberly G. Harkins, MD

PATIENT 25

A 72-year-old man with hypertension and renal insufficiency

A 72-year-old man presents to clinic with hypertension. He monitors his blood pressure at home, with average readings around 170/80 mmHg. He exercises regularly, follows a low sodium diet, and adheres to his medical regimen of amlodipine and hydrochlorothiazide. He takes no over-the-counter medications, does not use tobacco or alcohol, and has no other medical problems.

Physical Examination: Temperature 98.0°F, pulse 80, respiratory rate 14, blood pressure 165/80. BMI 23. Funduscopic: moderate narrowing of the arterioles and arteriovenous nicking. Cardiac: point of maximum impulse displaced laterally and inferiorly. Chest: clear. Abdomen: no bruits or masses. Extremities: bilateral pitting edema to mid-calf.

Laboratory Findings: Hemogram: hematocrit 33%. Electrolytes, glucose: normal; BUN 18 mg/dl, creatinine 1.8 mg/dl. Urinalysis: 50 mg/dl protein. Fasting lipid profile: total cholesterol 220 mg/dl, triglycerides 260 mg/dl, HDL-C 34 mg/dl, LDL-C 160 mg/dl. Renal ultrasonography: bilateral kidneys 8.5 cm in length, no hydronephrosis, echogenicity consistent with chronic renal disease.

Question: What is the cause of this patient's elevated creatinine?

Diagnosis: Hypertensive nephrosclerosis

Discussion: This patient demonstrates several features of benign hypertensive nephrosclerosis. Chronic hypertension exaggerates and exacerbates nephrosclerosis, a normal consequence of aging. Risk for nephrosclerosis from hypertension is increased in African Americans, and in patients with extreme elevations of blood pressure and for underlying renal disease.

As a protective mechanism, hypertension induces a hypertrophic response in renal vascular beds. Luminal narrowing in large and small renal arteries and afferent glomerular arterioles prevents systemic hypertension from being transmitted to the renal capillaries. Over time, ischemic changes lead to glomerulosclerosis, which may be focal and segmental or focal and global. Through poorly understood mechanisms, these vascular and glomerular changes lead to chronic interstitial nephritis.

Hypertensive nephrosclerosis is frequently associated with excretion of small amounts of protein, usually less than one gram per day. Patients with diabetes, other kidney disease, or renovascular disease may have more pronounced proteinuria. This patient also manifests other findings that are common in patients with nephrosclerosis, including retinopathy, left ventricular hypertrophy, small kidneys, and a nearly normal urine sediment. Although nephrosclerosis is the second leading cause of end-stage renal disease, most patients will show a slow, gradual decline in kidney function over the course of years.

The timing of onset of hypertension is important, as patients with primary renal disease frequently develop hypertension. With nephrosclerosis, the hypertension precedes the renal insufficiency. It is also important to distinguish bilateral renal artery stenosis from hypertensive nephrosclerosis. The two processes have similar clinical features, but, unlike nephrosclerosis, renal artery disease is potentially reversible.

Therapy of hypertensive nephrosclerosis centers on control of blood pressure. The African American Study of Kidney Disease (AASK) compared an angiotensin-converting enzyme (ACE) inhibitor (ramipril) a beta-blocker (metoprolol) and a calcium channel antagonist (amlodipine) in patients with hypertensive renal disease. Patients treated with ramipril showed a significant improvement in time to first renal event or death. Many patients in AASK were treated with a thiazide diuretic in addition to the study drug. The Antihypertensive and Lipid-Lowering Treatment to Prevent Heart Attack Trial (ALLHAT) demonstrated a reduction in cardiovascular events in high-risk hypertensive patients treated with a thiazide diuretic. Initial therapy of hypertension in patients with nephrosclerosis should include a thiazide diuretic and an ACE inhibitor if proteinuria is present. An angiotensin receptor blocker (ARB) would be a reasonable alternative in patients who develop cough while taking ACE inhibitors, although this class of agents has not been specifically tested in nephrosclerosis.

Blood pressure goal in renal disease has been evaluated in several studies, including AASK and the Modification of Diet in Renal Disease (MDRD) study. No additional benefit from aggressive blood pressure lowering was demonstrated in patients with mild proteinuria; therefore, these patients should be treated to a goal blood pressure of < 130/80 mmHg.

Clinical Pearls

1. Hypertensive nephrosclerosis presents as mild renal insufficiency and proteinuria in patients with hypertension.
2. Nephrosclerosis must be differentiated from primary renal disease and bilateral renal artery stenosis.
3. Diuretics and ACE inhibitors are the drugs of choice for treatment of hypertensive nephrosclerosis.
4. Blood pressure goal in patients with renal disease is < 130/80 mmHg.

REFERENCES

1. Major outcomes in high-risk hypertensive patients randomized to angiotensin-converting enzyme inhibitor or calcium channel blocker vs diuretic: The Antihypertensive and Lipid-Lowering Treatment to Prevent Heart Attack Trial (ALLHAT). JAMA 288:2981–2997, 2002.
2. Remuzzi G, Schieppati A, Ruggenenti P: Nephropathy in patients with type II diabetes. N Engl J Med 346:1145–1151, 2002.
3. Agodoa LY, Appel L, Bakris GL, et al: African American study of kidney disease and hypertension. JAMA 285: 2719–2728, 2001.
4. Bianchi S, Bigazza R, Campese VM: Microalbuminuria in essential hypertension: Significance, pathophysiology, and therapeutic implications. Am J Kid Dis 34:973–995, 1999.
5. Lazarus JM, Bourgoignie J, Buckalew V, et al: Achievement and safety of a low blood pressure goal in chronic renal disease. Hypertension 29:641–650, 1997.
6. Peterson, JC, Adler S , Burkhart JM, et al: Blood pressure control, proteinuria and the progression of renal disease: The Modification of Diet in Renal Disease Study. Ann Intern Med 123:754–762, 1995.

George E. Habeeb, Jr., MD
Kimberly G. Harkins, MD

PATIENT 26

A 60-year-old man with hematuria and flank pain

A 60-year-old man presents to his physician with ongoing chronic bilateral flank pain and right upper quadrant pain over the past year as the primary complaint. He states he noticed mild gross hematuria on two occasions. He reports decreased appetite and early satiety. He reports a past history of chronic urinary tract infections and borderline hypertension (untreated). The patient now reports developing edema of both legs. Family history reveals several relatives who died of brain aneurysms or kidney failure.

Physical Examination: Temperature 99.2°F, pulse 90, respirations 18, blood pressure 160/90. HEENT: stage II hypertensive retinopathy, no neck masses. Cardiac: regular rhythm. Chest: clear. Abdomen: bilateral palpable tender flank masses. Extremities: edema 1^+ legs and feet.

Laboratory Findings: WBC 14,000/μl, Hct 28%, Platelets normal. Chemistries: glucose 110 mg/dl, Na^+ 130 mmol/L, K^+ 5.5 mmol/L, Cl^- 105 mmol/L, BUN 32 mg/dl, creatinine 3.5 mg/dl. Liver panel: ALT 82 U/L, AST 75 U/L, total protein 7.1 g/dl, albumin 1.7 g/dl, total bilirubin and direct bilirubin normal, alkaline phosphatase 172 U/L. Spot urinalysis: protein > 300 mg/dl, many bacteria, WBCs 20/hpf, RBCs 15 hpf.

Question: What diagnostic tests should be ordered to elucidate the cause of this patient's symptoms?

Answer: Ultrasonography, CT scans, and MRI for radiographic confirmation.

Discussion: Autosomal dominant (adult) polycystic kidney disease (ADPKD) may affect 1/1000 persons. It causes 9–10% of end-stage renal disease in the United States. The inheritance is autosomal dominant with nearly 100% penetrance. The defective gene is related to the alpha globin gene of short arm chromosome 16, exclusively. Usually both kidneys are involved, but unilateral involvement relates to multicystic dysplasia. Renal function is preserved for many decades if the cysts involve only portions of the nephrons.

The kidneys can reach extreme sizes of up to 30 cm in length and weigh as much as 4 kg per kidney. The cysts displace the parenchyma, yet functioning nephrons are found between the cysts. Cyst fluid can range from clear to turbid, and red to brown, depending on hemorrhage or infection. The cyst epithelium can resemble proximal or distal tubule cells and has functional ability.

Clinical manifestations and symptoms may present from early childhood to as late as 80 years of age. Classic symptoms and signs are flank pain, abdominal pain, hematuria, with renal colic, infection of the urinary tract, hypertension, renal stones, proteinuria, and polyuria. Forty percent of ADPKD patients have polycystic liver disease. Cysts may be found in other organs, but most significantly, berry aneurysms in the circle of Willis are present in up to 30% of patients. The risk of subarachnoid hemorrhage is 10%. Hypertension occurs in 60% of cases.

Clinical diagnostic tests include renal ultrasonography, computed tomographic scans, and MRI for radiologic confirmation. Patients with infected cysts will require antibiotic therapy. Hemorrhagic cysts are treated conservatively in most cases. Very large symptomatic cysts with chronic pain may respond to cyst decompression, drainage, or sclerosis. For the hypertension, it is thought that these patients have increased intrarenal angiotensin effect, reduced renal blood flow, increased filtration fraction, and abnormal sodium balance—all leading to expanding extracellular fluid volume and hypertension.

Paradoxically, as the disease progresses there is excessive sodium loss and resulting volume contraction. Diuretics should be used with extreme caution as they may have negative effects on the course of the disease. Therefore, angiotensin-converting enzyme (ACE) inhibitors or dihydropyridine calcium channel blockers may be used.

For the patient progressing to end-stage renal disease (ESRD), dialysis or renal transplantation are potential options. For ADPKD and ESRD with chronic pain, one small series offered laparoscopic nephrectomy for relief of pain and included some patients with improved or resolved hypertension.

In the present patient, abdominal and renal ultrasonography revealed massive renal and hepatic cysts (see figure). One large cyst was thought to contain either hemorrhage or abscess. There was no evidence of hydronephrosis, and the kidney lengths were approximately 25 cm. The patient was treated with a combination of an ACE inhibitor and calcium channel blocker, with good control of his blood pressure.

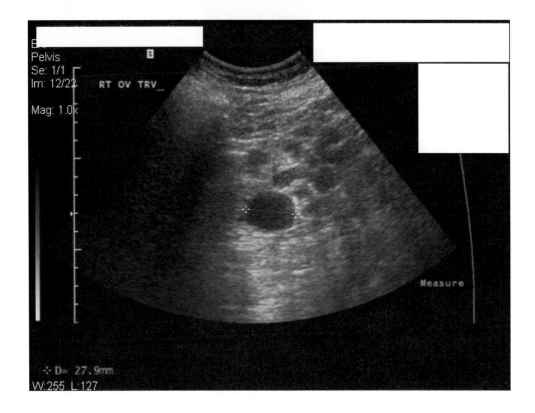

Clinical Pearls

1. Autosomal dominant (adult) polycystic kidney disease (ADPKD) may present in early, middle, or late life.
2. ADPKD often presents with flank pain, hematuria, and urinary tract infection.
3. ADPKD complications relate to infected or hemorrhagic cysts, berry aneurysms, hypertension, and end-stage renal disease.
4. The hypertension with ADPKD may be treated with ACE inhibitors or dihydropyridine calcium channel blockers. Diuretics should not be used routinely, and if necessary, should be used only with extreme caution.

REFERENCES

1. Kaplan NM: Clinical Hypertension, 8th ed. Philadelphia, Lippincott Williams & Wilkins, 2002.
2. Dunn MD, Portis AJ, Elbahnasy AM, et al: Laparoscopic nephrectomy in patients with end-stage renal disease and autosomal dominant polycystic kidney disease. Am J Kidney Dis 35:720–725, 2000.
3. Robbins SL, Cotran RS, Kumar V (eds): Robbins Pathologic Basis of Disease, 4th ed. Philadelphia, W.B. Saunders, 1989.
4. Tornes VE: Cystic disease of the kidney. In Glassock RJ (ed): Current Therapy in Nephrology and Hypertension, 4th ed. St. Louis, Mosby, 1998.

PATIENT 27

A 35-year-old woman with hypertension, morning nausea and vomiting, and some weight gain

A 35-year-old woman with a 4-year history of hypertension presents to the clinic for a follow-up appointment. The patient had recently noted some weight gain despite early morning nausea and vomiting. She also reported missing her monthly menstruation. Her hypertension had been successfully controlled with hydrochlorothiazide and ramipril.

Physical Examination: Height 5 feet 6 inches, weight 155 pounds, blood pressure 138/82, otherwise normal. General: appears fatigued. HEENT: normal fundi bilaterally. Chest: clear. Cardiac: normal. Extremities: no edema.

Laboratory Findings: Hemoglobin 14 g/dl, hematocrit 38%, serum creatinine 1.0 mg/dl, beta-hcg 50 IU/L, 24-hour urinary protein 8 mg/dl.

Question: How does pregnancy influence hypertension management?

Topic: Chronic hypertension in pregnancy

Discussion: Chronic hypertension in pregnant women is defined as hypertension present and detected prior to pregnancy or diagnosed before the 20th week of gestation. The National Institutes of Health National High Blood Pressure Education Program Working Group on High Blood Pressure in Pregnancy (NHBPEP) has four classifications of hypertensive disorders in pregnancy. In addition to chronic hypertension in pregnancy there is also preeclampsia-eclampsia, preeclampsia superimposed upon chronic hypertension, and gestational hypertension. This patient's history of hypertension prior to conception classifies her in the category of chronic hypertension in pregnancy, which carries a 2–5% risk of clinical complications with her pregnancy.

Pregnancy is associated with numerous compensatory mechanisms allowing a woman's body to create an environment that is highly conducive to fetal growth. These compensatory changes affect blood pressure through vasodilation, extracellular fluid expansion, activation of the renin-angiotensin-aldosterone system, and increased glomerular filtration rate (GFR). Vasodilation is a result of such changes as placental-induced arteriovenous shunt on the maternal circulation, endothelial cell production of nitric oxide and prostaglandin, and elevations in progesterone and estrogen levels. Vasodilation is followed by a decrease in peripheral vascular resistance, or afterload. The combination of decreased afterload with elevations in heart rate and stroke volume will produce a rise in cardiac output by 30–40%.

In pregnancy, stroke volume rises as extracellular fluid volume expands from the activation of the renin-angiotensin-aldosterone system. Physiological changes that trigger this complex system include vasodilatory effects to induce renin production from juxtaglomerular cells of the kidney, estrogen-induced stimulation of prorenin from the ovaries, and the uterine and placental sources of prorenin. These changes cause a series of conversions that change angiotensinogen into the potent vasoconstrictor angiotensin II. The normally elicited vasoconstrictor response is dulled in pregnancy, but angiotensin II additionally functions as a feedback mechanism to the adrenal gland, thereby increasing the release of aldosterone. Aldosterone will then cause retention of sodium and water by the kidney, which causes an increase in the patient's blood volume. Increased blood flow and GFR will also affect renal function. Renal blood flow can increase to the extent that it surpasses the glomerular filtration capacity of the kidney. The GFR can initially climb by 50%, followed by a gradual return to normal levels. Overall, pregnancy-induced cardiovascular changes typically cause an initial decrease in blood pressure. This is credited to four key physiological changes: (1) marked vasodilation producing a decrease in peripheral vascular resistance, (2) increased fluid volume leading to an increase in stroke volume, (3) activation of the renin-angiotensin-aldosterone system, and (4) increased renal blood flow with elevations in glomerular filtration rate.

Initially during the first weeks of pregnancy, the patient can expect to experience a fall in blood pressure. This decrease will be more drastic in patients with preexisting hypertension than in their normotensive counterparts. Generally, the diastolic pressure is affected to a greater extent than the systolic pressure. Diastolic pressure will fall to its lowest level during the middle or second trimester of the pregnancy and then will begin to rise to pre-pregnancy levels by term. This initial fall in the patient's blood pressure may allow for a reduction in antihypertensive medication use. During the third trimester, or postdelivery, the patient's blood pressure will return to its previous hypertensive level.

The third trimester also carries a greater risk for the development of superimposed preeclampsia, which leads to a number of maternal and fetal complications. There is no evidence supporting the use of antihypertensive treatment for the purpose of decreasing superimposed preeclampsia that can present earlier and progress more rapidly in hypertensive pregnancies. In addition to the inherent risk of preeclampsia during pregnancy, chronic hypertension will predispose patients to further complications such as the development or the progression of target organ damage including renal disease, ventricular hypertrophy, and retinopathy. There is a greater incidence of low birth weight and growth retardation of the fetus in the hypertensive patient population, as well as the premature separation of the placenta, or abruptio placentae. Increased fetal risks are accompanied by maternal risks such as cerebral hemorrhage, which carries an even greater incidence of maternal mortality than preeclampsia. The potential for adverse outcomes in both mother and child makes adequate blood pressure control imperative to minimize complications from chronic hypertension.

Clinicians must distinguish among chronic hypertension, gestational hypertension, or preeclampsia when evaluating hypertension in pregnancy. The key consideration when making this differential diagnosis is the time of onset of elevated blood pressures. As with this patient, chronic hypertension is most obvious when the patient develops the elevations in blood pressure prior to conception or within 20 weeks of gestation. Only in very rare circumstances does preeclampsia present this early. A more difficult diagnosis occurs when the patient presents with elevated blood pressures during or after the second trimester, taking into account the normal physiological adaptations that tend to produce a drop in blood pressure. Before making the diagnosis of preeclampsia, clinical features of preeclampsia such as proteinuria, thrombocytopenia, and elevated serum creatinine should be present. If these key laboratory abnormalities are not present, as in this patient, the diagnosis of chronic hypertension should be strongly considered over preeclampsia. The physician must also strongly consider the case of superimposed preeclampsia, which carries an incidence of up to 25% in the chronic hypertensive pregnant patient.

Management of chronic hypertension in pregnancy includes both nonpharmacologic and pharmacologic strategies. Nonpharmacological treatment such as weight loss and exercise are not recommended for pregnant patients, but rather the restriction of activity should be emphasized. The patient should also be encouraged to perform home blood pressure monitoring. Controlling mild to moderately high blood pressure with antihypertensive medications should be considered with caution. Excessively lowering blood pressure holds its own risks for the fetus, such as reduction in placental blood flow. An algorithm may be used when considering antihypertensive therapy (see figure). Guidelines issued by the NHBPEP states that antihypertensive medication can be safely withheld in patients without target-organ damage and with systolic blood pressure < 150–160 mmHg and diastolic blood pressure of < 100–110 mmHg.

When choosing the appropriate antihypertensive treatment, it is important to consider both the efficacy of the pharmacologic agent as well as any potential effects on the fetus. Methyldopa is considered the agent of choice when treating hypertension in pregnant women due to the numerous studies in this patient population and the absence of negative fetal effects found in long-term follow-up studies. One major drawback of methyldopa use is the potential to cause depression, sedation, and postural hypotension, leading to poor compliance rates.

Other antihypertensive agents should be considered if there is a response failure or poor patient tolerance of methyldopa. One such class of antihypertensive agents, beta-blockers, have shown overall good efficacy and safety profiles. The majority of studies involving beta-blockers, primarily the beta-1 selective agent atenolol, investigated their use in the third trimester and found effective control without significant adverse consequences. Although safety issues were not a significant concern with atenolol during the third trimester, atenolol use in gestational weeks 12 to 24 did show adverse effects such as growth restriction and decreased placental weight. This may be a unique feature of atenolol and not other beta-blockers. In general, beta-blocker use is secondary to methyldopa and reserved for later stages of pregnancy. Studies using primarily nonselective beta-blockers demonstrated a greater negative fetal-effect profile, such as bradycardia, when compared to those using selective beta-blockers. Labetalol, a combined alpha/beta-blocker, is one of the most frequently used agents in this class and as a parenteral treatment for severe hypertension.

Diuretics, such as the thiazides, are not recommended for patients with preeclampsia, but they may be employed in the management of chronic hypertension. Diuretics work to address the physiologic volume expansion that women experience during pregnancy. If the patient has been successfully managed with a diuretic prior to conception, diuretics may be continued through gestation, possibly at a lower dose or used in combination regimens with methyldopa or beta-blockers. As with any patient treated with diuretics, there is the theoretical risk of hyponatremia, hypokalemia, volume depletion, and thrombocytopenia.

Calcium channel blockers have been used to treat several hypertensive disorders in pregnancy including chronic hypertension, mild preeclampsia, and urgent hypertension in preeclampsia. Very few studies exist with calcium channel blockers in pregnancy, but those that do exist primarily focus on nifedipine use. Other agents include nicardipine, isradipine, and verapamil. Many clinicians are actually using amlodipine and felodipine as first-line agents in place of methyldopa. Although these agents seem relatively safe and effective, there is the potential for negative fetal effects. One of the major concerns with calcium-channel-blocker use is in combination with magnesium for the urgent control of preeclampsia with the potential to cause neuromuscular blockade or circulatory collapse.

Angiotensin-converting enzyme (ACE) inhibitors and angiotensin receptor blockers (ARBs) are contraindicated in pregnancy, not due to teratogenicity but rather to neonatal renal failure. Most of the harm caused by agents that affect the renin-angiotensin-aldosterone system occurs when the agents are used in the latter stages of pregnancy.

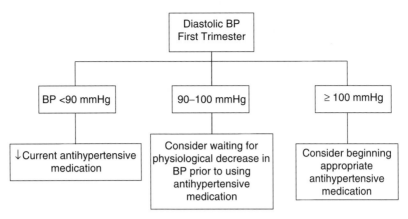

```
                    ┌─────────────────┐
                    │  Diastolic BP   │
                    │ First Trimester │
                    └─────────────────┘
        ┌───────────────────┼───────────────────┐
┌──────────────┐   ┌──────────────┐    ┌──────────────┐
│ BP <90 mmHg  │   │ 90–100 mmHg  │    │ ≥ 100 mmHg   │
└──────────────┘   └──────────────┘    └──────────────┘
```

Algorithm for instituting antihypertensive therapy in chronic hypertensive patients based on first-trimester diastolic blood pressure.

Therefore, there is little risk to the fetus if the mother conceives while receiving treatment with these agents, but they should be immediately discontinued once pregnancy is known.

Patients with chronic hypertension who are treated with medication must also be informed of concerns related to breast-feeding. If the patient's blood pressure is only mildly elevated, the choice may be to withhold pharmacological treatment during the breast-feeding period. Lack of data for antihypertensive use in lactating women has resulted in many clinicians advocating the avoidance of breast-feeding when pharmacological treatment is necessary. Overall it has been found that neonatal exposure to methyldopa is very low and use of the agent is generally regarded as safe. Atenolol exposure to the fetus is high, since the drug is concentrated in breast milk. Although atenolol is considered safe, labetalol is the preferred beta-blocker to use in breast-feeding women. There are insufficient data concerning breast-feeding and calcium channel blockers. Diuretics are discouraged because they reduce milk volume and cause suppression of lactation.

This patient should expect her blood pressure to drop initially due to physiological changes occurring in pregnancy, with an eventual rise to pre-pregnancy levels towards the end of her pregnancy. The patient is currently maintained with an ACE inhibitor requiring immediate discontinuation to avoid negative renal effects on the fetus. The patient may continue diuretic therapy, since she has been successfully managed on hydrochlorothiazide prior to pregnancy, but may not need the drug due to the expected fall in blood pressure. Antihypertensive pharmacologic therapy will be essential if the patient's diastolic blood pressure remains consistently elevated above 100 mmHg. Methyldopa is advocated by the NHBPEP as the drug of choice for treating hypertension in pregnancy. Other options or add-on agents include beta-blockers and calcium channel blockers. Appropriate therapy of this patient's hypertension while she is pregnant will help her avoid complications while preventing potential long-term risks to the fetus.

Clinical Pearls

1. Chronic hypertension in pregnancy is determined by the time of onset. Chronic hypertension is present prior to pregnancy or before the 20th week of gestation.
2. Blood pressure can be expected to drop initially, which may allow for the reduction or discontinuation of antihypertensive medications.
3. First-line treatment for chronic hypertension in pregnancy is methyldopa. Beta-blockers and calcium channel blockers are currently considered second line.
4. ACE inhibitors and ARBs are contraindicated in all pregnant patients due to the potential to cause neonatal renal failure.
5. Antihypertensives may be discontinued during breast-feeding in patients with mild elevations in blood pressure. If pharmacological intervention is necessary, preferred agents in breast-feeding women include methyldopa and labetalol.

REFERENCES

1. Zamorski MA, Green LA: NHBPEP report on high blood pressure in pregnancy: A summary for family physicians. Am Fam Physician 64(2):263–270, 2001.
2. National Institutes of Health National Heart, Lung, and Blood Institute: National High Blood Pressure Education Program Working Group Report on High Blood Pressure in Pregnancy NIH Publication No. 00-3029, 2000, pp 3-15.
3. Churchill D, Beevers DG: Treatment of the hypertensive disorders of pregnancy. In Churchill D, Beevers DG (eds): Hypertension in Pregnancy. London, BMJ Books, 1999.
4. Umans JG, Lindheimer MD: Antihypertensive treatment. In Lindheimer MD, Roberts, JM, Cunningham FG (eds): Chesley's Hypertensive Disorders in Pregnancy, 2nd ed. Stamford, Connecticut, Appleton & Lange, 1999.

Sara L. Noble, PharmD
James A. Cloy, MD
Sharon B. Wyatt, RN, CANP, PhD

PATIENT 28

A 68-year-old man with multiple medications

A 68-year-old man presents to his health care provider with only a complaint of "foot problems." He reports swelling and inflammation of his great toe from an ingrown toenail. This is his first visit to the health care provider since his wife died 9 months ago. At that time, the daughter had called to report the coping difficulties he was having and diazepam was prescribed by phone. Since then he has missed three appointments without canceling. Previously he had shown regular attendance but had complained about "taking so many medications." The daughter actually made today's appointment, informing the receptionist that her father is sleeping too much during the day and that she is worried about him. Today he admits to increased daytime fatigue and sleepiness and early morning headaches most days for the past week or so. Before that, he was beginning to feel better, the best he had felt since his wife died. He stopped taking his blood pressure medications about 3 weeks ago because he felt better and thought his blood pressure was low. Prior to stopping his medication altogether, he admits to not taking the medicine on some days. Also, he shares some of his medications with his sister when her pension check runs out. His health care costs are partially covered by Medicare, but he has no prescription benefits. He does have some trouble affording his medications. He accurately reports his prescribed medications as lisinopril 20 mg twice daily, hydroclorothiazide 25 mg daily, potassium chloride 20 mEq daily, Norvasc 5 mg daily, niacin 750 mg four times daily, diazepam 10 mg two to three times a day, and ranitidine 150 mg twice daily. He smokes one pack of cigarettes daily and has for 40 years. He has a family history of atherosclerotic heart disease and morbid obesity.

Physical Examination: Temperature 98.2°F, pulse 72, respiratory rate 16, blood pressure 190/87. Height 73 inches, weight 244 pounds, BMI 32. General: obese, appears sedated. Funduscopic: normal. Chest: clear. Cardiac: normal S_1, prominent S_2, no murmurs or gallops. Extremities: ingrown nail right great toe, no edema.

Laboratory Findings: WBCs 13,000/μl with 7% neutrophils (normal 3–5%). Potassium 5.4 mEq/L with all other electrolytes, glucose, BUN and creatinine: normal. Total cholesterol 198 mg/dl, triglycerides 180 mg/dl, HDL-C 40 mg/dl and LDL-C 122 mg/dl. AST and ALT: normal. EKG: left ventricular hypertrophy.

Question: To what do you attribute this patient's hypersomnolence and intermittent medication taking?

Diagnoses: Ingrown toenail, hypertension, obesity, dyslipidemia, hypersomnolence, nicotine addiction, and medication non-adherence.

Discussion: Treating hypertension should be simple, but it is not. Multidrug regimens and taking medications incorrectly, inconsistently, or not at all are major factors in poor blood pressure control. The latest NHANES data reveal that only 27% of patients with hypertension have their blood pressure controlled to below a target level of 140/90 mmHg. The easiest rationalization for these poor control rates is to blame our patients and assume they are not taking their prescribed medications. In fact, approximately 40% of patients with hypertension do not consistently take medications as prescribed. Although this noncompliance is certainly a part of the problem, we must also consider the health care providers and the health care system in which we operate. Poor provider–patient relationships, inadequate explanations of complex regimens, and the substantial cost of multidrug regimens together with limited prescription insurance benefits further contribute to this difficult problem. Whatever its etiology, poor compliance contributes to poor clinical outcomes that cost more than $100 billion annually in the United States.

The definition of adherence in relation to health care includes not only the degree to which a patient's actual medication dosing schedule matches the prescribed regimen, but also encompasses delays in seeking care, nonparticipation with recommended behavior changes, failure to keep appointments, and failure to follow medical instructions. In addition, major components of adherence include the degree to which the patient participated in decision-making and whether the regimen is congruent with the patient's attitudes, beliefs, motivations and lifestyle. Although accurate measures for adherence are lacking, simple measures such as directly questioning patients (e.g., "Many people find it difficult to take medications exactly as prescribed all of the time. Have you missed any pills this week?") and monitoring

appointment-keeping behaviors and treatment response provide ample evidence of problems. "Missing appointment" behavior is highly correlated with lower adherence to prescribed regimens. Table 1 provides a summary of practical and objective measures of adherence.

Medication adherence and persistence with antihypertensive medication have been studied extensively. About half of the people treated for high blood pressure stop taking their medications during the initial year of treatment, with 90 days as the median time to discontinuation. Persistence rates for individual drugs vary, with adverse effects being a main contributing factor for nonpersistence. However, antihypertensive drug compliance is better in older patients, women, and in those who are prescribed fewer medicines. Many factors contribute to lack of adherence. Adherence problems affect both women and men regardless of age, level of education, socioeconomic status, or disease severity. Adherence generally decreases over time, particularly with chronic illnesses. Depression, smoking, excessive alcohol intake, and other unhealthy behaviors are associated with nonadherence. Improved use of medication and resultant blood pressure control is correlated with the frequency of office visits for blood pressure monitoring. In addition, social support from family members and friends, employment, and having health insurance have also been shown to contribute to improved high blood pressure control. Patients' knowledge of hypertension, the benefits of treatment, and the outcomes if left untreated are important but do not necessarily translate into increased adherence. Nonadherence may be a rational choice from the patient's perspective, since other priorities in daily life may take precedence. It is important to determine what individual barriers exist for patients in addressing compliance. Concerns about side effects, not believing the medication is

---

Table 1. Measures of Adherence

Practical:
• Ask the patient using nonjudgmental technique
• Monitor treatment response
• Monitor attendance of appointments
Objective:
• Drug levels, if applicable
• Check pharmacy refills
• Pill counts
• Medication event monitors (electronic pill monitors)

Modified from Haynes, McDonald, and Garg, 2002.

truly beneficial, feeling that the condition has improved, medication costs, and dosing frequency should also be taken into account. Compliance is inversely related to the total daily doses of medication. Increasing the number of daily doses is related to a decline in compliance.

The expert panel on compliance has promoted the importance of recognizing a multilevel approach to the compliance challenge, suggesting a focus on the patient, provider, and organization. For long-term treatments such as antihypertensive therapy, a combination of cognitive, behavioral, and educational interventions are needed to assist persons with adherence to treatment regimens. Such interventions require significant effort on the part of providers. Table 2 summarizes the best evidence available from randomized clinical trials of adherence interventions. In all instances, it is imperative to respect the ethical principle regarding the patient's right to refuse treatment. Further, attempts to coerce adherence by threatening dire consequences are unethical and may result in total withdrawal from care.

Signs of nonadherence are clear in this patient. He admits to routinely missing medication doses and to stopping all medications recently. Further, he has failed to keep regular appointments, is possibly depressed or overmedicated, and is a smoker. He has inadequate health insurance coverage and takes multiple medications with a complex dosing schedule. The health care provider involved the patient in deciding the best course of action to address his headaches, hypersomnolence, and long-term blood pressure control. Together they decided to wean him from the diazepam over the next couple of weeks, reduce the dose of hydrochlorothiazide to 12.5 mg, stop the potassium supplementation, and institute a combination ACE inhibitor and calcium channel blocker dosed once daily. A pharmaceutical assistance program available to persons on Medicare was contacted to provide assistance with the cost on the combination pill, and the medication was mailed directly to his home. Further, they changed his regular niacin to a long-acting niacin dosed twice daily. He was provided with written information on each medication including indication, side effects, dose, and timing. He agreed to have his daughter assist him with organizing his medications in a weekly dispenser, and he placed it in a convenient location to remind him of his morning and evening medications. His daughter also brought him to appointments scheduled at bimonthly intervals for 2 months while all changes were initiated and monitored. To assist the patient's sister in obtaining her medications, information for patient medication assistance was provided to the family (1-800-PMA-INFO or http://www.phrma.org or www.needymeds.com). By the end of the 2 month period his blood pressure had normalized, his lipid levels remained stable, and he was again sleeping 6–7 hours a night without daytime somnolence. He had joined a local widows' group and was making regular outings.

Table 2.   Summary of Evidence-Based Adherence Interventions

Combinations of:
- Partnership with patient to achieve outcomes
- Education and educational materials
- Simplify regimen (less-frequent dosing, combination medications, controlled-release dosage forms)
- Supportive counseling
- Peer support groups
- Appointment reminders (computer and manual)
- Cuing medications to daily events
- Reminder packaging (using multidrug dose dispensers, blister packs, calendars)
- Explicitly acknowledging efforts to adhere
- Self-monitoring of outcome parameters with health care provider review and reinforcement
- Involving family members and significant others

Adapted from McDonald, Garg, and Haynes, 2002.

Clinical Pearls

1. Medication noncompliance is a major factor in poor blood pressure control; close to 100% of patients have some difficulty in adhering to regimens at some point.
2. Monitoring of adherence is an important but time-consuming part of routine clinical practice.
3. Enhance adherence by considering patient, provider, and health care system factors.
4. Use combinations of cognitive, behavioral, and education strategies including simplifying regimens, providing written explanations and reminder packaging, and scheduling frequent follow-up visits to assess outcomes.
5. Patients always have the final say and their right to refuse treatment must be respected at all times.

REFERENCES

1. Hansson L: 'Why don't you do as I tell you?' Compliance and antihypertensive regimens. Int J Clin Pract 56:164–166, 2002.
2. Haynes RB, McDonald HP, Garg AX: Helping patients follow prescribed treatment: Clinical applications. JAMA 288:2880–2883, 2002.
3. McDonald HP, Garg AX, Haynes RB: Interventions to enhance patient adherence to medication prescriptions: Scientific review. JAMA 288:2868–2879, 2002.
4. Claxton AJ, Cramer J, Pierce C: A systematic review of the associations between dose regimens and medication compliance. Clin Ther 23:1296–1310, 2001.
5. Vermeire E, Hearnshaw H, Van Royen P, Denekens J: Patient adherence to treatment: Three decades of research. A comprehensive review. J Clin Pharm Ther 26:331–342, 2001.

Dena W. Jackson, MD
Kimberly G. Harkins, MD

PATIENT 29

A 22-year-old woman with dizziness

A 22-year-old woman with no medical problems presents to a clinic with a 3-week history of episodic dizziness. She has recently married and works in a preschool. Her dizziness occurs indoors and outdoors, lasting about 15 minutes and resolving when she sits quietly. She has had some headache and nausea with the dizziness, but no chest pain, palpitations, diaphoresis, or dyspnea. She does not use tobacco, alcohol, or drugs. Her only medication is an oral contraceptive, which she started taking about 3 months prior to presentation.

Physical Examination: Temperature 98°F, pulse 75, respiratory rate 18, blood pressure 152/93 in both arms. General: well developed, slightly anxious appearing. Funduscopic, cardiac, respiratory, and abdominal: normal.

Laboratory Findings: Hemogram: normal. Electrolytes, BUN, creatinine: normal. Urine pregnancy test: negative.

Question: What is the etiology of this patient's high blood pressure?

Diagnosis: Hormone-induced hypertension, related to use of OCPs

Discussion: Since their introduction in the 1960s, oral contraceptive pills (OCPs) have been known to raise both systolic and diastolic blood pressure in some patients. Early studies found that between 4% and 18% of patients taking oral contraceptives developed hypertension. This incidence of hypertension was among patients taking preparations that contained high doses of estrogen ($\geq$ 50 g) and progesterone (1–4 mg). Oral contraceptives in use today contain much smaller doses of hormones. The relative risk of hypertension in OCP users compared to those who have never used oral contraceptives is 1.5 for current use and 1.1 for previous use. There appear to be no modifying effects of age, family history of hypertension, ethnicity, or body mass index (BMI). Most often this increased blood pressure returns to normal after cessation of the drug. The concern is that, if present, the persistent increase in blood pressure may increase the risk of further cardiovascular disease.

The exact mechanism of this elevation in blood pressure is unclear. The renin-angiotensin-aldosterone system has been implicated because estrogen stimulates increased levels of angiotensin. This increase could lead to increased levels of aldosterone, causing sodium and water retention and elevating blood pressure. However, women taking oral contraceptives who do not have hypertension have also demonstrated an increase in renin substrate. Estrogen-induced salt and water retention has also been suggested as a mechanism, but has not been borne out by further study. There appears to be a genetic susceptibility to oral contraceptive–induced hypertension, but the mechanisms are complex.

As in this patient, the elevation in blood pressure generally appears within 4 months of beginning oral contraceptives. When prescribing oral contraceptives, the patient's blood pressure and other cardiovascular risk factors should be considered. After initiation of oral contraceptives, patients should be scheduled for a follow-up blood pressure check within 4–6 months. If blood pressure is found to be elevated at that visit, the patient should be offered alternative birth control methods. If no alternative methods are suitable and the risk of pregnancy outweighs the potential risk of cardiovascular disease, the blood pressure can be lowered with appropriate therapy. Thiazide diuretics or beta-blockers may be appropriate initial therapy for hypertension in patients who choose not to discontinue oral contraceptives.

When patients choose to discontinue oral contraceptives, monitoring for a return of blood pressure to a normal level is important. Hypertension caused by oral contraceptives should normalize within 3 months of discontinuing the medication. If this does not occur, evaluation for essential hypertension or secondary hypertension from another cause is indicated. This patient elected to discontinue her oral contraceptive pills, and her blood pressure was 130/72 mmHg at a follow-up visit 8 weeks later. Her symptoms of dizziness completely resolved.

Clinical Pearls

1. Oral contraceptive use is a cause of hypertension in susceptible patients; blood pressure should be checked within 6 months of initiating OCPs.
2. When possible, contraceptive use should be discontinued, and blood pressure should normalize within several months.
3. Patients who continue oral contraceptives may require antihypertensive agents. Thiazide diuretics or beta-blockers may be used unless compelling indications for use of other agents exist.

REFERENCES

1. Mulatero P, Rabbia F, Morra di Cella S, et al: Angiotensin-converting enzyme and angiotensinogen gene polymorphisms are non-randomly distributed in oral contraceptive-induced hypertension. Hypertension 19:713–719, 2001.
2. Kaplan NM: Systemic Hypertension; Mechanisms and Diagnosis. In Braunwald E , Zipes DP, Libby P (eds.): Braunwald: Heart Disease: A Textbook of Cardiovascular Medicine, 6th ed. Philadelphia, W.B. Saunders, 2001.
3. Ribstein J, Halimi JM, duCailar G, et al: Renal characteristics of angiotensin suppression in oral contraceptive users. Hypertension 33:90–95, 1999.
4. Chasan-Taber L, Willett WC, Manson JE, et al: Prospective study of oral contraceptives and hypertension among women in the united states. Circulation 94:483–489, 1996.
5. Woods J: Oral Contraceptives and Hypertension. Hypertension 11 [Suppl II]: II-11-II-15, 1988
6. Clezy TM, Foy BN, Hodge RL, et al: Contraceptives and hypertension. An epidemiological survey. Br Heart J. 34:1238–1243, 1972.

Holly E. Rogers, PharmD
Kimberly G. Harkins, MD

PATIENT 30

A 32-year-old woman with newly diagnosed hypertension

A 32-year-old woman with no medical problems presents to a clinic with headache, dizziness, and palpitations of 3-week duration. She has no history of heart disease and this is her first experience with these symptoms. For the past 6 months, she has been dieting and exercising in effort to lose the weight she gained during her three pregnancies. She originally lost approximately 20 pounds, but she hit a plateau about 2 months ago. She recently began using an over-the-counter supplement to help her in her weight-loss efforts and reports an additional 10-pound weight loss since starting use of the product. She has a family history of type 2 diabetes mellitus, dyslipidemia, and obesity.

Physical Examination: Temperature 98.4°F, respiratory rate 14, pulse 115 (sitting), blood pressure 180/105 mmHg, weight 150 pounds (decreased from 180 pounds 6 months ago), height 5 feet 6 inches, BMI 24 (decreased from 29 6 months ago). Funduscopic: normal. Cardiac: tachycardic, no murmurs. Lungs: clear breath sounds throughout. Abdomen: no tenderness, no masses, hypoactive bowel sounds. Neurological: pupils 4 mm in diameter bilaterally; responsive to light, sensory, and motor normal.

Laboratory Findings: Hemogram: normal. Electrolytes, glucose, BUN, creatinine: normal. EKG: sinus tachycardia, rate 110, no changes suggestive of ischemia.

Question: To what do you attribute this patient's hypertension?

Diagnosis: Drug-induced hypertension

Discussion: This patient's hypertension was caused by the use of an herbal weight-loss supplement. The number of Americans who are overweight or obese has risen dramatically in the last decade. The use of products marketed for weight loss, specifically those containing herbal constituents, has escalated. These products are available without a prescription and are often marketed as "all natural." However, they may contain compounds known to increase blood pressure, heart rate, and the risk of adverse cardiovascular events. Unfortunately, these products are often combined with other substances, such as caffeine, that affect the central nervous system and greatly increase the risk of serious adverse events.

Ephedra, a primary ingredient in many weight-loss products, is a potent central nervous system stimulant with amphetamine-like actions. Its systemic effects are mediated through nonselective activation of alpha, beta-1, and beta-2 receptors. Ephedra also releases norepinephrine from body stores. The effects of ephedra include mydriasis, increased myocardial contraction and heart rate, bronchodilation, decreased gastrointestinal tract motility, and peripheral vasoconstriction (see figure). Products containing ephedra are promoted to increase metabolism, suppress appetite, suppress sleep, improve concentration, increase endurance, and "burn fat" through thermogenesis. The cardiovascular effects of ephedra compounds can last ten times longer than the effects of epinephrine.

The use of ephedra has been associated with an increased risk of myocardial infarction, stroke, and hyperglycemia in patients with preexisting conditions such as hypertension, coronary artery disease, and diabetes. Unfortunately, many patients may be unaware of existing medical conditions.

The most serious adverse events associated with the use of ephedra are cardiac arrhythmias and arrest, myocardial infarction, seizure, and stroke. Other adverse reactions associated with use may include anxiety, confusion, constipation, dizziness, headache, insomnia, psychosis, and uterine contractions. As of 2000, the U.S. Food and Drug Administration (FDA) had received over 800 case reports, including 22 deaths, associated with ephedra-containing products. In February 2003, as part of an effort to address safety concerns associated with dietary supplements containing ephedra, the FDA proposed a warning label for all ephedra-containing supplements. This label will warn of the risks of adverse cardiovascular events; emphasize the increased risk with higher doses; strenuous exercise, and other stimulants; specify groups (such as pregnant women) who should never use these products; and list conditions that rule out the use of ephedrine alkaloids.

Ephedra is known by numerous herbal names, most commonly Ma Huang. However, it may also appear as Mexican tea, natural ecstasy, sea grape, squaw tea, yellow astringent, yellow horse, and

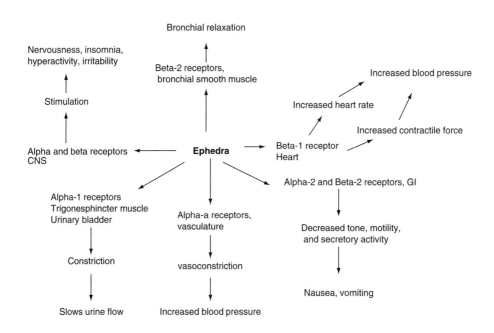

epitonin. The pharmaceutical properties of this evergreen come from components found within the seeds and stems. Numerous alkaloids such as ephedrine, methylephedrine, and pseudoephedrine are commonly found within the species.

The most serious drug–drug interactions known to occur with concomitant use of ephedra are those associated with beta-blockers, monoamine oxidase inhibitors, phenothiazines, and theophylline. The use of ephedra with beta-blockers may result in hypertension due to the unopposed alpha agonist effect and enhanced sympathomimetic effects on the vasculature. Conversely, the concomitant use of phenothiazines produces hypotension and tachycardia secondary to blockade of the alpha effects of ephedra by the phenothiazine.

It is imperative to question all patients at each encounter about the use of over-the-counter products, including herbal dietary supplements. Patients are often hesitant to reveal the use of these products; however, this should not discourage providers from inquiring. This patient was instructed to discontinue the use of the herbal weight-loss product immediately and to resume her previously successful diet and exercise program. She was educated extensively about the potential dangers of these products. Within 3 days, her heart rate and blood pressure returned to normal, and over the next 3 months she was able to lose an additional 10 pounds.

Clinical Pearls

1. Ephedra-containing compounds cause hypertension through activation of the sympathetic nervous system.
2. Serious adverse events including death and stroke have been associated with the use of ephedra-containing weight-loss products.
3. Hypertension caused by ephedra should resolve within 72 hours of discontinuing use of the product.
4. All patients with hypertension or other cardiovascular disease risks should be counseled to avoid herbal weight-loss products that contain ephedra.

REFERENCES

1. Shekelle P, Morton S, Maglione M, et al: Ephedra and ephedrine for weight loss and athletic performance enhancement: Clinical efficacy and side effects. AHRQ Publication no. 03-E022. Rockville, MD, Agency for Healthcare Research and Quality, 2003.
2. Bent S, Tiedt TN, Odden MC, Shlipak MG: The relative safety of ephedra compared with other herbal products. Ann Intern Med 138:468–471, 2003.
3. Boullata JI, Nace AM: Pharmacotherapy 20:257–269, 2000. www.fda.gov: Federal Register / Vol. 65, No. 64 / Monday, April 3, 2000 / Notices: 17510–13.
4. Fetrow CW, Avila JR (eds): Complementary and Alternative Medicines, 1st ed. Springhouse, PA, Springhouse Corporation, 1999.
5. Robbers JE, Tyler VE (eds): Tyler's Herbs of Choice: The Therapeutic Use of Phytomedicinals. Binghamton, NY, The Haworth Herbal Press, an imprint of the Haworth Press, Inc, 1999.

Fleetwood Loustalot, RN, NP-C, MSN
Sharon B. Wyatt, RN, CANP, PhD

PATIENT 31

A 52-year-old woman with nausea, vomiting, and epigastric pain

A 52-year old devout Seventh Day Adventist with a 10-year history of essential hypertension presents to the outpatient department of a local medical center with nausea, epigastric pain, and vomiting of 3-day duration. The outpatient department follows the patient regularly and she indicates that she is currently taking hydrochlorothiazide and aspirin but stopped taking her ramipril about a month ago, preferring to rely on God to take care of her blood pressure. She reports praying privately one or more times daily for about 15 minutes. She denies taking any other medications. After confirming her mildly elevated blood pressure, the health care provider inquires about her use of any herbs or other nonprescription therapies. Only then does she report taking coenzyme Q 10 for the past several weeks to "help my heart." She says the epigastric pain "feels like knots in my stomach" and is slightly worsened with food intake. The patient reports the pain as a 4 on a scale from 0 to 10, 0 being no pain and 10 being the worse pain conceivable. Pain is mildly reduced by resting in a recumbent position and taking an over-the-counter antacid. The nausea and vomiting occur after meals, and the vomit is reported as a small amount, with no blood. The patient reports no recent travel, changes in diet, or being in proximity to others with similar symptoms. She also reports a positive family history of high blood pressure and a strong tendency of her family members to rely on prayer for healing.

Physical Examination: Temperature 99.0°F, pulse 80, respirations 14, blood pressure 145/90 (second check 148/84). General: overweight, calm. Oropharynx: mildly erythematous. Lymphatic: no significant nodules. Cardiac: regular rate, no murmurs. Abdominal: no tenderness. Extremities: no edema.

Laboratory Findings: WBCs 10,000/μL, with normal differential. Hct: 49.1%. Hgb: 14.0 g/dl. Electrolytes, BUN, creatinine: within normal limits. ALT and AST: within normal limits. Abdominal ultrasonography: no significant findings.

Question: What are the possible reasons for the new-onset gastrointestinal distress and elevated blood pressure in this patient?

Diagnosis: Poor blood pressure control; nonadherence to prescribed medical regimen; side effects from complementary treatment for hypertension

Discussion: Complementary and alternative medical (CAM) therapies are widely used by adults in the United States and are rarely reported to health care providers. The majority of patients who use CAM therapies report that they did not inform the provider because they did not think it was important for the provider to know or because the provider did not inquire about use of the therapies. Data gathered from a national sample estimate 629 million visits to alternative medical practitioners in 1997, which is greater than the number of visits of the U. S. population to all primary care providers. CAM therapies can include yoga, meditation, prayer, biofeedback, herbal medicines or dietary supplements, massage, homeopathy, and other nonconventional medical regimens. This patient was relying on two CAM therapies to manage her blood pressure: coenzyme Q 10 and prayer, and she was not taking her prescribed antihypertensive agent.

Most data on the efficacy of CAM dietary supplements are based on small-sample trials, and there are few large randomized controlled trials. CAM dietary supplements are exempt from the U.S. Food and Drug Administration (FDA) regulations through the Dietary Supplement Health and Education Act of 1994, and, therefore, they have not been required to undergo the rigors of controlled trials. Coenzyme Q10 was discovered in 1957, and it has been indicated for cardiovascular-related disorders since 1974. Coenzyme Q10 is a strong antioxidant, and is one of the primary components of the mitochondria. Endogenous coenzyme Q10 is found in the heart, liver, kidneys, and pancreas. After the administration of exogenous coenzyme Q10, it is slowly absorbed through the gastrointestinal wall, and the majority is transmitted to the liver where it is distributed to the very low density lipoproteins. The exogenous supplementation for the deficiency of coenzyme Q10 may enhance antioxidant effects as well as improve the functioning of the mitochondria. Several studies have also noted the effects on platelet aggregation and decreased blood viscosity as potential mechanisms of action. One of the proposed benefits of the supplement is the low toxicity reported; however, doses >300 mg daily place the patient at a higher risk for potential side effects. This patient was experiencing some of the possible side effects of coenzyme Q10.

CAM therapies are not limited to dietary supplements. In addition to experiencing the gastrointestinal side effects, this patient had also stopped taking ramipril for blood pressure control. Patients who use one form of CAM therapy may also be participating in other activities outside of conventional therapy. The use of prayer as a CAM therapy has been demonstrated to lower anxiety scores, to elicit greater life satisfaction and well-being, cancer adaptation, and positive religious coping. The connection with the transcendent and the development of meaning and purpose in life, leading to reduced anxiety, may be the mechanisms though which prayer promotes health and lowers blood pressure. There are also several religiousness instruments used in health research that include private prayer. Participation in nonorganized religious activities such as prayer and Bible study were significantly related to lower diastolic blood pressure in a bivariate analysis; however, the statistical significance was lost after controlling for covariates. The same study combined religious attendance with prayer and Bible study participation and found a statistically significant difference between the high attenders and Bible study participants and low attenders and participants. Although most instruments do not specify which type of prayer was used, a categorical understanding of prayer types will aid in their understanding.

Meditative or repetitive prayer has been examined through Transcendental Meditation (a Buddhist mind-focusing technique), the Relaxation Response (the repetition of a word or phrase while clearing the mind of other distractions), and through relaxation-assisted biofeedback (which assists persons in reacting to the signals from the body). Three months of Transcendental Meditation significantly lowered systolic blood pressure and diastolic blood pressure in older African Americans with mild hypertension. The Relaxation Response may also incorporate ritualistic prayer through the incorporation of a religious phrase or word from the participant's religious affiliation. The Relaxation Response has shown to significantly reduce blood pressure levels in certain clinical situations. A recent meta-analysis of randomized controlled trials showed that relaxation-assisted biofeedback significantly reduced both diastolic and systolic blood pressure. Although prayer should not be prescribed to patients, health care providers should encourage activities that may elicit positive coping mechanisms for their patients.

The use of CAM therapies continued to rise during the previous decade. Patients have increased access to both sound and questionable medical advice via the Internet. Health care providers need to become more familiar with CAM therapies to understand potential side effects, interactions, and contraindications, and to provide patients with advice about their use.

This patient was advised to stop her coenzyme Q10, which she agreed to do. The health care provider also supported her continuing use of prayer as a meditative strategy that may have an impact on blood pressure. Together, they decided to monitor her blood pressure for the next month without restarting the ramipril with the understanding that if her blood pressure remained elevated, they would again discuss pharmacotherapy.

Clinical Pearls

1. Ask patients specifically about the use of CAM dietary supplements because many patients do not consider this part of their pharmacological treatment.
2. Promote stress reduction and social support mechanisms through which patients can cope and manage their chronic conditions.
3. CAM users traditionally have been framed as well-educated women of higher socioeconomic status, but new research shows that a wide variety of individuals use CAM therapies.

REFERENCES

1. Seeman TE, Dubin LF, Seeman M: Religiosity/spirituality and health: A critical review of the evidence for biological pathways. Am Psychol 58(1):53–63, 2003.
2. Sarter B: Coenzyme Q10 and cardiovascular disease: A review. J Cardiovasc Nurs 16(4):9–20, 2002.
3. Koenig H, McCullough M, Larson D: Handbook of religion and health. New York, Oxford University, 2001.
4. Eisenburg D, Kessler R, Van Rompay M, et al: Perceptions about complementary therapies relative to conventional therapies among adults who use both. Ann Intern Med 135(5):344–351, 2001.
5. Serebruany V, Ordonez J, Herzog W: Dietary coenzyme Q10 supplementation alters platelet size and inhibits human vitronectin (CD51/CD61) receptor expression. J Cardiovasc Pharmacol 29:16–22, 1997.
6. Greenberg S, Frishman W: Coenzyme Q10: A new drug for cardiovascular disease. J Clin Pharmacol 30:596–608, 1990.

Nancy L. Campbell, MD
Marion R. Wofford, MD, MPH

PATIENT 32

A 69-year-old woman with hypertension, hypercalcemia, renal insufficiency, and hypokalemia

A 69-year-old woman with hypertension is admitted to the hospital after sustaining an unwitnessed fall. She says she tripped on a rug and denies any loss of consciousness, jerking movements, aura, or post-ictal confusion associated with the fall. She admits to recent fatigue, weakness, and low-back and left flank pain with radiation to the groin. She also experienced several episodes of incontinence, which she attributes to new-onset polydipsia and polyuria. Her prior medical history includes an unknown heart arrhythmia, status-post pacemaker placement, and hypertension diagnosed 10 years ago and treated with oral twice daily, enalapril 20 mg and isosorbide dinitrite 10 mg three times daily.

Physical Examination: Temperature 99.2°F, pulse 71, respiratory rate 22, blood pressure 182/106. General: obese, slow to answer questions but oriented times 4. Chest: crackles and expiratory wheezes in bilateral lung bases. Cardiac: regular rate and rhythm with no murmurs, rubs, or gallops. Abdomen: obese, soft, nontender, normoactive bowel sounds. Extremities: no cyanosis, clubbing, or edema.

Laboratory Findings: WBCs 8500/μl with 12% monocytes, Hct 34%, platelets 271. Sodium 145 mEq/L, potassium 3.4 mEq/L, chloride 109 mEq/L, bicarbonate 26 mEq/L, BUN 57 mg/dl, creatinine 2.7 mg/dl, calcium 12.9 mg/dl, total protein 10.4 g/dl, albumin 2.8 g/dl. Ionized calcium 1.30 (normal, 1.05–1.30 mmol/L). Urinalysis: urine protein 100, urine blood. Peripheral smear: rouleaux (see figure). Chest radiograph: enlarged cardiac silhouette. Kidneys, ureter, and bladder (KUB): no free air, no calcifications.

Question: What diagnosis can explain this patient's polyuria and polydipsia, low-back pain, hypertension, laboratory findings, and the peripheral smear?

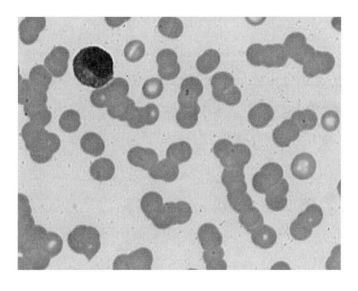

Diagnosis: Multiple myeloma

Discussion: Calcium is involved in many of the body's physiological processes, most notably muscle contraction, enzyme and energy production, and the release of neurotransmitters and hormones.

This patient has several signs and symptoms of hypercalcemia, including hypertension. Thirty percent of patients with hypercalcemia have hypertension, but the pathophysiology is not well-understood. One mechanism proposed is that long-standing hypercalcemia and hypercalciuria lead to tubular atrophy and interstitial fibrosis within the kidney with resultant polyuria, salt-wasting, and hypertension. Another thought is that hypercalcemia leads to hypertension through calcification of the myocardium and blood vessels. A newer theory proposed for patients with hypercalcemia is that they have an increased sympathetic drive to the heart during the night, leading to hypertension and arrhythmia. Finally, studies of patients with primary parathyroidism show increased calcium uptake within vascular smooth muscle and increased intracellular calcium levels. However, the pathophysiologic mechanism that would explain this finding is unclear as the hypertension does not correct with parathyroidectomy, and, therefore, it is likely that a mechanism apart from increased parathyroid hormone (PTH) or its attendant hypercalcemia is responsible.

There are many other signs and symptoms of hypercalcemia exhibited by this patient. Polydipsia, polyuria, and signs of dehydration are common and are thought to result from hypercalcemia-induced osmotic diuresis, type 2 renal tubular acidosis (RTA), and/or nephrogenic diabetes insipidus. The latter is thought to be caused by calcium-induced tubulointerstitial damage and resultant impaired generation of the interstitial osmotic gradient. This patient's flank pain could be from calcium-induced nephrolithiasis. Low-back pain is probably related to a lytic lesion in the lumbar or sacral spine associated with multiple myeloma. She reports abdominal pain, fatigue, and weakness, all of which are associated with hypercalcemia, as are confusion and slow mentation.

Other signs and symptoms of hypercalcemia, which this patient did not exhibit include osteopenia, anorexia, constipation (from decreased smooth muscle tone and/or decreased autonomic function), pancreatitis (secondary to deposition of calcium into the pancreatic duct or calcium activation of trypsinogen within the pancreatic parenchyma), peptic ulcer disease (via calcium stimulation of gastrin secretion), depression,

decreased deep tendon reflexes, and short QT segment on EKG.

When investigating hypercalcemia, one must be aware of factors that can give false readings of the body's calcium level. Pseudohypercalcemia is a laboratory artifact that occurs when there is increased protein in the blood. Fifty to sixty percent of calcium is bound to protein, so when the total amount of protein within the body is high, measurements of calcium will be recorded as high, but physiologic (ionized) calcium may be within the normal range. Pseudohypercalcemia is found in dehydration and multiple myeloma. To obtain correct levels of calcium when high protein levels are present, order an ionized calcium level. Second, since most calcium is bound to albumin, correct for albumin levels with the following formula:

$$\text{calcium concentration} = [0.8 \times (4 - \text{albumin level})] + \text{measured calcium level.}$$

Third, be aware that alkalosis leads to more calcium being bound to albumin; therefore, ionized levels will be lower than the serum levels indicate. In contrast, acidosis leads to less calcium being bound to protein with ionized calcium levels higher than expected.

This patient had an ionized calcium level that was at the high end of normal. Because she had several signs and symptoms of hypercalcemia, she was considered to have true hypercalcemia.

Determining the etiology of hypercalcemia first involves determining the source of increased levels of calcium within the body. Calcium enters the circulation from either the gastrointestinal tract or bone and exits via the urine or by being deposited into bone. Most hypercalcemia is caused by increased calcium absorption from the gastrointestinal tract and/or increased calcium reabsorption from bone. Calcium levels are regulated primarily by three substances: vitamin D, parathyroid hormone, and calcitonin.

Increased calcium absorption within the gastrointestinal tract occurs by both active and passive transport in the small intestine. Active transport is stimulated by vitamin D, whereas passive transport occurs only when calcium intake exceeds 1–2 g/day. Increased levels of vitamin D result from ingestion of vitamin D (mainly in vitamin D–fortified milk), production of calcitriol (the most active metabolite of vitamin D) in granulomatous disease, malignant lymphoma, and acromegaly, or in spontaneous idiopathic excess production of calcitriol via increased angiotensin-converting enzyme (ACE) or idiopathic bodily production of calcitriol. Vitamin D also stimulates decreased renal excretion of calcium.

Increased bone resorption is usually caused by osteoclast activation from increased parathyroid hormone or from paraneoplastic processes associated with malignancy, such as (but not limited to) the production of parathyroid hormone–related peptide (PTHrP).

The two most common etiologies associated with hypercalcemia are hyperparathyroidism in ambulatory patients, and, as in this patient, malignancy in hospitalized patients.

Malignancies associated with hypercalcemia include osteolytic cancers (breast, melanoma, and multiple myeloma), solid tumors that secrete PTHrP (squamous cell lung, renal cell, pheochromocytoma, ovarian, head and neck, bladder), and hematologic cancers (B-cell lymphoma, human T-cell leukemia virus I [HTLV-I]).

Other etiologies of hypercalcemia include diseases associated with increased bone turnover: hyperthyroidism, immobilization, Paget's disease, acromegaly, and adrenal insufficiency (via increased bone resorption, volume contraction, increased proximal tubular calcium resorption, and increased binding of calcium to serum proteins).

Medication use can also lead to hypercalcemia: antacids (via milk-alkali syndrome in which increased calcium and vitamin D lead to hypercalcemic nephropathy, which then causes decreased glomeuklar filtration rate [GFR] with retention of the alkali in the antacid and resultant metabolic alkalosis), thiazides (usually only in patients with mild hyperparathyroidism), lithium (via change in the calcium-induced set point for parathyroid hormone [PTH] release), vitamin A (via increased bone resorption), theophylline ingestion, and estrogen or anti-estrogen treatment of patient's with bone metastases.

Miscellaneous etiologies include rhabdomyolysis and acute renal failure (from calcium mobilized from injured muscles), familial hypocalciuric hypercalcemia, metaphyseal chondrodysplasia, and congenital lactase deficiency.

Since most hypercalcemia is due to primary hyperparathyroidism, the work-up of hypercalcemia begins with a serum parathyroid level. If elevated, the differential is most likely primary hyperparathyroidism or lithium ingestion. If the PTH is not elevated, step two is to obtain a PTHrP level as a marker for malignancy and consider other signs and symptoms of malignancy. Third, if neither the PTH nor PTHrP is elevated and there is no obvious malignancy, look at calcidiol and calcitriol levels as evidence of vitamin D intoxication from granuloma, lymphoma, or PTH-induced renal production. Fourth, if PTH, PTHrP, and vitamin D are all normal, consider other causes of bone resorption, such as thyrotoxicosis, immobilization, or Paget's disease.

Multiple myeloma was strongly suspected in this patient because of the her symptoms of back and flank pain, polydipsia and polyuria, and her laboratory findings of borderline pseudohypercalcemia, elevated total protein, and large protein in the urine. Therefore, her next tests were serum protein electrophoresis and urine protein electrophoresis with immunofixation and quantification of immunoglobulins and a radiologic skeletal bone survey, all of which supported the diagnosis of multiple myeloma. A bone marrow biopsy followed, confirming the diagnosis with 15% plasma cells.

Clinical Pearls

1. Use the following to distinguish among the laboratory results associated with hyperparathyroidism, malignancy, and vitamin D ingestion:

	PTH	Vit D
Hyperparathyroidism	↑↑	↑ or normal
Malignancy	↓	↓
Increased vitamin D	↓	↑↑

2. Be sure to measure physiologic calcium when considering hypercalcemia.
3. The most common causes of hypercalcemia are primary hyperparathyroidism in ambulatory patients and malignancy in hospitalized patients. In hyperparathyroidism, the calcium level is usually < 12 mg/dl; in cancer, calcium is usually > 12 mg/dl. The following is a step-wise approach to the work-up of hypercalcemia:
   - Start with a PTH level.
   - If PTH is negative, look for malignancy with PTHrP and other studies appropriate for a malignancy work-up.
   - If results of previous studies are negative, order calcitriol and calcidiol levels to look for vitamin D intoxication from granulomatous disease, lymphoma, or acromegaly.
   - If the first three steps do not give an answer, search for the etiology among the rarer causes of hypercalcemia.

REFERENCES

1. Agus Z: Clinical manifestations of hypercalcemia. UptoDate 1–5, 2003, http://www.uptodateonline.com.
2. Agus Z: Diagnostic approach to hypercalcemia. UptoDate 1–5, 2003, http://www.uptodateonline.com.
3. Agus Z: Etiology of hypercalcemia. UptoDate, 2003, pp 1–7, http://www.uptodateonline.com.
4. Agus Z, Savarese DMF: Treatment of hypercalcemia. UptoDate 1–7, 2003, http://www.uptodateonline.com.
5. Barletta G, DeFeo ML, Del Bene R, et al: Cardiovascular effects of parathyroid hormone: A study in healthy subjects and normotensive patients with mild primary hyperparathyroidism. J Clin Endocrinol Metab 85(5):1815–1821, 2000.

Jon Hubanks
Betsy Andrews
Kimberly G. Harkins, MD

PATIENT 33

A 56-year-old man with nausea, diaphoresis, and extreme hypertension

A 56-year-old man presents to the emergency department with complaints of nausea, abdominal pain, diaphoresis, and anxiety. He began experiencing these symptoms after a change in his blood pressure medication. His current daily medical regimen includes atenolol 50 mg, ramipril 2.5 mg, and hydrochlorothiazide 25 mg. He also brings in an empty bottle of clonidine 0.2 mg, which he takes twice daily. Recently the primary care physician instructed him to discontinue the clonidine. Ramipril was recommended instead "because my BP was still too high." He had been taking the clonidine for more than 6 months prior to discontinuing.

Physical Examination: Temperature 99.2°F, pulse 98, respirations 18, blood pressure 172/98 g. General: well-developed well-nourished, diaphoretic, anxious. Funduscopic: arteriovenous nicking present. Skin: normal. Cardiac: regular rate and rhythm. Abdomen: bowel sounds positive. Neurological: brisk reflexes.

Laboratory Findings: All laboratory results, including a thyroid stimulating hormone, normal.

Question: What phenomenon is contributing to the elevation of blood pressure?

Diagnosis: Abrupt discontinuation of clonidine with concomitant use of beta-blockers

Discussion: "Overshoot hypertension" is defined as a sudden increase in blood pressure that exceeds the patient's pre-treatment level. "Rebound hypertension" is defined as a sudden increase in blood pressure that returns to a patient's pre-treatment level. One should consider overshoot or rebound hypertension in a patient who has recently had an alteration in antihypertensive therapy, especially if the patient was receiving clonidine.

The concurrent administration of a beta-blocker with clonidine may decrease the antihypertensive effect of the alpha-2 agonist. When arterial beta-2 receptors are antagonized, peripheral blood flow is decreased due to vasoconstriction. This vasoconstriction could blunt the effect of clonidine-induced vasodilation that is a result of decreased alpha-1 stimulation. Therefore, combination therapy with a beta-blocker and clonidine should not have a significant additive effect on blood pressure reduction. This patient's blood pressure was poorly controlled, possibly due to the mechanism described.

When clonidine therapy is abruptly withdrawn, discontinuation syndromes can readily appear, such as rebound or overshoot hypertension, which may present with or without signs and symptoms of sympathetic overactivity. This is most likely attributed to a return of catecholamine release that was suppressed by the clonidine therapy. Increased plasma catecholamines are free to stim-ulate unopposed alpha-1 receptors in the vascular smooth muscle causing vasoconstriction. In this patient, the discontinuation syndrome is exacerbated by concurrent beta-blocker therapy. If a patient remains on beta-blocker therapy when clonidine is suddenly withdrawn, beta-receptors in the vasculature are not free to mediate vasodilation. Consequently, a patient is more susceptible to discontinuation syndrome if receiving beta-blocker therapy when clonidine is withdrawn. To avoid this situation, clonidine should be slowly tapered over a period of 3 or more days. To address discontinuation syndrome due to clonidine withdrawal, the reinstitution of clonidine should resolve signs and symptoms rapidly. However, labetalol can be administered to reduce elevated blood pressure if required. To avoid complications when changing a patient's regimen on a combination of beta-blocker and clonidine, clinicians should slowly taper and discontinue beta-blocker therapy before tapering clonidine.

This patient's signs, symptoms, and medical history are suggestive of overshoot hypertension with sympathetic overactivity due to clonidine withdrawal and concomitant use of beta-blockade. The patient presented with nausea, abdominal pain, anxiety, diaphoresis, and markedly elevated blood pressure. Once clonidine therapy was reinstated, the patient's blood pressure decreased and signs and symptoms of sympathetic activity resolved.

Clinical Pearls

1. Consider the potential for overshoot or rebound hypertension in patients prescribed clonidine or beta-blockers.
2. Concurrent administration of a beta-blocker with clonidine may decrease the antihypertensive effect of the alpha-2 agonist.
3. Abrupt discontinuation of clonidine and beta-blockers may cause symptoms of sympathetic overactivity.
4. Treatment for rebound due to clonidine withdrawal is with reinitiation of clonidine. This should resolve the signs and symptoms.

REFERENCES
1. Marsh CB, Mazzaferri EL: Internal Medicine Pearls. Hanley & Belfus, Philadelphia, 1993.
2. Mehta JL, Lopez LM: Rebound hypertension following abrupt cessation of clonidine and metoprolol. Arch Intern Med 147:389–390, 1987.
3. Lilja M, Jounela AJ, Juustila HJ, Paalzow L: Abrupt and gradual change from clonidine to beta-blockers in hypertension. Acta Med Scand 211:374–380, 1982.

Michael Mohundro, PharmD
George E. Habeeb, Jr., MD

PATIENT 34

A 50-year-old man with proteinuria and a renal mass

A 50-year-old man presents to his physician for an annual physical examination. He feels well with no symptoms or complaints. He would like a detailed check-up because of his age. He has never had medical problems or taken any medications. He does not use tobacco and drinks alcohol socially. His parents are still living and healthy; at 75 years of age his father takes one medication for hypertension.

Physical Examination: Temperature 99.0°F, pulse 74, respiratory rate 18, blood pressure 148/94. General: healthy, in no distress. Skin: color and turgor normal. Cardiac: regular rhythm with normal heart sounds. Chest: clear. Abdomen: nondistended, no bruits, no hepatosplenomegaly, and no palpable masses. Genitourinary: prostate normal size, no mass, fecal occult blood test negative.

Laboratory Findings: Hemogram: normal. Blood chemistries, BUN, creatinine: normal. Liver panel: normal. Fasting total cholesterol 180 mg/dl, HDL-C 41 mg/dl, triglycerides 150 mg/dl, LDL-C 109 mg/dl. Urinalysis: protein > 100 mg/dl, WBC 3/hpf, RBC 2/hpf. 24-hour urine: protein 800 mg, creatinine clearance 110 mL/min. Renal ultrasonography: suggestion of solid left renal mass. Computed tomographic (CT) scan of abdomen with contrast: mass in left kidney (see figure).

Question: What is the etiology of the proteinuria and renal mass?

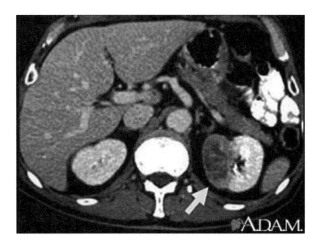

Diagnosis: Renal cell carcinoma

Discussion: Approximately 30,000 people are diagnosed with renal cell carcinoma in the United States each year, and around 12,000 patients die of this disease annually. Renal cell carcinoma affects men more than women, and is most commonly seen in those over 55 years of age. Renal cell carcinoma is associated with several risks including cigarette smoking, family history, obesity, well-cooked meat, and occupational exposures. Studies suggest that workplace exposure to asbestos, the heavy metal cadmium, and organic solvents (particularly trichloroethylene), increase the risk of developing renal cell carcinoma.

As in this patient, renal cell carcinoma is often an insidious disease process. Few patients present with the classic triad of flank pain, palpable abdominal mass, and hematuria. Symptoms are nonspecific and may develop very slowly. Often patients do not develop flank or back pain, weight loss, hematuria, abdominal distention, or hypertension until the disease becomes advanced. Subtle clues such as this patient's isolated proteinuria can lead to further investigation and subsequent diagnosis of renal cell carcinoma in the early stages.

Although rare, systemic or para-neoplastic syndromes can raise the suspicion of the presence of renal cell carcinoma. Patients may develop hypercalcemia, anemia, amyloidosis, hepatic dysfunction, fever, cachexia, anorexia, erythrocytosis, or thrombocytosis. Tumors may overproduce hormones such as erythropoietin, parathyroid hormone–related protein (PTHrP), gonadotropins, human chorionic somatomammotropin (an adrenocorticotropic hormone ACTH–like substance), renin, glucagon, or insulin.

When renal cell carcinoma is suspected in a patient, renal ultrasonography is a useful diagnostic tool. If a mass is noted to be round and sharply demarcated, with smooth walls and a strong posterior wall echo, the chance of malignancy is considered to be low. If a complex cyst or solid mass is seen, computed tomography of the abdomen with contrast can further characterize the mass. Neoplastic lesions have thickened, irregular walls, thickened or enhanced septae within the mass, and may enhance with contrast. Most malignant renal masses are > 4 cm. For patients with contrast allergies or renal insufficiency in whom a contrasted CT scan is contraindicated, magnetic resonance imaging (MRI) of the abdomen with gadolinium contrast is useful and nontoxic.

Treatment depends on tumor stage and classification of the type of renal cell carcinoma. In early-stage disease, partial or total nephrectomy is effective in eliminating the cancer without a high incidence of recurrence. Once metastasis has occurred (most commonly to lungs, lymph nodes, bones, liver, or the contralateral kidney), surgery is no longer an effective modality. Nonsurgical treatments, including radiation, hormonal therapy, immunotherapy, and chemotherapy, have limited success rates. Ongoing research into development of a vaccine for immunotherapy and unique detection methods offer hope for improved survival in renal cell carcinoma.

Hypertension associated with renal cell carcinoma is caused by renal parenchymal damage in the involved kidney. Removal of the malignant kidney generally resolves the hypertension. In some cases, the contralateral kidney has sustained damage from chronic hypertension, and continued medical therapy is necessary. Management then follows the same guidelines as for other patients with essential hypertension and renal parenchymal disease. This patient had a total left nephrectomy and recovered with no complications or recurrence of cancer. His blood pressure normalized after surgery.

Clinical Pearls:

1. Renal cell carcinoma may present with subtle changes; clinicians should be alert for symptoms such as flank pain, hematuria, and proteinuria in patients with risk factors.
2. Renal ultrasonography is a useful screening test; CT scan of the abdomen can be used in patients with suspicious masses.
3. Surgical resection of the malignancy in the early stages provides the best prognosis and should eliminate or reduce the need for antihypertensives.

REFERENCES

1. Mickisch G, Carballido J, Hellsten S, et al: Guidelines on renal cell cancer. Eur Urol 40:252–255, 2001.
2. Gold PJ, Fefer A, Thompson JA: Paraneoplastic manifestations of renal cell carcinoma. Semin Urol Oncol 14:216–222, 1996.
3. Curry NS: Small renal masses (lesions smaller than 3 cm): Imaging evaluation and management. Am J Roentgenol 164:355–362, 1995.
4. Bosniak, MA. The small (less than or equal to 3.0 cm) renal parenchymal tumor: Detection, diagnosis, and controversies. Radiology 179:307–317, 1991.
5. Laski ME, Vugrin D. Paraneoplastic syndromes in hypernephroma. Semin Nephrol 7:123–30, 1987.
6. Chisholm GD, Roy RR: The systemic effects of malignant renal tumors. Br J Urol 43:687, 1971.

Angela Stubbs, RN, CFNP, MSN
Marion R. Wofford, MD

PATIENT 35

A 52-year-old woman with declining visual acuity

A 52-year-old woman presents as a new patient to a clinic for a routine physical examination. She expresses concern that she has been experiencing a decline in her vision over the last several months. She has never required eyeglasses. There is no history of hypertension, coronary artery disease, or diabetes. She presents a history of smoking one pack of cigarettes per day for the last 25 years and denies alcohol consumption. She is currently taking no prescription. She admits to taking over-the-counter antihistamines and decongestants for frequent sinusitis. Significant is a strong family history of hypertension, diabetes, and heart disease.

Physical Examination: General: obese, no acute distress. Temperature 98.2°F, pulse 86, blood pressure 170/98 both arms. Weight 165 pounds, height 64 inches, BMI 28.3. Cardiac: regular rhythm, I/VI systolic murmur at left lower sternal border. No gallops, thrills, or bruits. Point of maximum intensity (PMI) at sixth intercostal space, midclavicular line. No jugular venous distention or edema. Lungs: clear to posterior and anterior auscultation. No tactile fremitus. Neurological: all cranial nerves intact. Pupils equal and reactive to light. Funduscopic examination: diffuse narrowing of arterioles with copper wire changes; early venous tapering; optic disc margins sharp without edema (see figure).

Laboratory Findings: CBC normal. Electrolytes, BUN, creatinine: normal. Thyroid-stimulating hormone normal. Other diagnostic findings: EKG: normal sinus rhythm and left ventricular hypertrophy (LVH). ECG: an enlarged left ventricle with mild mitral valve prolapse. Ejection fraction 45%.

Question: What is the significance of this patient's funduscopic examination?

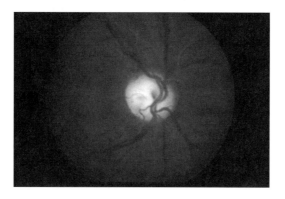

Diagnosis: Hypertensive retinopathy

Discussion: Retinopathies are pathologic conditions of the retina that occur in conjunction with certain systemic disorders such as hypertension, nephritis, toxemia of pregnancy, and diabetes mellitus. The Atherosclerosis Risk in Communities (ARIC) clinical study suggests that microvascular retinal changes may precede the onset of ischemic stroke. The retina is the light-sensitive portion of the eye, containing cones, which are responsible for night vision. The retinal circulation is derived from branches of the ophthalmic artery and is composed of the central retinal artery, the central retinal vein, and their branches. In hypertensive retinopathy, the light reflex from the arteriolar wall is abnormal and constriction of the venous wall appears at sites of arteriovenous crossing. A reliable sign of hypertensive retinopathy is variation in the caliber of the renal arterioles. The retinal circulation is highly sensitive to local tissue metabolic needs, specifically glucose and oxygen metabolism, and is susceptible to damage from circulatory dysfunction. Changes in retinal blood vessels are the most common vascular lesions of systemic hypertension in the eye.

The ocular lesions of systemic hypertension reveal important information about the duration and severity of the hypertensive state. The retinal changes observed during the funduscopic examination of this patient are indicative of end-organ hypertensive damage. Initial visible changes in the retinal vessels in hypertension are narrowing of the arteries and arterioles. The ratio of retinal artery-to-vein diameter is noted to be subjective and variable in the literature with the most common suggestion of 2:3. The arterial-wall changes seen in hypertension are indicative of arteriosclerosis and represent chronic moderate hypertension. Collagen replaces the muscle layer, which results in progressive thickening of the arterial wall.

The "copper wire" change (see figure) seen in this patient is indicative of hypertensive retinal changes. Arteriosclerotic changes produce an increase in the central light reflex and a decrease in the width of the blood column seen on either side of the light reflex. With progression, the light reflex becomes reddish brown instead of the normal yellow–white appearance. As the wall continues to thicken, the blood-column width diminishes and eventually disappears. At this point, the artery appears as a white thread and is referred to as a "silver wire" change.

Arteriovenous nicking, sometimes referred to as venous tapering, is also a visible change that this patient has that may indicate retinal vessel damage related to chronic hypertension or arteriosclerosis. The thick-walled artery with its increased luminal pressure, as well as the proliferation of perivascular glia, compress the thin-walled, low pressure veins at the point of their crossing. The vein may change direction at this point of crossing producing a right-angle bend. Arteriovenous nicking can lead to retinal vein occlusion, which is characterized by sudden, severe loss of vision. The funduscopic examination would reveal dilated and tortuous veins with a wedge-shaped cluster of hemorrhages pointing toward the responsible arteriovenous crossing.

Other findings that are associated with severe hypertension include soft exudate ("cotton wool spots") that appear as round white patches with soft irregular borders and indicate a reduced blood flow from sclerosis and infarction of the small retinal arteries. Hard exudates appear as creamy or yellowish lesions with well-defined borders. These lesions may combine to form larger lesions and often occur in clusters, or in circular, linear, or star-shaped patterns. Hemorrhages may occur as a result of the disruption of the blood–retina barrier from prolonged hypertension, occasionally seen as flame-shaped. Capillary microaneurysms are usually associated with diabetic retinopathy, but they may also occur in hypertensive retinopathy. The funduscopic examination reveals a berry-shaped (fusiform) outpouching of the retinal capillaries. Arteriolar macroaneurysms are characterized by berry-shaped outpouching of the retinal artery or arteriole and may be surrounded by a ring of lipid exudate. These aneurysms are benign in that they thrombose spontaneously.

This patient has stage 2 (moderate) essential hypertension. Randomized prospective clinical trials have shown that aggressive treatment of high blood pressure decreases the occurrence and extent of end-organ damage that can result from uncontrolled hypertension. The goal for treating hypertensive retinopathy is to aggressively control the blood pressure. This patient is also at high risk for cardiovascular disease. She was instructed on lifestyle modifications such as a low-salt, low-fat diet, smoking cessation, and exercise. Pharmacological therapy is based on the severity of hypertension and the presence or absence of end-organ damage. Prescribed pharmacological therapy for this patient includes a thiazide diuretic, hydrochlorothiazide 12.5 mg daily, and an ACE inhibitor, trandolapril 2 mg daily. The patient was also prescribed aspirin 325 mg daily because of her high risk factor for heart disease. She returned to the clinic 2 weeks later for follow-up evaluation. Her blood pressure at that time had decreased significantly to 130/84 mmHg, close to goal. This patient's funduscopic examination revealed no further retinal changes.

Clinical Pearls

1. A thorough funduscopic examination should be included in the initial evaluation of all hypertensive patients.
2. The ocular lesions of systemic hypertension reveal important information about the duration and severity of the hypertensive state.
3. With prolonged uncontrolled hypertension, retinal changes include soft and hard retinal exudates, retinal hemorrhages, and papilledema.
4. The goal for treating hypertensive retinopathy is to aggressively control the blood pressure.

REFERENCES

1. Wong TY, Klein R, Sharrett AR, et al: Aric Investigators. Atherosclerosis Risk in Communities Study. JAMA 288(1):67–74, 2002.
2. Kaplan NM: Kaplan's Clinical Hypertension, 8th ed. Philadelphia, Publisher 2002.
3. Sobel BJ, Bakris GL: Hypertension: A clinician's guide to diagnosis and treatment, 2nd ed. Philadelphia; Hanley & Belfus, 1999.
4. Sapira JD: The eye: In The Art and Science of Bedside Diagnosis. Baltimore; Williams & Wilkins, 1990.

Barbara Boss, RN, CFNP, PhD
Pamela Helms, RN, CFNP, MSN
Sharon B. Wyatt, RN, CANP, PhD

PATIENT 36

A 44-year-old man with too much stress at work

A 44-year-old man walks into the clinic asking to be seen. He has been employed for several years as a clerk in a local convenience store. His chief complaint is "I have too much stress at work and have been feeling bad for weeks. I am getting worse." For several weeks he has experienced nervousness, anxiety, and headaches. He admits to being under increasing stress on his job since a promotion to night supervisor, which resulted in working more consecutive days with less time off. The patient denies any significant health problems, is not taking any prescription medication, and does not have a health care provider. For 20 years he has smoked a pack of cigarettes daily. He reports that his mother, father, and brother have been diagnosed with hypertension.

Physical Examination: Temperature 98°F, pulse 94, respiratory rate 24, blood pressure 170/110 sitting, 164/100 standing, height 6 feet, weight 160 pounds, BMI 22. Eyes: normal funduscopic. Neck: normal thyroid, no jugular venous distension or bruits. Chest: clear. Cardiac: loud S_2 but otherwise normal. Abdomen: normal, scaphoid. Neurological: normal. Peripheral vascular: normal.

Laboratory Findings: Electrolytes, BUN, and creatinine normal. ECG normal.

Question: What is the relationship of the patient's stress to his elevated blood pressure?

Diagnosis: Primary hypertension potentially related to stress/anxiety

Discussion: The adverse reactions of individuals to their environments in terms of their blood pressure has been examined via (1) epidemiological field studies that investigated the effects of environmental stressors, (2) research on personality differences between normotensive and hypertensive persons, (3) laboratory studies in humans to examine the influence of individual differences regarding susceptibility or reactivity to standardized stressors, and (4) animal models of stress-induced hypertension.

Epidemiological data including a 30-year observational study of Italian nuns and observational studies of persons who migrate from stable traditional societies to a westernized society, support that elevation in blood pressure is environmentally and culturally determined. Age-related increases in blood pressure do not occur in all societies. Something about modern society elevates blood pressure in a short period of time and sustains that rise in blood pressure even though heart rate and body weight increases are not sustained. Sodium retention and increased sympathetic nervous system activity are the suspected pathophysiologic explanations.

A growing body of evidence supports an increased sympathetic nervous system activity in early hypertension. In animal studies that examine control, dominant animals have higher blood pressures, but the highest blood pressures are seen in subdominant animals seeking dominance. Likewise in humans, prisoners in isolation have lower blood pressure than those living in dormitories. Activation of the sympathetic nervous system, known by several names—a flight or fight response, a defense reaction to challenges, or a neurogenically mediated pressor response— releases catecholamine neurotransmitters from postsynaptic nerve endings. From 15 to 25% of the catecholamine released is norepinephrine, which is known to mediate vasoconstriction of arteriolar smooth muscle, resulting in narrowing of the vessels. Subsequently norepinephrine, the hormone, is released from the adrenal medulla. Norepinephrine at physiologic concentration binds primarily to the adrenergic receptors. Fortunately, very little adrenal medullary norepinephrine actually reaches the vessels themselves. No evidence exists that supports this as the mechanism for sustained hypertension.

However, epinephrine release as the mechanism for sustained blood pressure elevation, called stress-linked hypertension, is supported by evidence. A possible mechanism for sustained hypertension is the secretion of epinephrine from the adrenal medulla, called the "adrenaline hypothesis" of essential hypertension. The blood-pressure changes are far greater and last longer than could be explained by the flight or fight mechanism. Part of the epinephrine is believed to enter the sympathetic nerve endings to be released into the synapse during subsequent sympathetic nervous system stimulation. Epinephrine also affects the presynaptic B2 receptors to further additional epinephrine release. Cardiac norepinephrine spillover is higher in hypertension and has been correlated directly with the release of epinephrine. There is a hemodynamic pattern of high cardiac output created. In addition, neuronal reuptake of norepinephrine has been found to be impaired in hypertension. There is also increasing evidence that environmental stress promotes sodium retention via renal sympathetic nerve activity that increases renin release.

Further, individuals often respond to prolonged or chronic stress with behaviors that further elevate the blood pressure. Tobacco use may start, resume, or increase in response to the stressor. Alcohol, caffeine, or illegal drug use may also start, resume, or increase. Eating is often a way of coping with stressors, causing weight gain. If the person exercises, this health practice may fall by the wayside in times of chronic stress. Under the influence of cortisol, the sleep–wake cycle is disturbed and the individual often becomes sleep deprived, a physical stressor further intensifying the stress response. A prolonged blood pressure elevation may be the result of combining the above factors with the final common pathway mediating the sustained blood pressure with the sympathetic nervous system.

The end result of persisting blood pressure elevation is permanent arteriolar damage. Prolonged vasoconstriction and high pressures stimulate blood vessels, especially arteries and arterioles, to thicken and strengthen in order to withstand the pressure. Arteriolar smooth muscles undergo hypertrophy (cellular enlargement) and hyperplasia (cell proliferation). The tunica intima and tunica media of the blood vessel experience fibromuscular thickening, which narrows the blood vessel lumen. The vessels are permanently narrowed. Peripheral vascular resistance is permanently increased, so the blood pressure becomes chronically elevated. The hemodynamic pattern of high cardiac output changes resulting from decreased cardiac compliance, decreased beta-adrenergic responsiveness, and decreased cardiac output to a high resistance pattern in late hypertension due to the increased vascular resistance.

Work-related stress has been studied as a source of chronic stress that may exacerbate the development of high blood pressure. Of particular interest is the level of individual control over the work situation. The most substantive data linking chronic stress to hypertension as well as increased left ventricular mass are found in studies examining "job strain," i.e., high demand with little control. High job strain lasting over 3 years yielded a 11/7 mmHg higher blood pressure. Neither demand nor control independent of the other elevates blood pressure.

This patient knew that the night supervisor position was his primary stressor and that he had a strong family history of hypertension. He clearly understood that stress, specifically job stress, was causing his symptoms including his hypertension. He was aware that he was smoking more. He admitted that all he had time to eat was junk food. The long work hours had caused sleep deprivation and there was no time for him to relax or exercise. He agreed to accept a medical excuse ordering him to work only 5 days a week. He was willing to walk several times a week as exercise and actively seek out nutritious foods such as salads with low-fat dressings. He was referred to a smoking cessation program. The next week his blood pressure was falling and he was talking about quitting his supervisor position. Within a month he had resigned the supervisor position and was working a 40-hour week. This allowed him time to exercise, eat better, and work on his smoking cessation. His blood pressure was averaging 150–155/90–95 mmHg. He was placed on hydrochlorothiazide (HCTZ) 12.5 mg daily, which normalized his blood pressure to 130–135/75–80 mmHg. He is still struggling with eliminating the cigarettes completely.

Clinical Pearls

1. Environmental stressors including social, economic, and cultural factors influence blood pressure.
2. Dysregulation of renal sympathetic activity is an important contributor to the pathogenesis of hypertension.
3. Catecholamines account for both the pressor mechanism that mediates early hypertension and the trophic mechanism that mediates late hypertension
4. Increasing control over work-related stress can moderate negative blood pressure effects of excess job strain.

REFERENCES

1. Kivimaki M, Leino-Arjas P, Luukkonen R, et al: Work stress and risk of cardiovascular mortality: Prospective cohort study of industrial employees. BMJ 325(7369):857, 2002.
2. Kaplan NK: Kaplan's Clinical Hypertension, 8th ed. Philadelphia, Lippincott Williams & Wilkins, 2002.
3. Esler M, Rumanter M, Lambert G, Kaye D: The sympathetic neurobiology of essential hypertension: Disparate influences of obesity, stress and noradrenaline transporter dysfunction. Am J Hypertens 14:139S–146S, 2001.
4. Webber M: Hypertension Medicine. Totowa, New Jersey, Humana Press, 2001.
5. Izzo JL, Black HR: Hypertension Primer. The Essentials of High Blood Pressure, 2nd ed. Dallas, American Heart Association, 1999.

Michelle M. Horn, MD
Marion R. Wofford, MD, MPH

PATIENT 37

A 41-year-old woman with hypertension, obesity, and hirsutism

A 41-year-old obese woman with hypertension for the past 10 years as well as hirsutism since her late adolescent years was evaluated in the clinic for hypertension. The patient was not currently taking any antihypertensive agents, although she had been on numerous therapies in the past. At the time of her visit, she was experiencing vaginal bleeding even though she had just had a normal menses 2 weeks earlier. Other than dysfunctional uterine bleeding, the patient reported no other problems. Four of her eight pregnancies resulted in live births, and four in miscarriages. She underwent menarche at the age of 13 with normal menses until recently. Her first pregnancy occurred at the age of 20. Her past surgical history was pertinent for left ovarian removal secondary to a "nonmalignant tumor." Her family history was significant for hypertension in both parents diagnosed when they were in their 50s.

Physical Examination: Temperature 97.2°F, pulse 79, respirations 16, blood pressure 180/95, BMI 32. General: obese, no acute distress. Chest: clear to auscultation bilaterally. Cardiac: regular rate and rhythm with normal S_1, prominent S_2, 3/6 systolic murmur at lower left sternal border with radiation to the left axilla. Extremities: no edema of bilateral lower extremities. Skin: male-pattern terminal hair growth on chin and sides of face, white comedones and acne scars on the forehead and nose.

Laboratory Findings: Electrolytes normal, glucose 132 mg/dl, BUN 19 mg/dl, creatinine 1.3 mg/dl. Urinalysis: > 300 protein, small blood with three RBCs. Reflexive TSH 0.795 μIU/mL. Testosterone level 144 ng/dl (normal 60–86 ng/dl), dehydroepiandrosterone sulfate (DHEAS) 450 μg/dl (normal 44–352 μg/dl). Progesterone level 9 ng/dl (normal 50 ng/dl), 17-OH progesterone 58 ng/dl (normal 20–100 ng/dl). Insulin 79.8 μIU/mL (normal 1.9–23 μIU/mL), HgbA1c 5.6% (normal 4.3–6.1%). Follicle stimulating hormone (FSH) 4.4 mIU/mL (normal 0–9.0 mIU/mL). Luteinizing hormone (LH) 20 mIU/mL (normal 1.0–12 mIU/mL). EKG: left axis deviation with left ventricular hypertrophy (LVH) and left atrial enlargement (LAE). Transthoracic echocardiogram: moderate mitral regurgitation with left atrial dilation, moderate concentric LVH with overall normal left ventricular systolic function and a left ventricular ejection fraction of 55%. Transvaginal ultrasonography (see figure): right ovary measured 3.6 × 3.5 cm with multiple peripheral cysts.

Question: What is the most likely diagnosis given this patient's hirsutism and hypertension?

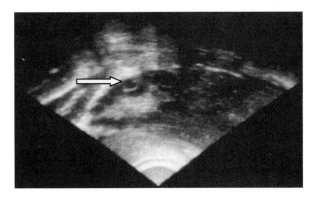

Diagnosis: Polycystic ovary syndrome

Discussion: Polycystic ovary syndrome (PCOS) is one the most common endocrinopathies in women of reproductive age and occurs in 2–10% of such women. In the past, no clear definition for this entity was available until a 1990 National Institutes of Health (NIH) conference on PCOS established two criteria used in making the diagnosis of PCOS. These criteria include menstrual irregularity and evidence of hyperandrogenism. The menstrual irregularity can be in the form of oligo- or anovulation. The evidence of hyperandrogenism can be either clinical in the form of hirsutism, acne, or male pattern balding or biochemical in the form of elevated testosterone levels. Other clinical findings associated with PCOS include virilization, which occurs in 20% of these patients, amenorrhea in 50% of patients, dysfunctional uterine bleeding in 30%, and normal menstruation in 20%.

In order to have a better understanding of this syndrome and its associated clinical findings, it is important to discuss the pathophysiologic basis of this disorder. The fundamental defect in PCOS patients is inappropriate signals to the hypothalamus and pituitary glands. Increased formation of extraglandular estrogen by peripheral conversion of androgen to estrogen leads to decreasing levels of FSH, which acts on the ovary to decrease follicle maturation and thus lead to chronic anovulation in some patients. The increased estrogen levels also cause increasing levels of LH, which acts on the ovary to stimulate stromal and thecal cells to secrete more androgen. The adrenal gland also secretes androgens, thereby contributing to androgen excess. Androgens are converted peripherally to estrogens, leading to continuation of the cycle. Obesity plays a key role in this cycle, in that the peripheral conversion of androgen to estrogen also occurs in adipose tissue. Therefore, the more obese the patient, the more the cycle is perpetuated.

One of the key PCOS clinical features present in this patient is hypertension. Several mechanisms establishing the relationship between PCOS and hypertension have been proposed, but no single mechanism has been discovered. One of these proposed mechanisms is enhancement of sympathetic activity due to insulin resistance, which most of these patients also have. This enhanced sympathetic activity leads to increased cardiac output, vasconstriction leading to increased peripheral resistance, and increased sodium resorption by the kidney. All of these factors may cause elevated blood pressure. Increased adrenal catecholamine and glucocorticoid release along with elevated testosterone levels may also exacerbate hypertension and insulin resistance in patients with PCOS.

Another feature of PCOS that was also manifested in this patient is hirsutism. Hirsutism occurs in 70% of PCOS patients and is secondary to increased androgen production. Other possible diagnoses associated with hirsutism are idiopathic hirsutism, congenital adrenal hyperplasia, ovarian tumors, and adrenal tumors, to name a few. Idiopathic hirsutism was ruled out given this patient's multiple findings associated with PCOS, such as menstrual irregularity with dysfunctional uterine bleeding, acne, and elevated testosterone levels. Congenital adrenal hyperplasia is an unlikely diagnosis as this patient has been pregnant. The patient had normal progesterone and 17-OH progesterone levels, making this diagnosis unlikely. Ovarian tumor was excluded given the patient's ultrasonographic findings (see figure). Adrenal tumor is unlikely given the patient's normal electrolyte levels.

Obesity occurs in 40–60% of patients with PCOS and plays a significant role in PCOS, along with the other key clinical features. In PCOS patients, obesity enhances the peripheral conversion of androgens to estrogens in adipose tissue, a key element in the pathophysiology of PCOS. Obesity is clearly linked to the development of the insulin resistance syndrome, which is closely associated with hypertension.

In 50–90% of PCOS patients, the serum testosterone level is increased with the DHEAS level being elevated in 30% of patients; both were elevated in this patient. An LH to FSH ratio > 2 is also consistent with a diagnosis of PCOS. Although not part of the diagnostic criteria, in 80–100% of patients, ultrasonography of the ovaries shows a peripheral array of small follicles (8–10 per ovary).

In order to treat PCOS, all of the key clinical features associated with this syndrome must be treated, so many different treatment modalities must be enlisted. Weight loss is a key therapy, since obesity is a key feature in PCOS patients. Hypertension associated with PCOS can be treated with the usual measures required to treat hypertension. Certain classes, such as angiotensin-converting enzyme (ACE) inhibitors, may be appropriate in patients with type 2 diabetes mellitus and proteinuria. Weight loss and dietary changes are recommended. Metformin suppresses hepatic gluconeogenesis, thereby decreasing insulin levels and providing benefit in the patient with impaired glucose tolerance.

Hirsutism treatment focuses on changing or minimizing the effects of excess androgens. The response rate to treatment for hirsutism ranges from 20 to 95% depending on the type of treatment used and individual response to such therapy. The response may not be evident for 6–12 months. Treatment may prevent further terminal hair development but effects little change on the number of hairs already present. Spironolactone, an aldosterone antagonist and potent antiandrogen, is frequently used in the treatment of hirsutism with improvement in 70–75% of hirsute females after 6 months. Oral contraceptives may decrease hirsutism and the endometrial hyperplasia found in some PCOS patients. Oral contraceptives ensure endometrial shedding and decrease the risk of endometrial cancer. PCOS patients are at increased risk for endometrial cancer and breast cancer due to unopposed estrogen.

This patient was started on spironolactone, quinapril, and furosemide with improvement in her blood pressure into the 150–160/80–90 mmHg range. Many months of therapy may be required before reduction of hirsutism is seen.

Clinical Pearls

1. Polycystic ovary syndrome is defined by two criteria established by a 1990 NIH conference on PCOS. These criteria include menstrual irregularity due to oligo- or anovulation and evidence of hyperandrogenism, whether clinical or biochemical.
2. Other key features found in patients with PCOS are hirsutism, virilization, infertility, amenorrhea or normal menstruation, dysuterine bleeding, insulin resistance secondary to hyperinsulinemia, obesity, hypertension, and dyslipidemia.
3. Laboratory findings in patients with PCOS include an elevated androgen level, normal or elevated DHEAS, and a LH to FSH ratio > 2 with either a normal or decreased FSH level.
4. Ultrasonography of the ovaries shows a peripheral array of many, small follicles on one or both ovaries.
5. Treatment of PCOS involves drug therapy consisting of spironolactone, metformin, oral contraceptives, and/or ACE inhibitors. Lifestyle modification to achieve weight reduction is recommended.

REFERENCES
1. McPhee SJ, Papadaris MA, Tierney LM: Current Medical Diagnosis and Treatment, 41st ed. New York, McGraw-Hill, 2002.
2. Homburg R: Polycystic Ovary Syndrome. United Kingdom, Martin Dunitz Ltd, 2001.
3. Amowitz LL: Cardiovascular consequences of polycystic ovary syndrome. Endocrinol Metab Clin North Am. 28(2):439–458, 1999.
4. Carr BR, Bradshaw KD: Disorders of the ovary and female reproductive tract. In Fauci AS, Braunwald E, Isselbacher KJ, et al (eds): Harrison's Principles of Internal Medicine, 14th ed. New York, McGraw-Hill, 1998.

Jinna M. Shepherd, MD
Marion R. Wofford, MD, MPH

PATIENT 38

A 56-year-old man with palpitations and sedentary lifestyle

A 56-year-old man presents to the outpatient clinic for a comprehensive physical examination. He describes a long history of palpitations and chest tightness, worsened by emotional upset. He also notes progressive anxiety with airplane travel and riding in elevators over the last several years. He denies a past history of medical problems. He has siblings with hypertension controlled on medication. He is a former runner whose lifestyle has become sedentary related to a knee injury. He is a former smoker and consumes two fifths of alcohol per week. He denies illicit drug use.

Physical Examination: Temperature 98.4°F, pulse 88, blood pressure 155/89, BMI 27. General: overweight, slightly anxious. Funduscopic: normal. Neck: no bruits. Chest: clear. Cardiac: normal S_1 and S_2, no murmur or gallop. Abdomen: no bruits. Extremities: no edema, pulses normal.

Laboratory Findings: Electrolytes, BUN, creatinine, glucose: normal. Liver panel: ALT 48 U/L, AST 138 U/L. CBC normal, increased mean cell volume (MCV) 100 fL. r TSH: normal. Lipid panel: total cholesterol 242 mg/dl, triglycerides 362 mg/dl, HDL-C 58 mg/dl, LDL-C 121 mg/dl. EKG: normal. Exercise stress test: negative for ischemia.

Question: What is the most likely etiology for the patient's hypertension?

Diagnosis: Alcohol abuse

Discussion: Several laboratory values suggest that this patient consumes excessive alcohol. Hepatic transaminases are elevated as a result of effect of alcohol on hepatic function. Macrocytosis demonstrated by a high MCV may also result from continuous insult to hepatic function. Alcohol abuse must be considered in the etiology of hypertension and hypertension control in this patient.

The relationship between alcohol and hypertension has long been established. Even as early as 1915, hypertension was noted in French servicemen who drank three or more liters of wine daily. The evidence supports an association between blood pressure and quantity of alcohol intake, which suggests a "threshold" level above which elevation in blood pressure occurs. Although this threshold level has not been defined, higher levels of alcohol consumption ($\geq$ 3 drinks per day) have been associated with approximate doubling of the prevalence of hypertension in men. Among drinkers, elevations of the systolic pressures are greater than diastolic pressures. Most studies have found a 3–4 mmHg elevation in systolic blood pressure and a 1–2 mmHg elevation in diastolic blood pressure in individuals consuming three drinks per day compared to nondrinkers. According to the Atherosclerosis Risk in Communities (ARIC) data, even low-to-moderate alcohol consumption by African American men was associated with a greater risk of hypertension. Excessive alcohol intake, an independent risk factor, may be the most common reversible cause of hypertension, as reduction of intake has been shown to decrease blood pressure. Continued alcohol use may also lessen the effectiveness of other modes of hypertension management.

Several mechanisms for alcohol-induced hypertension have been proposed, based on the direct and indirect physiologic and pharmacologic effects of alcohol. Proposed mechanisms focus on the effects of alcohol on renin, aldosterone, cortisol, insulin, and catecholamine secretion. Other hypotheses include the direct effects of alcohol on vascular smooth muscle through calcium transport, impaired insulin sensitivity, impaired baroreflex response, or magnesium depletion. None of these hypotheses have been confirmed. The interaction is obviously complex, and it seems unlikely that a single mechanism will be found responsible for the relationship between alcohol and hypertension.

In addition to the relationship between alcohol and hypertension, there are other cardiovascular conditions affected by alcohol use. The Honolulu Heart Program, which studied Japanese-American men, found a positive correlation between heavy alcohol intake and the development of hemorrhagic stroke, but an inverse correlation between alcohol and coronary artery disease. Alcoholic cardiomyopathy develops in susceptible patients with persistent use of large amounts of alcohol. In areas where malnutrition is prevalent, thiamine deficiency may play a role in the development of alcoholic heart disease.

This patient's history and presentation suggest alcohol-induced hypertension. The patient was counseled to reduce his alcohol intake to less than three drinks per day, as well as to initiate an exercise program and salt restriction. He was placed on an antidepressant for generalized anxiety and underwent counseling for stress management. After successful lifestyle modification, the patient's blood pressure and laboratory study results normalized.

Clinical Pearls

1. The quantity of alcohol intake correlates with hypertension and hypertension treatment.
2. Heavy alcohol use correlates with the risk for stroke and cardiomyopathy.
3. Excessive alcohol intake is a common reversible cause of hypertension.

REFERENCES

1. Kawano Y, Abe H, Imanishi M, et al: Pressor and depressor hormones during alcohol-induced blood pressure reduction in hypertensive patients. J Hum Hypertens 10(9):595–599, 1996.
2. MacMahon S: Alcohol consumption and hypertension. Hypertension 9:111–121, 1987.
3. Klatsky AL, Friedman GD, Siegelaub AB, Gerard MJ: Alcohol consumption and blood pressure Kaiser-Permanente Multiphasic Health Examination data. N Engl J Med 296(21):1194–1200, 1977.

George Joshua Blair, MD
Marion R. Wofford, MD, MPH

PATIENT 39

A 48-year-old man with extremely elevated blood pressure, nausea/vomiting, and mental status changes

A 48-year-old man is brought to the emergency department by his wife after she witnessed him having a seizure. For the previous 24 hours, he had been sleeping and difficult to arouse. He has vomited several times. His mental status has failed to improve since the seizure, and she has noticed that he is not moving his right side. She thinks he may have had a stroke. The patient is somnolent and unable to give much of a history. According to the wife, the patient has complained of a dull headache and blurry vision for several days. He has no history of prior seizures. His previous medical history is significant only for hypertension for which he takes "two or three" medicines. His wife admits that he ran out of his medicines over a week ago. A nitroprusside infusion is started upon his arrival to the emergency department.

Physical Examination: Temperature 96.9°F, pulse 104, respiratory rate 20, blood pressure 245/130. General: well-developed, somewhat somnolent. Chest: rales in bilateral lung bases. Cardiovascular: tachycardic rate with a normal S_1, prominent S_2, and an audible S_3. II/VI systolic ejection murmur heard best at right sternal border without radiation to the carotids, mildly elevated jugular venous pressure. Radial and dorsalis pedis pulses present. Extremities: trace bilateral lower extremity edema. Neurological: aphasic, pupils sluggishly reactive, right-sided hemiparesis with hemisensory loss, cranial nerves intact, deep tendon reflexes hyperreflexive on the right, normal on the left. Direct ophthalmoscopy (see figure): arteriovenous nicking, copper wiring, and papilledema.

Laboratory Findings: WBC 9300 µl, normal differential. Hgb 13 g/dl, Hct 39%, platelets 220. Electrolytes normal, BUN 12, creatinine 2.3. Glucose normal, PTT 36, PT 14; CK 350, CKMB 1.1, troponin I 0.15. Routine urinalysis: 2+ protein, large blood, 25 RBCs. Urine drug screen: negative. EKG: normal sinus rhythm with evidence of left ventricular hypertrophy (LVH), ST-segment depression in anterior leads. Chest radiograph: prominent cephalization of pulmonary vasculature, mild pulmonary edema, mild cardiomegaly. Noncontrast CT of head: moderate-sized acute hemorrhage in left thalamus with significant surrounding edema, no evidence of midline shift or herniation.

Question: In a patient with severe hypertension and seizures, what diagnosis should be considered?

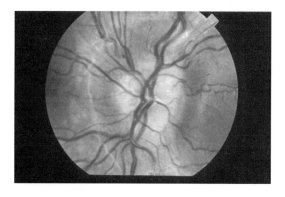

Discussion: This patient obviously has malignant hypertension and a hemorrhagic stroke. Severely elevated blood pressure is often grouped into two categories: hypertensive emergencies and urgencies. The presence or absence of signs and symptoms of end-organ damage is used to differentiate and categorize the presentation. Hypertensive *emergencies* include elevated blood pressures along with end-organ damage involving the cerebral, cardiac, or renal circulations. In hypertensive *urgencies,* blood pressure is severely elevated without evidence of organ damage. The former requires more immediate treatment to prevent further end-organ damage. This patient represents a further subset of hypertensive emergencies that involves the neurological system. Malignant hypertension is a hypertensive emergency defined as severely elevated blood pressure with associated acute neurological end-organ damage represented by papilledema or focal neurological deficits.

A stroke is defined as any injury involving the vascular system that reduces blood flow to a specific region of the brain causing neurological damage. Stroke represents the third leading cause of death in the United States and is the leading cause of disability in adults. Nearly one million people experience a stroke each year, 80% of which are ischemic and 20% hemorrhagic. There are many risk factors for intracerebral hemorrhage (ICH) including hypertension, cocaine use, anticoagulant use, tumors, arteriovenous malformations, amyloid angiopathy, and ruptured aneurysms. Hypertension is the most common risk factor for ICH. Patients with hypertension have more than double the risk as normotensive patients. This case represents a common scenario in which antihypertensive therapy is discontinued or therapy is inadequate for treatment of long-standing hypertension.

The pathophysiologic basis of hypertensive emergencies involves alterations in the autoregulation of vital organ vascular beds. Under normal conditions, blood vessels dilate as blood pressure falls, to sustain stable blood flow to vital organs. When blood pressure rises, vessels constrict. This autoregulatory mechanism is only effective in a specific range of blood pressures. When pressures rise above the capacity of this autoregulation, vessels dilate in response to increasing pressure. This process is mediated by fibrinoid necrosis and causes injury to the vascular endothelium, leading to increased vascular permeability. With acute rises in blood presssure, breakdown of the blood–brain barrier allows leakage of blood into surrounding tissue with ensuing hemorrhage.

Hypertensive hemorrhages occur in the territory of penetrator arteries that branch off major intracerebral arteries. The presenting neurological deficits depend on the involved area. Brain injury and subsequent symptoms are related to the edema that develops around the area of hemorrhage. This edema increases intracranial pressure leading to papilledema.

When a patient presents with severely elevated blood pressure, immediate determination of acute end-organ damage is required to differentiate hypertensive urgency from emergency. A focused medical history and physical assessment can help with differential diagnosis. As with this man, patients with neurological emergencies often present with severe headache, vomiting, a decreased level of consciousness, somnolence, stupor, seizures, stiff neck, or meningismus. Patients presenting with any of these findings should undergo a thorough neurological examination including examination of optic fundi by direct ophthalmoscopy. Any patient with papilledema, new retinal hemorrhages or exudates, or focal neurological deficits should be considered as a neurological emergency.

Neurological emergencies, which include ischemic stroke, intracerebral hemorrhage, and hypertensive encephalopathy, are the most difficult to distinguish from one another. Correct diagnosis is critical because treatment is dramatically different. Hypertensive encephalopathy is a diagnosis of exclusion. Stroke or other etiologies must be excluded. This patient likely had encephalopathy for several days prior to the acute stroke.

Ischemic and hemorrhagic strokes are diagnosed by demonstrating focal neurological deficits with corresponding lesions on a computed tomographic (CT) scan. The physical examination can be indistinguishable between an ischemic stroke and an ICH. The gold standard for differentiation is the noncontrasted CT scan. A CT scan can show the size and location of the hemorrhage as well as information about extension or surrounding edema. It allows accurate detection of any midline shifts or herniation. Hyperacutely, blood will appear hyperdense, in contrast to chronic blood which will become isodense and gradually become hypodense. Although CT scan is most commonly used, recent studies suggest that MRI can also be used to diagnoses acute ICH.

Mortality after ICH is extremely high, and in those who survive, only a minority will function independently after the event. All patients presenting with malignant hypertension should be hospitalized with close monitoring of blood pressure. The treatment involves the judicious lowering of blood pressure, while avoiding excessive drops in pressure that can cause end-organ damage by hypoperfusion.

This patient's mental status and aphasia improved within 2 days of blood pressure reductions. Unfortunately, he has a severe residual right-sided neurologic deficit.

Clinical Pearls

1. Hypertensive emergencies differ from hypertensive urgencies by having signs and symptoms of end-organ damage.
2. Hypertensive emergencies result from an alteration in the autoregulation of important vascular beds of vital organs.
3. Hypertensive encephalopathy presents with mental status changes and is diagnosed after excluding other etiologies.
4. Any patient presenting with severely elevated blood pressures should have their optic fundi inspected by direct ophthalmoscopy to rule out papilledema.
5. Hyperacute blood is hyperdense on a CT scan, whereas chronic blood may be either isodense or hypodense.

REFERENCES

1. Phillips RA, Greenblatt J, Krakoff LR: Hypertensive emergencies: Diagnosis and management. Prog Cardiovasc Dis 45(1):33–48, 2002.
2. Kaplan NM: Hypertensive crises. In Kaplan NH, Lieberman E, Neal W (eds): Kaplan's Clinical Hypertension, 8th ed. Philadelphia, Lippincott Williams & Wilkins, 2002.
3. Elliott WJ: Hypertensive emergencies. Crit Care Clin 17(2):435–451, 2001.
4. Gebel JM, Broderick JP: Intracerebral hemorrhage. Neurol Clin 18(2):419–438, 2000.
5. Varon J, Marik PE: The diagnosis and management of hypertensive crisis. Chest 118(1):214–227, 2000.

PATIENT 40

A 60-year-old woman with weight loss, palpitations, and nervousness

A 60-year-old woman presents to a local emergency department with complaints of epigastric pain that radiates to her chest for the past week. The pain occurs mostly at night and is worse when she eats spicy food or drinks beverages containing caffeine. She gets relief by taking antacids. Occasionally she has nausea, vomiting, and diarrhea. She reports a 50-pound weight loss over the past year, 10 pounds of which occurred over the past month, despite a good appetite. She began experiencing palpitations a few months ago that are intermittent but not associated with chest pain. She has also had difficulty swallowing food for the past few months and has been unable to sleep for the past 3 days. She has noticed edema in her legs for approximately 3 weeks and she states she is "more nervous than usual." She notes that her hair has become more fine and seems to be getting thinner recently. She reports no significant medical history and states that she is 10 years postmenopause. She does not take any medications. She lives with her husband and has smoked one-half pack of cigarettes daily for the past 20 years. She does not use alcohol. She has a daughter who was recently diagnosed with hyperthyroidism and a sister with Graves' diseases. Her father had arthritis and died of a stroke when he was 56. Her mother had breast cancer and her grandmother died of leukemia.

Physical Examination: Temperature 98.8°F, pulse 114, respirations 18, blood pressure 150/82, height 5 feet 2 inches weight 118 pounds. General: thin, appears anxious. Skin: hyperpigmented on upper back and lower extremities. Hair: fine and sparse. Eyes: lid lag and mild proptosis, normal funduscopic. Neck: supple, smooth, symmetrically enlarged thyroid with thyroid bruit and jugular venous distension to jaw line. Chest: clear. Cardiac: hyperdynamic S_1 and S_2 with tachycardia and irregularly irregular rhythm; no murmurs. Abdomen: flat with palpable aortic pulsations. Extremities: 2^+ pitting edema to the knees, fingernails and toenails flaking with prominent ridges on thumbnails.

Laboratory Findings: CBC normal. Electrolytes, BUN, and creatinine normal. Thyroid panel: total T_4 24.3 µg/dl, TSH < 0.018 µU/mL, T_3 resin uptake (RU) 49%, total T_3 720 ng/dl. EKG: atrial fibrillation with ventricular response of 118.

Question: What diagnosis can explain this patient's symptom complex?

Diagnosis: Graves' disease, hyperthyroidism, hypertension, and new-onset atrial fibrillation.

Discussion: Thyrotoxicosis has many causes, but the most common cause of hyperthyroidism is Graves' disease. A triad of effects including high levels of circulating thyroid hormone, diffusely enlarged goiter, and either ophthalmopathy or dermopathy usually characterizes Graves' disease. The etiology of the disease is unknown, but is likely an autoimmune response. Graves' disease affects mostly women (5:1 ratio) and its onset occurs most commonly during the third decade of life. Symptoms of hyperthyroidism include heat intolerance, increased sweating, increased appetite, thinning of hair, prominence of the eyes, lid lag, palpitations, fatigue, weakness, nervousness, irritability, and insomnia.

Hyperthyroidism, especially overt thyrotoxicosis, may have significant effects on the cardiovascular system. Thyroid hormone acts on the heart and systemic vasculature directly by exerting a vasodilatory effect on the vascular smooth muscle. This results in decreased systemic vascular resistance as much as 50–70%, and increased blood flow to the skin, muscles, liver, and heart. Consequently, these events lead to a reflex tachycardia, increased stroke volume, and increased cardiac output. The increased shunting of blood to peripheral tissues causes the perfusion pressure to the kidneys to decrease. This leads to the release of renin and activation of the renin-angiotensin system. Thus, elevated levels of angiotensin-converting enzyme (ACE) have been demonstrated in hyperthyroidism. The end result of this cascade is increased sodium resorption and expanded plasma and blood volumes. Thyroid hormone also acts directly on cardiac myocytes that modulate cardiac contractility. The end result of cardiac and peripheral vascular changes on blood pressure is an increase in systolic pressure, a decrease in diastolic pressure, and thus a widened pulse pressure.

Initial therapy is directed at reversing the cardiac effects of thyrotoxicosis to prevent damage to the heart. Beta-blockers are effective at improving symptoms of hyperthyroidism including anxiousness, tremulousness, muscle weakness, and heat intolerance, together with the cardiac effects of tachycardia, widened pulse pressure, increased stroke volume, increased cardiac output, hyperdynamic precordium, and palpitations. They have no effect on goiter size or weight loss. Beta-blockers are also the treatment of choice for atrial fibrillation in the face of hyperthyroidism. Parenteral beta-blockers are reserved for patients with thyroid storm or those who are hemodynamically compromised. Propranolol is the beta-blocker most commonly used in the treatment of hyperthyroidism. Doses of 20 to 40 mg, three to four times daily often improve symptoms, but severely toxic patients may require 240 to 480 mg per day to control symptoms and decrease heart rate. All beta-blockers, both selective and nonselective, appear equally efficacious in symptomatic treatment. Beta-blockers with intrinsic sympathomimetic activity are not recommended because they do not have as much effect on heart rate as other beta-blockers.

Ultimate treatment involves re-establishing of a euthyroid state through radioiodine therapy (radiolabeled iodine 131 [^{131}I]), or antithyroid medications such as propylthiouracil or methimazole, or surgery. In the United States, the treatment of choice for patients with Graves' disease is radioiodine therapy. Generally, radioactive iodine is quick, easy, painless, and effective. The most common complication with radioiodine therapy is hypothyroidism, which occurs in 30–70% of patients. The patients then require lifelong thyroid hormone replacement therapy. Alternative therapy for hyperthyroidsim is usually antithyroid drugs; propylthiouracil or methimazole. These drugs are thioamides that inhibit the oxidation binding of iodide and its coupling to tyrosine. In addition, propylthiouracil inhibits the peripheral conversion of T_4 to T_3 and also has a faster onset than methimazole. It is also the drug of choice for hyperthyroidism in pregnancy. Methimazole, however, can be used as a single daily dose of 30 to 40 mg, compared to propylthiouracil which must be dosed at 400 to 600 mg, divided in three-to-four doses per day. Both drugs have demonstrated similar efficacy. Adverse effects of both drugs are similar and include skin rashes, gastrointestinal symptoms, and, less commonly, hepatitis and agranulocytosis. Because of the risk of agranulocytosis it is recommended that patients receive a baseline WBC count, and periodic monitoring of WBC counts, especially if a patient exhibits symptoms of high fever, malaise, gingivitis, and sore throat. Thioamide therapy is usually empirical, used for 12 to 18 months, although remission rates have a wide range from 15–80% after discontinuation of therapy. Antithyroid drugs may be used as "pretreatment" to radioiodine therapy in elderly or cardiac patients to deplete the thyroid gland of hormone and to decrease the risk of excessive posttreatment hyperthyroidism. The antithyroid drugs are also preferred by some endocrinologists in childhood Graves' disease.

Because of the cardiovascular effects of thyroid hormone, hyperthyroidism can cause new-onset or worsening atrial fibrillation or heart failure. Atrial fibrillation may be difficult to control until a euthyroid state is reached. Beta-blockers and calcium channel blockers are often used as rate controllers, and anticoagulation with warfarin is recommended in those at highest risk for systemic emboli. Once a euthyroid state is reached, spontaneous conversion to normal sinus rhythm may occur, but is less likely if the duration of atrial fibrillation persists longer than 4 months of euthyroidism.

This patient exhibits classic symptoms of Graves' disease and new-onset atrial fibrillation. She was noted to have dermopathy but no visual problems. Her thyroid panel revealed high free T_4 levels, low TSH, high total T_3 levels, and a high T_3RU. These are all indicative of hyperthyroidism. The patient was treated with propranolol and methimazole initially, and eventually was treated with radioiodine and subsequent levothyroxine. Her blood pressure normalized with beta-blocker therapy, and she remained normotensive following radioactive ablation of her thyroid, without further need for antihypertensive therapy. Beta-blockers were discontinued over a 3-week period following radioiodine therapy, and she has had no further bouts of atrial fibrillation.

Clinical Pearls

1. Hyperthyroidism may cause increased systolic pressures and decreased diastolic pressures, and may thus cause an increase in pulse pressure.
2. Hyperthyroidism may cause a new-onset or worsening of atrial fibrillation and although the atrial fibrillation is difficult to control until an euthyroid state occurs, beta-blockers are used for both rate control and symptoms.
3. Beta-blockers may be used in hyperthyroidism and can reduce symptoms including blood pressure, heart rate, and tremor.
4. Blood pressure may decrease once a person with hypothyroidism is treated with thyroid hormone replacement therapy.
5. Because thyroid hormone has significant cardiovascular effects, thyroid hormone replacement therapy should be used cautiously in patients with known cardiovascular disease.

REFERENCES
1. Brent G: Thyroid Hormones (T4, T3). In Conn PM, Melmed S (eds): Endocrinology: Basic and Clinical Principles, Totowa, NJ: Humana Press 1997.
2. Klein I: Thyroid hormone and blood pressure regulation. In Laragh JH, Brenner BM (eds): Hypertension, Pathophysiology, Diagnosis and Management, 2nd ed. New York, Raven Press, 1995.
3. Franklyn JA: The management of hyperthyroidism. N Engl J Med 330:1731–1738, 1994.
4. Thyroid Guidelines Committee. AACE medical guidelines for clinical practice for evaluation and treatment of hyperthyroidism and hypothyroidism. Endocr Pract 8:457–469, 2002.
5. Geffner DL, Hershman JM: Beta-adrenergic blockade for the treatment of hyperthyroidism. Am J Med 93:61–68, 1992.

James K. Glisson, MD, PharmD
Marion R. Wofford, MD, MPH

PATIENT 41

A 45-year-old man with headaches for 2 weeks

A 45-year-old man presents with his wife who is concerned about his recently elevated blood pressure readings and his use of dietary supplements. His chief complaints include daily frontal headaches for 2 weeks and what he describes as "male menopause." He denies a history of chest pain, shortness of breath, dyspnea on exertion, palpitations, dizziness, or syncope. He was diagnosed with hypertension 14 months ago, with an average blood pressure of 150–160/90–100 mmHg. He tried salt restriction and increased the frequency of his exercise program in an attempt to avoid antihypertensive medications. He does maintain a low-fat, low-salt diet and checks his blood pressure with an automated home monitor three times a week in the midmorning. His blood pressures at home have gradually increased over the past few months. During the past 2 weeks his blood pressures have been 180–200/100–115 mmHg. He swims 20 laps three times weekly in addition to lifting weights four times each week. He has a Ph.D. in microbiology and reads many alternative medicine books and journals.

Six months ago his physician prescribed Ziac (bisoprolol 2.5mg / hydrochlorothiazide 6.25 mg) once daily. His blood pressure at that time was 155/95 mmHg. His wife states that he quit taking the Ziac after only one month of therapy. He is afraid of side effects related to synthetic drugs and he wanted to take something natural for his blood pressure and his "male problems." He is currently taking pregnenolone and DHEA (dehydroepiandrosterone) for a decreased libido and reports improvement in "male function" and energy level with these supplements. He is a nonsmoker and drinks one glass of red wine each night before bed. He takes a garlic supplement and vitamin C for blood pressure control.

Physical Examination: Temperature 98.7°F, respiratory rate 12, pulse 70, blood pressure (sitting) in dominant arm 190/110. Weight 155 pounds, BMI 24.

General: thin, no distress. Funduscopic: no papilledema, otherwise normal. Skin: no rashes or discolorations, temporal regions nontender. Cardiac: normal. Lungs: clear bilaterally. Abdomen: soft, no masses or bruits. Neurological: normal.

Laboratory Findings: Chemistries, CBC, urinalysis normal. Spot microalbumin/creatinine ratio normal. EKG sinus mechanism, rate 65, no ST changes or left ventricular hypertrophy (LVH) criteria.

Question: What diagnosis describes the severity and management of hypertension in this patient?

Diagnosis: Hypertensive urgency secondary to noncompliance

Discussion: Both hypertensive urgency and hypertensive emergency are classifications of hypertensive crisis according to the Seventh Report of the Joint National Committee on the Prevention, Detection, Evaluation and Treatment of High Blood Pressure (JNC VII). The primary difference between hypertensive urgencies and hypertensive emergencies is whether progressive target-organ damage (TOD) is present. Hypertensive urgencies require blood pressure reduction over several hours to days; however, hypertensive emergencies require immediate blood pressure reduction. Untreated hypertensive urgencies will likely result in acute TOD.

A common cause of hypertensive urgency is patient noncompliance with prescribed antihypertensives. In addition, dietary supplements containing stimulants or illicit drugs may also contribute to acute or long-term elevations in blood pressure. Ephedra alkaloids (Ma Huang) are commonly implicated dietary supplements. Dietary supplements with mineralocorticoid activity may also lead to elevations in blood pressure. Steroid precursors such as pregnenolone, which this patient was taking, are readily available in a variety of retail outlets. Pregnenolone may be converted into active metabolites with mineralocorticoid effects and may interfere with prescription antihypertensives.

Patients with hypertensive urgency are usually asymptomatic. Hypertensive urgency is, therefore, somewhat of a diagnosis of exclusion. Evidence of TOD should be pursued via a thorough physical examination in order to rule out hypertensive emergency. Specifically, the neurologic examination may be helpful in this endeavor (evidence of retinal hemorrhages, papilledema, or mental status changes). Furthermore, physical signs and symptoms that suggest myocardial infarction, cerebrovascular accident, or acute renal failure suggest hypertensive emergency. When evaluating a patient with severely elevated blood pressure and no obvious signs or symptoms of hypertensive emergency, the following diagnostic studies should be obtained: EKG, urinalysis, complete blood count, serum chemistries, and a toxicology screen, if appropriate. Renal insufficiency and electrolyte abnormalities may suggest secondary causes of hypertension or TOD. Microangiopathic hemolytic anemia as seen on peripheral blood smear also suggests hypertensive emergency. A toxicology screen may be positive for cocaine or other stimulants and thus reveal the etiology of a hypertensive urgency or emergency. An EKG may reveal long-standing LVH, but a close examination for any findings that suggest unstable angina or myocardial infarction should be undertaken.

Many patients may "carry on with their normal lives" for days while having hypertensive urgency, based upon blood pressure measurement of 180/120 mmHg. All patients presenting with blood pressure values in this range without evidence of progressive TOD who do not have the diagnosis of hypertension should undergo a thorough physical evaluation and laboratory analysis. Patients with such blood pressure measurements who have previously been diagnosed with hypertension and who are currently noncompliant with their antihypertensive medications should resume treatment. For patients who have not been diagnosed with hypertension, many authorities suggest the use of a fast-acting angiotensin-converting enzyme inhibitor (ACEI) such as captopril or other oral agents, such as labetolol or a loop diuretic. A precipitous drop in blood pressure should be avoided, as well as the practice of giving sublingual nifedipine. Optimally, patients with hypertensive urgency should be observed for several hours after an oral agent is given to reduce blood pressure. Most hypertensive urgency can be managed as an outpatient with oral agents and rapid follow-up visits to ensure adequate blood pressure reduction.

This patient presents with hypertensive urgency, based upon history, physical examination, and laboratory analysis. His recent noncompliance with previously prescribed antihypertensives is the primary etiology of his elevated blood pressure. Furthermore, the possible mineralocorticoid effects of the dietary supplement pregnenolone may have further contributed to his hypertension.

This patient discontinued the use of garlic, DHEA, and pregnenolone after counseling by his physician. He was also advised of the importance of adequate blood pressure control and monitoring. He was given 25 mg of captopril in the clinic, and after 2 hours his blood pressure had decreased to a reasonable level and he was sent home with a prescription for bisoprolol 2.5 mg/hydrochlorothiazide 6.25 mg (Ziac) once daily and instructed to take the first dose on the day of his clinic visit. He returned for weekly follow-up visits and after one month his average blood pressure was 145/90 mmHg after increasing the Ziac to 10 mg/6.25 mg.

Clinical Pearls

1. Patients who present with hypertensive urgency do not have evidence of acute target-organ damage.
2. Each patient should undergo a thorough history and physical to determine possible etiologies.
3. Patient noncompliance must always be considered as a contributing factor.
4. Dietary supplements and illicit drugs are often an unconsidered cause of increases in blood pressure and hypertensive urgency.

REFERENCES

1. Jellin JM, Gregory P, Batz F, et al: Pharmacist's letter/prescriber's letter natural medicines comprehensive database, web version. Stockton, CA: Therapeutic Research Faculty. Available from http://www.naturaldatabase.com. (Accessed October 23, 2002.)
2. Kaplan NM: Hypertensive crises. In Kaplan NM, Lieberman E (eds): Kaplan's Clinical Hypertension, 8th ed. Philadelphia, Lippincott Williams & Wilkins, 2002.
3. Blumenfeld JD, Laragh JH: Management of hypertensive crises: The scientific basis for treatment decisions. Am J Hypertens 14:1154–1167, 2001.
4. Bales A: Hypertensive crisis: How to tell if it's an emergency or an urgency. Postgrad Med 105:119–126, 130, 1999.
5. Chobanian AV, Bakris GL, Black HR, et al: National Heart, Lung, and Blood Institute Joint National Committee on Prevention, Detection, Evaluation, and Treatment of Blood Pressure; National High Blood Pressure Education: The Seventh Report of the Joint National Committee on Prevention, Detection, Evaluation, and Treatment of High Blood Pressure: the JNC VII report, JAMA 289(19):2560–2572, 2003.

Karen Winters, RN, MSN
Sharon B. Wyatt, RN, CANP, PhD

PATIENT 42

A 47-year-old woman with inconsistent blood pressure measurements

A 47-year-old woman presents to the clinic to follow up on an elevated blood pressure reading obtained at a community screening. Both her parents and one of her brothers have hypertension, and her father had a heart attack at age 62. She has no history of diabetes and reports no chest pain, palpitations, dyspnea, orthopnea, or paroxysmal nocturnal dyspnea. She rarely engages in exercise. She is obese and admits to eating a diet that is high in fat and sugar. She does not smoke or drink alcoholic beverages.

Physical Examination: Temperature 99.2°F, pulse 72 and regular, respiratory rate 18, initial blood pressure 166/108 (taken by nursing assistant using regular adult cuff), repeat 136/84 (taken by nurse practitioner using large adult cuff). BMI 39. Cardiac: normal with no gallops or murmurs; peripheral pulses palpable, no carotid bruits, no peripheral edema. Lungs: breath sounds clear, respiratory effort unlabored. Abdomen: soft and nondistended, liver not palpable. Funduscopic: unremarkable. Neurologic: unremarkable.

Laboratory Findings: Hemogram: normal. Electrolytes: normal, thyroid-stimulating hormone (TSH) 3.4, fasting glucose 88. Urinalysis: negative for glucose and protein.

Question: What is the cause of inconsistency in blood pressure measurement?

Discussion: Accurate measurement of blood pressure is necessary for the appropriate diagnosis and treatment of hypertension. Falsely high measurements increase health care costs by unnecessarily treating those who do not have hypertension. Obtaining falsely low measurements of blood pressure puts patients at risk for morbidity and mortality as a result of prolonged periods of uncontrolled hypertension. Inconsistent readings confuse the patient and the provider, resulting in sporadic treatment.

The indirect measurement of blood pressure is the most common and costeffective way of monitoring the blood pressure, and is the most appropriate method for a clinic setting. Errors in the measurement of blood pressure can occur as a result of inherent variability of the blood pressure, problems with equipment, or poor adherence to proper technique.

The equipment needed for indirect measurement of the blood pressure includes a stethoscope or sensing microphone for auscultation of the Korotkoff sounds and a sphygmomanometer. The sphygmomanometer consists of an inflation system and a mercury or aneroid manometer with a calibrated scale for measuring pressure. The inflation system includes an inflatable bladder enclosed in a cuff that wraps around the patient's arm, a valved rubber bulb for inflation and deflation of the bladder, and tubing that connects the bulb and the manometer to the bladder. Equipment problems include cracks in bladder or tubing, poor connections between various parts, decalibration of the manometer, and faulty valves. When the manometer is properly calibrated, the pressure in the cuff reflects the pressure on the column of mercury or the location of a needle on a dial scale (aneroid). The mercury manometer is more accurate, easier to maintain, and less likely to become decalibrated than the aneroid manometer. However, the use of a mercury manometer has been discouraged due to concerns of exposure to mercury from accidental spills. The aneroid manometer is prone to decalibration and requires maintenance every 6 months to ensure accuracy. For both the mercury and aneroid manometers, the reading on the scale should rest at zero when the cuff is not inflated.

The size of the inflation bladder and cuff are very important. A cuff or bladder that is too small will cause the measurement to be higher than the actual pressure (see figure). A cuff or bladder that is too large will cause the measurement to be lower than the actual pressure. The width of the bladder should be at least 40% of the upper arm circumference at the midpoint. The length of the bladder should be long enough to encircle at least 80% of the arm in adults. In children the bladder should be long enough to encircle the arm completely. The cuff that encases the bladder should be long enough to completely encircle the limb so that the noninflatable portion overlaps that containing the bladder. Table 1 displays common cuff

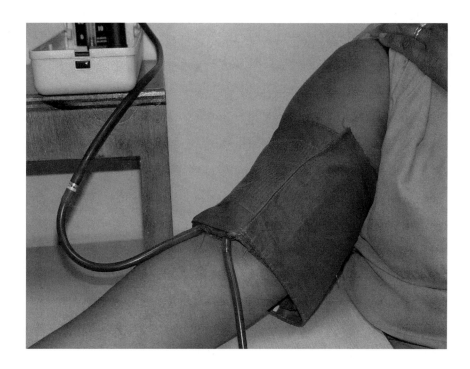

Table 1. Recommended Blood Pressure Cuff Size by Arm Circumference

Cuff	Bladder Width (cm)	Bladder Length (cm)	Arm Circumference Range at Midpoint (cm)
Infant	5	15	6–15
Child	8	21	16–21
Small adult	10	24	22–26
Adult	13	30	27–34
Large adult	16	38	35–44
Adult thigh	20	42	45–52

sizes and the appropriate arm circumferences for which they should be used.

Automated devices are available to measure the blood pressure by the auscultory or oscillometric technique. The oscillometric method is based on detecting the oscillations in the occluded artery that begin when the cuff has been deflated to a level that approximates the systolic pressure. The oscillations reach their peak at the level of the mean arterial pressure. The systolic pressure is fairly accurate, but the diastolic pressure is a derived value, and may not be as accurate. Automated devices that use the auscultory technique employ an electronic device to detect the Korotkoff sounds in a manner similar to the manual technique. All automated devices must be maintained and calibrated to ensure accuracy of measurement.

The American Heart Association Council for High Blood Pressure Research has established standards for the accurate measurement of blood pressure, as outlined in Table 2. Errors in the measurement of blood pressure occur frequently in clinical practice. Many heath care workers are unaware of these recommendations. Furthermore, most health care workers do not participate in regular training programs to improve and reassess their skills in blood pressure measurement. Human errors that can lead to inaccurate BP measurements include selection of an inappropriate cuff size, improper positioning of the patient's limb, improper speed in inflation or deflation of the cuff, digit bias, and failure to maintain the equipment.

A longer and wider cuff is needed for obese or muscular patients with very large upper arms. If the upper arm is relatively short with a large circumference, it may be difficult to fit the standard large cuff over the arm. If the upper arm is so large that a thigh cuff will not fit, a properly sized cuff can be wrapped around the forearm and the radial pulse can be palpated to estimate the systolic blood pressure. Care should be taken not to deflate the cuff too rapidly when the patient has a slow or irregular pulse. Multiple blood pressure measurements should be made and the results averaged.

In this patient, the nurse practitioner correctly suspected that the blood pressure measurement may have been erroneous and rechecked it using the proper size cuff and technique. The repeat measurement showed a blood pressure in the high normal range. Lifestyle modification was recommended to this patient, and she was scheduled to return for blood pressure measurements every six weeks for the next several months. The inexperienced nursing assistant used a cuff that was too small for this obese patient. Without rechecking the blood pressure, the provider may have initiated pharmacotherapy in conjunction with lifestyle changes. Accurate blood pressure measurement assured initiation of appropriate therapy. In order to reduce inconsistency in blood pressure measurement, the nurse practitioner established formal training in blood pressure measurement for nursing assistants and other staff in the clinic to learn the proper technique and validate the accuracy of blood pressure measurement.

Table 2.   American Heart Association Guidelines for Blood Pressure Measurement

1. Have a paper and pen available so that the blood pressure can be immediately recorded.
2. Seat the patient in a calm, quiet environment.
3. Position the patient so that both feet rest on the floor and the upper arm is supported and positioned at the level of the heart.
4. Bare the arm by raising the sleeve or removing the arm from the garment. Care should be taken to avoid rolling up the sleeve so that it forms a tight tourniquet around the upper arm.
5. Estimate or measure the circumference of the bare upper arm at the midpoint and select an appropriately sized cuff. The length of the bladder inside the cuff should be 80% of the circumference of the arm in adults and 100% of the circumference in children. If in doubt, use a larger sized cuff.
6. Palpate the brachial artery and place the cuff so that the midline of the bladder is over the arterial pulsation and the lower edge of the cuff is 1 inch (2 cm) above the antecubital fossa.
7. Wrap the cuff around the arm and secure it snugly.
8. Place the manometer so that it is easily visible, at eye level, and the tubing is unobstructed.
9. Inflate the cuff rapidly to 70 mmHg and increase by 10-mmHg increments while palpating the radial pulse. Note level at which the pulse disappears and subsequently reappears during deflation. This procedure provides an approximation of the systolic blood pressure to ensure an adequate level of inflation during the actual measurement. This method is useful for avoiding underinflation in patients who have an ausculatory gap and overinflation in patients who have a very low blood pressure. Allow at least 30 seconds between this procedure and the inflation of the cuff for the actual blood pressure measurement.
10. Place the earpieces of the stethoscope in the ear and the bell of the stethoscope over the brachial artery.
11. Inflate the bladder rapidly and steadily to a pressure that is 20 to 30 mmHg above the estimated systolic pressure that was previously determined by palpation, then slowly (2 mm/sec) deflate the cuff while listening for the appearance of the Korotoff sounds.
12. Note the level of the pressure on the manometer at the first appearance of repetitive sounds (Phase I), at the muffling of these sounds (Phase IV), and when the sounds disappear (Phase V).
13. After the last sound is heard, continue deflating the cuff slowly for another 10 mmHg to ensure that no other sounds are audible, and then rapidly and completely deflate the cuff.
14. Immediately record the systolic (Phase I) and diastolic (Phase V) blood pressure measurement. If the Phase V sound can be heard at the level of 0 mmHg, then the Phase IV pressure should also be recorded.
15. Repeat the measurement after at least 30 seconds and average the two readings.

Clinical Pearls

1. The accurate measurement of blood pressure is crucial to diagnosis and treatment of hypertension.
2. Health care professionals who measure blood pressure should adhere to standards of performance established by the American Heart Association.
3. Mercury manometers remain the gold standard for blood pressure measurement
4. Use equipment that is regularly calibrated and properly maintained.
5. Use a cuff that has a bladder with a width that is at least 40% of the circumference of the arm and length that is at least 80% of the circumference.

REFERENCES
1. Jones DW, Appel LJ, Sheps SG, et al: Measuring blood pressure accurately: New and persistent challenges. JAMA 289:1027–1030, 2003.
2. National Institutes of Health: Working meeting on blood pressure measurement. Vol.1: National High Blood Pressure Education Program, National Heart Lung, and Blood Institute, American Heart Association, 2002.
3. National Institutes of Health: The Sixth Report of the Joint National Committee on Prevention, Detection, Evaluation, and Treatment of High Blood Pressure. Arch Intern Med 157:2413–2446, 1997.
4. Perloff D, Grim C, Flack J, et al: Human blood pressure determination by sphygmomanometry. Circulation 88:2460–2470, 1993.

Michael Shoemaker-Moyle, MD
Marion R. Wofford, MD, MPH

PATIENT 43

A 52-year-old woman with depression

A 52-year-old woman with no significant previous medical history presents to an outpatient clinic stating that she has "felt down" a good bit of the time for the past 4 to 5 months. She says that "all she wants to do is sleep." Despite sleeping 12 or more hours each day, she does not feel rested upon awakening. She has lost pleasure in most activities and has even lost her appetite. She also has been bothered by constipation for the last year. Her only medication is a selective serotonin reuptake inhibitor that her local doctor prescribed about 2 months ago. She says her feeling of depression is no better since starting this medication. She does not use tobacco, alcohol, or drugs.

Physical Examination: Temperature 97.4°F, pulse 65, respiratory rate 18, blood pressure 140/96 (equal in both arms). General: well developed in no apparent distress, affect blunted and appears tired. Funduscopic: normal. Cardiac: normal. Respiratory: clear. Abdominal: no bruits. Reflexes: Achilles tendon with slowing in relaxation phase.

Laboratory Findings: WBC count: normal with normal differential, Hgb 15 g/dl. Electrolytes, BUN, and creatinine normal. rTSH 72.

Question: What is the cause of her elevation in blood pressure?

Diagnosis: Hypothyroidism-induced blood pressure elevation.

Discussion: Hypothyroidism is one of the most commonly overlooked secondary causes of elevated blood pressure. The prevalence of hypertension in hypothyroid patients is a subject of considerable debate with rates reported between 0 and 50%. The large difference in the reported prevalence is due to the different criteria used to define hypertension and hypothyroidism and differences in the studied patient populations. Using the World Health Organization criteria, the prevalence of hypertension in hypothyroid patients is three times that of their euthyroid counterparts.

The mechanism of hypertension in hypothyroid patients is poorly understood. It is believed to involve increased sympathetic tone and changes in sodium transport. Higher plasma levels of catecholamines are found in hypothyroid patients. In addition, hypothyroid patients have a decreased number of beta-adrenergic receptors and an increase in alpha-receptor responsiveness. There is an increase in total body water in hypothyroidism related to a reduction in the glomerular filtration rate (GFR) and antidiuretic hormone secretion. Despite the decreased GFR, there are low aldosterone and plasma renin activity levels in the hypothyroid state, implying that the hypertension seen in hypothyroidism is not caused by activation of the renin-aldosterone system. It is likely that the hypertension associated with hypothyroidism is related to many factors.

The diagnosis of hypothyroidism should be entertained in any patient presenting with hypertension. Assessment of the signs and symptoms of this common condition are easily incorporated into the history and physical for the hypertensive patient. This patient demonstrates many of these findings, including depression, hypersomnia, constipation, and slowing of the relaxation phase of her reflexes. There are no current recommendations on screening for hypothyroidism in hypertensive patients. However, the presence of elevated blood pressure in a patient with suggestive symptoms should prompt assessment of the plasma TSH level.

The identification of hypothyroidism in the hypertensive patient is important because many patients will have considerable improvement in blood pressure readings with treatment of their thyroid hormone deficiency. A recent study demonstrated that half of hypertensive, hypothyroid patients started on hormone replacement therapy had complete resolution of their elevated blood pressure. As patient age increases, it is more likely that additional antihypertensive therapy will be necessary to achieve blood pressure goals.

This patient exhibited classic symptoms of hypothyroidism. She was started on thyroxine-replacement therapy with slow resolution of her symptoms. At the end of 8 weeks her TSH was 2.5 and her blood pressure had returned to normal.

Clinical Pearls

1. Hypothyroidism is a commonly overlooked secondary cause of hypertension.
2. Thyroid hormone replacement is often effective in reducing blood pressure in hypothyroid patients.
3. Older patients with hypothyroidism are more likely to require antihypertensive therapy in addition to thyroxine in order to reach blood pressure goals.

REFERENCES

1. Dernellis J, Panaretou M: Effects of thyroid replacement therapy on arterial blood pressure in patients with hypertension and hypothyroidism. Am Heart J 143:718–724, 2002.
2. Fletcher AK, Weetman AP: Hypertension and hypothyroidism. J Hum Hypertens 12:79–82, 1998.
3. Klein I, Ojamaa K: Thyroid hormone and blood pressure regulation. In Laragh JH, Brenner BM (eds): Hypertension Pathophysiology, Diagnosis, and Management, 2nd ed. New York, Raven Press, 1995.
4. Saito I, Saruta T: Hypertension in thyroid disorders. Endocrinol Metab Clin North Am 23:379–386, 1994.
5. Streeten DHP, Anderson GH, Howland T, et al: Effects of thyroid function on blood pressure, recognition of hypothyroid hypertension. Hypertension 11:78–83, 1988.

Spencer E. Harpe, PharmD, MPH
Marion R. Wofford, MD, MPH

PATIENT 44

A 53-year-old dialysis patient with recent blood pressure increase

A 53-year-old man with a history of focal segmental glomerulosclerosis has received hemodialysis three times a week for the last 2 years. Over the past few months, his hematocrit and hemoglobin levels have been decreasing. Approximately 4 weeks ago, erythropoietin (EPO) therapy was initiated. The patient has a history of well-controlled blood pressure since he has been on dialysis (136/89). The dialysis nurse notes a slight increase in blood pressure after the third week of EPO therapy. By the end of the fourth week of EPO therapy, the patient's blood pressure is averaging 147/98 mmHg. His other medications include an iron supplement and various dialysis-related medications. The patient and his wife report full compliance with all medications and dietary restrictions associated with hemodialysis.

Physical Examination: Temperature 98.4°F, pulse 78, blood pressure 142/100, respiratory rate 14, BMI 28. General: well-developed, no distress. Chest: clear. Cardiac: normal S_1, S_2. 2/6 systolic murmur at the left midsternal border, no S_3. Abdomen: obese, no masses or bruits. Extremities: left upper extremity graft is patent with thrill. Skin: normal.

Laboratory Findings: WBC 8500/ul, normal differential. Hct 31%. Electrolytes and glucose: normal. BUN 27 mg/dl, creatinine 6.5 mg/dl.

Question: What is the most likely explanation for the increase in this patient's blood pressure?

Diagnosis: Erythropoietin-induced hypertension

Discussion: Recombinant human erythropoietin, or epoetin, and the novel erythropoietin-stimulating protein darbepoetin, have significantly improved the treatment of anemia related to chronic renal failure. Use of these agents not only reduces the need for transfusions but also increases patient quality-of-life. In general, these agents are well-tolerated by patients. According to prescribing information, hypertension is one of the most highly reported adverse effects of use of both epoetin and darbepoetin, 24% and 23%, respectively. An estimated 25–30% of dialysis patients who are receiving erythropoietin therapy will develop hypertension. Interestingly, increases in blood pressure have not been associated with erythropoietin therapy for anemia related to other medical causes (e.g., AIDS and cancer chemotherapy).

Blood pressure increases may occur from a few weeks to a few months after initiation of EPO therapy in patients with chronic renal failure. The mechanism of EPO-induced hypertension is not well understood. Originally, the increase in erythrocyte mass, and the resultant increase in blood viscosity, was thought to be the main factor associated with increases in blood pressure. However, blood pressure elevations have not been observed in patients receiving transfusions, which would increase hematocrit more quickly than epoetin therapy does. Recent research on this subject has focused on the possibility of increased vascular resistance due to the presence of epoetin. Nitric oxide resistance and increased intracellular concentrations of calcium are likely explanations for the increase in peripheral vascular resistance, based on current research in animal mod-els. The calcium theory has been further supported by reductions in blood pressure after administration of a calcium channel blocker in animal experiments. In addition, in vitro evidence points to the possible proliferative effects of EPO on smooth muscle and vascular endothelial cells. Further research is needed to determine if this vascular remodeling is a contributor to EPO-induced hypertension.

According to the Kidney Disease Outcomes Quality Initiative (K/DOQI), blood pressure monitoring should be performed in all patients with chronic kidney disease, especially when EPO therapy is initiated. In the event of increases in blood pressure, antihypertensive therapy may need to be initiated or intensified, or the dose of EPO may need to be reduced to maintain a more gradual rise in hemoglobin/hematocrit. Because there is insufficient evidence supporting special treatment of EPO-induced hypertension, the recommended target blood pressure in these patients is < 130/80 mmHg. However, the J-curve phenomenon may be of concern in this population, given the high occurrence of ischemic cardiovascular disease in these patients. This phenomenon suggests that reducing diastolic blood pressure too much may result in an increased risk for coronary events secondary to decreased perfusion pressure in the coronary circulation. Therefore, blood pressure goals should be set according to the patient's clinical status and achieved gradually to avoid further clinical complications.

This patient was started on a calcium channel blocker with resulting blood pressures averaging 126/78 mmHg. The EPO was continued at the previous doses with a resulting increase in hematocrit to 34%.

Clinical Pearls

1. Blood pressure should be monitored closely in all patients with chronic renal failure who are receiving erythropoietin therapy.
2. Patients with high normal blood pressure or existing hypertension appear to be at increased risk for erythropoietin-induced hypertension.
3. Erythropoietin therapy should be discontinued until the patient is clinically stable if hypertensive encephalopathy (with or without seizures) develops.
4. Due to the suspected role of intracellular calcium in erythropoietin-induced hypertension, blood pressure control with calcium-channel blockers may be a logical treatment option.

REFERENCES

1. Product Information: Aranesp®, darbepoetin alfa. Amgen, Thousand Oaks, CA, 2002.
2. NKF-K/DOQI clinical practice guidelines for anemia of chronic kidney disease: update 2000. Am J Kidney Dis 37(1 Suppl 1):S182–238, 2001.
3. Product Information: Epogen®, epoetin alfa. Amgen, Thousand Oaks, CA, 1999.
4. St. Peter WL, Lewis MJ: Chronic renal insufficiency and end-stage renal disease. In DiPiro JT, Talbert RL, Yee GC, et al (eds): Pharmacotherapy: A Pathophysiologic Approach, 4th ed. Stamford, CT, Appleton & Lange, 1999.
5. Vaziri ND: Mechanism of erythropoietin-induced hypertension. Am J Kidney Dis 33:821–828, 1999.
6. Ni Z, Wang XQ, Vaziri ND: Nitric oxide metabolism in erythropoietin-induced hypertension: Effect of calcium channel blockade. Hypertension 32:724–729, 1998.
7. Chobanian AV, Bakris GL, Black HR, et al: National Heart, Lung, and Blood Institute Joint National Committee on Prevention, Detection, Evaluation, and Treatment of Blood Pressure; National High Blood Pressure Education: The Seventh Report of the Joint National Committee on Prevention, Detection, Evaluation, and Treatment of High Blood Pressure: the JNC VII report, JAMA 289(19):2560–2572, 2003.

George E. Habeeb, Jr., MD
Kimberly G. Harkins, MD

PATIENT 45

A 44-year-old woman with hematuria

A 44-year-old woman presents to clinic with a 5-day history of severe dyspnea on exertion, weight gain, and diffuse edema. She has been healthy other than recurrent episodes of cystitis for which she takes antibiotics every few months. She does not drink alcohol or use tobacco. She takes amlodipine for hypertension and levothyroxine for hypothyroidism. Her bladder infections are sometimes preceded by blood in her urine and she occasionally has pain in her side with these episodes.

Physical Examination: Temperature 98.6°F, pulse 95, respiratory rate 24, blood pressure 190/110. General: facial swelling. Neck/Thyroid: normal. Cardiac: regular rhythm, S_3 gallop. Lungs: bilateral lower lobe rales. Extremities: pitting edema in both upper and lower extremities.

Laboratory Findings: WBC: normal. Hemoglobin 8.0 g/dl, hematocrit 24%. Sodium 138 mmol/L, potassium 5.8 mmol/L, CO_2 18 mmol/L, BUN 55 mg/dl, creatinine 3.4 mg/dl. Serum albumin 2.1 g/dl. Urinalysis: > 300 mg/dl protein, RBC 2/hpf, and WBC 2/hpf. 24-hour urine: 8 g protein, creatinine clearance 32 mL/min. Chest x-ray: pulmonary edema. EKG: sinus tachycardia, left ventricular overload pattern.

Question: What is the cause of this patient's renal insufficiency and hypertension?

Diagnosis: Immunoglobulin (Ig) A nephropathy with acute glomerulonephritis

Discussion: This patient demonstrates some classic features of IgA nephropathy, the most common form of glomerulonephritis. Focal or diffuse glomerular disease may be present and eventually lead to glomerular sclerosis. Although idiopathic, IgA nephropathy can show a familial predilection. One proposed mechanism for developing IgA nephropathy is induction of a local IgA antibody response by a mucosal viral infection, leading to mucosal immunization. IgA-containing complexes are deposited in the glomeruli and cause damage through direct injury or by activation of other immunologic factors. Both cellular immunity and IgA-mediated injury are proposed.

The classic symptoms and signs of IgA nephropathy include active or recent viral infection of the respiratory or gastrointestinal tract, immediately followed by gross hematuria. Although this patient did not have a recent illness, she has been treated chronically for cystitis with intermittent microscopic hematuria. Upon this presentation to the clinic, the patient was hospitalized and treated with loop diuretics and antihypertensive agents. Symptomatically she improved, with resolution of pulmonary edema, but her renal function only partially improved. A renal biopsy revealed IgA nephropathy.

When patients have a history suggestive of IgA nephropathy, a renal biopsy is the diagnostic procedure of choice. Immunofluorescence reveals diffuse IgA and C3 in the mesangium; light microscopy shows increased matrix and cellularity. Polymorphism of the angiotensin-converting enzyme (ACE) gene may predict decline in renal function, outcomes, and response to ACE-inhibitor treatment.

Therapy is nonspecific. For both hypertension and proteinuria, ACE inhibitors are the drugs of choice. These agents may reduce proteinuria and glomerular fibrosis. The goal of therapy is to achieve blood pressures of < 130/80 mmHg. Other agents, such as nondihydropyridine calcium channel blockers may be necessary, along with diuretics. Sodium restriction and lifestyle modification are important adjuncts to pharmacologic therapy of hypertension. Even patients with normal blood pressure and IgA nephropathy may benefit from ACE inhibition.

Corticosteroids and immunosuppressive agents usually do not alter the course, except in some cases of acute nephrotic syndrome without hematuria, in which remission may occur. Although ACE inhibitors, steroids, and cytotoxic agents may reduce proteinuria, no agents have yet been proven to preserve renal function.

Progression to end-stage renal disease occurs in 20–50% of patients within 20 years of diagnosis. Patients with IgA nephropathy who undergo a renal transplant have a 50% chance of developing recurrent disease in the transplanted kidney. This patient eventually progressed to end-stage renal failure requiring dialysis.

Clinical Pearls

1. IgA nephropathy, the most common cause of glomerulonephritis, presents with hematuria following a viral respiratory or gastrointestinal illness.
2. Patients with nephropathy require strict blood pressure control.
3. ACE inhibitors are useful for both blood pressure control and management of proteinuria in IgA nephropathy.

REFERENCES
1. Janssen U, Bahlmann F, Kohl J, et al: Activation of the acute phase response and complement C3 in patients with IgA nephropathy. Am J Kidney Dis 35:21–28, 2000.
2. Glassock RJ: Current Therapy in Nephrology and Hypertension, 4th ed. St. Louis, Mosby, 1998.
3. Rose BD, Jacobs JB: Nephrotic syndrome and glomerulonephritis. In Rose BD (ed): Pathophysiology of Renal Disease, 2nd ed. McGraw-Hill, 1987.

Marion R. Wofford, MD, MPH

PATIENT 46

A 56-year-old man complaining of dyspnea and nocturia

A 56-year-old man presents to an acute care clinic for evaluation of shortness of breath. He has been noticing increasing dyspnea while cutting the grass and climbing stairs over the last 3 months. He has also experienced nocturia and is now sleeping on two pillows. He has a history of hypertension from the remote past but quit taking medications more than one year ago. He was not having any symptoms of hypertension so thought he did not need to take the medications previously prescribed.

Physical Examination: Blood pressure 170/105, pulse 70, respiratory rate 18. General: overweight, no apparent distress. Neck: normal jugular venous pressure, no bruits. Chest: faint rales in bilateral lower lung fields. Cardiac: point of maximal impulse is the size of a quarter and displaced laterally, normal S_1 and S_2, soft systolic murmur radiating to left axilla. Extremities: slight pitting edema in ankles.

Laboratory Findings: Hct 46%, electrolytes, BUN, creatinine normal. EKG: left ventricular hypertrophy (LVH). Echocardiogram: eccentric LVH with estimated ejection fraction 35%. Chest x-ray: blunting of the costophrenic angles.

Question: What diagnosis should be considered in the management of hypertension in this patient?

Diagnosis: Congestive heart failure (CHF) with systolic dysfunction

Discussion: This patient has mild symptoms of CHF although the echocardiogram confirms that he has a moderate degree of left ventricular systolic dysfunction and eccentric LVH, suggesting systolic dysfunction. Most likely the etiology of his CHF is hypertension, although other etiologies should be considered and managed.

Patients with longstanding hypertension are at risk for development of LVH and alterations of normal diastolic or systolic function known as CHF. The majority of patients with diastolic or systolic CHF have hypertension. Most patients with symptomatic CHF have systolic dysfunction, the leading cause of hospitalization in adults more than 65 years old. There are many etiologies of CHF, the most common being hypertension and ischemic heart disease. Elevated blood pressure may worsen the symptoms of CHF irrespective of the etiology. One of the primary goals in the management of CHF is blood pressure control.

CHF is a clinical syndrome that results from a continuum of alterations in myocardium. An excessive systolic load on the left ventricle results in myocyte hypertrophy and left ventricular hypertrophy. The increase in left ventricular mass and thickness causes diastolic tension. Although systolic function may still be normal at this stage, a patient may have symptoms of pulmonary congestion due to diastolic dysfunction.

Alterations in the myocardial structure evolve as the continuum of CHF progresses. Myocyte loss and replacement by connective tissues cause loss of compliance and stiffening of the left ventricle. The remaining myocytes undergo further hypertrophy and fibrosis, a process known as remodeling. If systolic load, as a result of elevated blood pressure, is maintained this process continues, causing left ventricular dilation and systolic failure.

Compensatory mechanisms for a decrease in cardiac output include an increase in heart rate, myocardial contraction, and volume expansion as a result of neurohumoral modifications. These neurohumoral adaptations, while important in maintaining normal perfusion of vital organs, play a major role in the progressive deterioration leading to left ventricular dysfunction. Activation of the renin-angiotensin system and the sympathetic nervous system are two major compensatory mechanisms of left ventricular failure. Increased levels of norepinephrine, renin, antidiuretic hormone, and atrial and brain naturetic peptides occur in patients with asymptomatic or symptomatic CHF.

The goals of hypertensive treatment are to decrease both preload to improve symptoms of pulmonary congestion and afterload to enhance cardiac contractility, thereby relieving symptoms and possible reversing myocardial remodeling.

Alteration in lifestyle should be recommended for all patients with CHF, as in patients with primary hypertension. Avoidance of excess sodium, cessation of tobacco products, and limitation of alcohol consumption should be discussed. Weight reduction in overweight or obese patients is encouraged. Exercise programs should be initiated, with caution in those with severe systolic dysfunction, but they are important to decreasing morbidity and mortality.

Angiotensin-converting enzyme inhibitors (ACEI) have been shown to improve survival of patients with CHF and are considered the standard of care. These agents decrease preload and afterload, and therefore improve symptoms of CHF and improve myocardial contractility. These medications should be increased to the maximal recommended and tolerated dose.

Angiotensin receptor blockers (ARBs) have not been shown to be superior to ACEI in the treatment of CHF. In those patients intolerant of ACEI due to cough, angioedema, or other side effects, valsartan, the only ARB thus far to receive an indication for treatment of CHF, may be added.

Beta-blockers were previously thought to be detrimental in patients with left ventricular systolic dysfunction. Three beta-blockers, carvedilol, metoprolol, and bisoprolol, improve survival in patients with New York Heart Association (NYHA) class II or III CHF. These drugs may cause a transient worsening of symptoms so should be initiated cautiously.

Loop diuretics are used to improve blood pressure control and symptoms of pulmonary and peripheral edema. Over-aggressive use of diuretics may cause renal failure, whereas an inadequate dose may not be beneficial in the augmentation of the effect of other drugs. Furosemide or torsemide are the most commonly used diuretics for CHF.

Spironolactone has also been shown to decrease hospitalization and mortality in patients who are receiving standard therapy for CHF. The mechanism by which this drug provides benefit is not related to its diuretic effect, but it may decrease myocardial fibrosis due to excess aldosterone. Spironolactone is recommended in patients with class III or IV CHF, without hyperkalemia, and in whom the serum creatinine level is < 2.5 mg/dl.

A combination of hydralazine and nitrates provides reduction of ventricular preload and afterload, so this treatment may be considered for those patients that cannot tolerate ACEI or ARBs.

It is not uncommon for patients with hypertensive cardiomyopathy, the likely diagnosis in this patient, to take a combination of four to five medications for the treatment of hypertension and CHF. Over time, aggressive treatment may preserve myocardial function and will often reverse cardiac remodeling if blood pressure control is achieved with lifestyle changes and appropriate therapy.

Clinical Pearls

1. Chronic hypertension leads to a continuum of myocyte hypertrophy and fibrosis, left ventricular remodeling, and ultimately may result in left ventricular systolic dysfunction and failure.
2. Activation of the renin-angiotensin and sympathetic nervous systems contributes to the deterioration of normal cardiac function in CHF.
3. Control of blood pressure in CHF decreases mortality, morbidity, and symptoms related to CHF and may result in reversal of cardiac remodeling.

REFERENCES

1. Gomberg-Maitland M, Baran DA, Fuster V: Treatment of contestive heart failure. Arch Intern Med 161:242–352, 2001.
2. Cohn JN. Drug therapy: The management of chronic heart failure. N Engl J Med 335:490–498, 1996.
3. Levy D, Larson MG, Vasan RS, et al: The progression from hypertrophy to congestive heart failure. JAMA 275:1557–1562, 1996.
4. Cohn JN. Structural bases for heart failure: Ventricular remodeling and its pharmacological inhibition. Circulation 91:2504–2507, 1995.

Kristi W. Kelley, PharmD, BCPS
Kimberly G. Harkins, MD

PATIENT 47

A 69-year-old woman with resistant hypertension

A 69-year-old African American woman with hypertension for 20 years presents to a hypertension specialist for management. Her primary care physician has ruled out secondary hypertension with a thorough evaluation. Her blood pressure is poorly controlled on four antihypertensive medications: trandolapril 4 mg daily, felodipine 5 mg daily, furosemide 20 mg twice daily, and doxazosin 2 mg daily. She reports adherence to her medical regimen. Her other medical problems include type 2 diabetes which she is managing with diet alone.

Physical Examination: Temperature 98.2°F, pulse 64, respiratory rate 16, blood pressure 164/90. Height 5 foot 2 inches, weight 146, BMI 26.7. General: overweight. Funduscopic: arteriolar narrowing. Chest: clear. Cardiac: regular rhythm, point of maximum impulse displaced laterally and inferiorly. Abdomen: no bruits or masses.

Laboratory Findings: WBC 8000/μl normal differential, hemoglobin 13.4 g/dl, hematocrit 38.7%. Electrolytes, glucose, BUN, creatinine: normal. 24-hour ambulatory blood pressure monitor: Daytime mean systolic reading 164 mmHg, mean diastolic reading 82 mmHg, mean heart rate 66; nighttime mean systolic reading 160 mmHg, mean diastolic reading 80 mmHg, mean heart rate 59.

Question: What pattern of hypertension is demonstrated in the ambulatory blood pressure monitor readings?

Diagnosis: Uncontrolled hypertension, nondipper

Discussion: The ambulatory blood pressure monitor (ABPM), extensively used in clinical trials, is infrequently utilized in clinical practice. Use of ABPM is recommended in patients with suspected "white-coat" hypertension, episodic hypertension, autonomic dysfunction, hypotensive symptoms, and apparent drug resistance. The World Health Organization-International Society of Hypertension (WHO/ISH) recommends ABPM for evaluation of office hypertension in subjects with low cardiovascular risk, variability of blood pressure, hypotensive symptoms, and resistant hypertension.

Most ABPM reports provide a printout of all readings as well as a summary, including maximum, minimum, and average blood pressure and heart rate during daytime, nighttime, and the entire duration of the monitoring period. Blood pressure is assessed during a patient's usual activities, with daytime and nighttime readings to assess diurnal blood pressure variations. An ABPM avoids measurement error and observer bias. White coat effect can be ruled out by evaluating blood pressure outside the physician's office. Blood pressure values obtained outside the office are expected to be lower than values obtained in the office. The American Society of Hypertension recommends an average daytime blood pressure < 135/85, with < 130/80 considered optimal.

Blood pressure readings are lower at night, when patients are sleeping, than during the day when patients are most active. The difference between daytime and nighttime readings, or diurnal variation, is termed "nocturnal dipping." Patients whose blood pressure does not decline at night are termed "nondippers." A traditional definition of a nondipper is < 10% reduction in nocturnal blood pressure compared to daytime readings. Some authorities suggest that this definition is arbitrary and that true nondippers are patients with nighttime blood pressure readings that are higher than daytime

readings. For this patient, there was very little difference between nighttime and daytime blood pressure readings.

A normal decrease of approximately 15% in nighttime blood pressure is primarily due to the patient's sleep and inactivity. Men and women show similar decreases in blood pressure. Smokers have a greater decrease in nocturnal blood pressure due to the absence of nicotine's vasopressor effects. Factors associated with nondippers include poor sleep quality, advanced age, diabetes, and secondary hypertension.

Complications associated with nondipping blood pressure include carotid artery thickening, carotid artery plaques, cerebrovascular disease, left ventricular hypertrophy, increased number and complexity of ventricular arrhythmias, microalbuminuria, and increased rate of progression of renal insufficiency. Race is a significant risk factor for lack of nocturnal decline in blood pressure, with African Americans showing less decline in both systolic and diastolic blood pressure at night compared to Caucasians. Excessive nocturnal declines in blood pressure, defined as a fall in blood pressure > 20%, have also been associated with cardiovascular complications such as myocardial ischemia in patients with left ventricular hypertrophy.

In this patient with apparent resistant hypertension, an ABPM documented that her blood pressure was uncontrolled and gave additional information about her lack of nocturnal variation in blood pressure. She is at high risk for cardiovascular complications from her hypertension. Her physician increased her felodipine to 5 mg dosed twice daily, and up-titrated the doxazosin, which was dosed at bedtime. In light of her normal renal function and lack of edema, her loop diuretic was changed to a once-daily thiazide. With improved adherence to a low sodium diet and healthy lifestyle, her new medication regimen lowered her blood pressure in the office to 138/82 mmHg.

Clinical Pearls

1. Ambulatory blood pressure monitoring is a useful tool to assess white coat effect, resistant hypertension, patients with hypotensive symptoms, and excess variability of blood pressure
2. Normal diurnal variability in blood pressure is defined as a 15% drop at nighttime
3. A nondipper pattern on ABPM (less than 10% decrease at night) signifies an increased risk for cardiovascular complications, particularly in diabetic, elderly, or African American patients

REFERENCES

1. Ernst ME, Bergus GR: Noninvasive 24-hour ambulatory blood pressure monitoring: Overview of technology and clinical applications. Pharmacotherapy 22:597–612, 2002.
2. Kaplan NM: Clinical hypertension. 8th ed. Baltimore (MD): Lippincott Williams & Wilkins, 2002.
3. Phillips RA, Sheinart KF, Godbold JH, et al: The association of blunted nocturnal blood pressure dip and stroke in a multiethnic population. Am J Hypertens 13:1250–1255, 2000.
4. Verdecchia P: Prognostic value of ambulatory blood pressure: Current evidence and clinical implications. Hypertension 35:844–851, 2000.
5. White WB: How well does ambulatory blood pressure predict target-organ disease and clinical outcome in patients with hypertension? Blood Press Monit 4 (suppl 2):S17–S21, 1999.
6. Pickering TG: What is the `normal' 24h, awake, and asleep blood pressure? Blood Press Monit 4:S3–S7, 1999.
7. Profant J, Dimsdale JE: Race and diurnal blood pressure patterns: A review and meta-analysis. Hypertension 33:1099–1104, 1999.
8. Zanchetti A: The role of ambulatory blood pressure monitoring in clinical practice. Am J Hypertens 10:1069–1080, 1997.

Kevin Lee Keeton
Marion R. Wofford, MD, MPH

PATIENT 48

A 36-year-old man with uncontrolled hypertension and a history of alcohol use

A 36-year-old man presents to the hypertension clinic upon recommendation by the company nurse. He has had his blood pressure checked several times in the last 6 months, each being elevated. The patient reports alcohol use on a regular basis "to help calm his nerves." He reports drinking about three to four beers on a regular day, but sometimes drinks up to eight beers per day.

Physical Examination: Temperature 98.9°F, pulse 72, respiratory rate 12, blood pressure 160/100. General: appears slightly intoxicated and breath smells of alcohol, obese. Cardiac: normal S_1 and S_2, S_3 and S_4 sounds present, no murmurs. Neurological: fails finger-to-nose test.

Laboratory Findings: CBC normal. BUN/creatinine normal, potassium 3.3 mg/dl. Urinalysis: normal. EKG: normal.

Question: What advice should be given to this patient?

Diagnosis: Binge drinking and need for reduction in alcohol intake.

Discussion: Alcohol use is responsible for an estimated 30% of essential hypertension. The use of three or more standard drinks per day is shown to correlate with hypertension in a large number of epidemiological studies. A standard drink is defined as approximately 14 grams of ethanol (12-oz beer, 5-oz wine, or 1.5-oz of distilled spirits). Studies examining the differences in blood pressure of nondrinkers (individuals consuming less than three drinks per day), and those consuming three or more drinks per day have shown very little difference. Changes in blood pressure correlate with the amount of ethanol consumed, rather than the type consumed.

The pressor effects of alcohol follow a J-shaped relationship. A beneficial effect on cardiovascular risk has been demonstrated in subjects who consume one to two standard drinks per day. This effect has been linked to increased HDL-C and decreased LDL-C levels associated with moderate alcohol intake. Studies have also demonstrated that the benefit may be associated with decreased platelet aggregation or antioxidant properties. However, when one consumes more than three drinks per day, the pressor effects of alcohol overcome the beneficial effects.

There are several proposed mechanisms for the pressor effects of alcohol. One mechanism involves the chronic drinker being in a constant state of withdrawal, resulting in elevated blood pressure. A more viable mechanism proposes that alcohol leads directly to an increase in blood pressure. Additional proposed mechanisms include increased intracellular calcium, stimulation of sympathetic catecholamines, inhibition of relaxing substances, calcium or magnesium depletion, and elevated acetaldehyde.

Increased intracellular calcium through direct cell membrane alteration may lead to enhanced vascular smooth muscle tone. With this, an increase in response to stimuli would be expected. However, in one study of normotensive men, a decrease in response to stimuli was seen with 7 days of regular alcohol use despite increases in systolic and diastolic blood pressure.

Alcohol has been shown to increase plasma epinephrine, norepinephrine, cortisol, and renin activity. However, several case-control studies have failed to identify a rise in plasma levels in drinking subjects when compared with nondrinking subjects. Ongoing studies are investigating the association between blood pressure, relaxing substances, and acetaldehydes with alcohol use.

Chronic alcohol use may also decrease the effectiveness of hypertensive treatment regimens. Treatment failure may be related to alcohol–medication interactions or noncompliance. The current recommendation for cardiovascular health is a reduction in alcohol to two or fewer drinks per day for men or one or no drink per day for women. Studies have shown that consuming one fewer drink per day, down to this recommended amount, will decrease both systolic and diastolic blood pressure by 1 mmHg. If hypertension remains uncontrolled, hypertension medications may be employed.

The current patient was counseled on the potential risk of increased blood pressure associated with alcohol use. He was advised to limit the use of alcoholic beverages.

Clinical Pearls

1. Chronic alcohol use causes approximately 30% of essential hypertension.
2. Use of more than three standard drinks per day eliminates the beneficial effects of alcohol on cardiovascular risk by causing an elevation of blood pressure.
3. A decrease in alcohol intake of one drink per day decreases diastolic and systolic blood pressure by approximately 1 mmHg.
4. Treatment includes reducing alcohol intake to two or fewer drinks per day for men and one or no drink per day for women.

REFERENCES
1. Kaplan NM: Clinical Hypertension, 8th ed. Philadelphia, Lippincott Williams & Wilkins, 2002.
2. Cushman WC: Alcohol use and blood pressure. In Izzo JL, Black HR (eds): Hypertension Primer, 2nd ed. Baltimore, Lippincott Williams & Wilkins, 1999.

Jonathan S. Caudill, MD
Jimmy L. Stewart, MD

PATIENT 49

A 16-year-old girl with obesity, hypertension, and hyperglycemia

A 16-year-old girl with type 2 diabetes mellitus presents to the general pediatric clinic for evaluation of hyperglycemia. She had been seen in the emergency department on the previous day with complaints of dizziness and increased urinary frequency, and she was subsequently found to have an elevated blood glucose of 285 mg/dl. Her antihyperglycemic regimen consisted of metformin and subcutaneous insulin. She reported recent medical and dietary noncompliance and admitted to a fairly sedentary lifestyle.

A thorough work-up of her obesity had been undertaken by a pediatric endocrinologist and type 2 diabetes mellitus was diagnosed in the past year. Elevated blood pressures ≥130/80 mmHg in the 95th percentile for age and sex were recorded on at least three occasions. Regarding her family history, only hypertension was reported. There were no family members with diabetes mellitus or heart disease. She was referred for further outpatient assessment and management.

Physical Examination: Temperature 98.4°F, pulse 77, respirations 14, blood pressure 154/95 (> 95th percentile for age and sex). Weight 150.8 kg (> 95th percentile for age and sex), BMI 58.9. General: morbidly obese. Funduscopic: sharp disc margins. Chest: clear. Cardiac: normal S_1, S_2, no murmurs. Abdomen: massive pannus, no palpable organomegaly. Extremities: no edema. Skin: hyperpigmented region involving most of posterior neck.

Laboratory Findings: Serum chemistries: sodium 138 mmol/L, potassium 4.5 mmol/L, chloride 93 mmol/L, CO_2 24 mmol/L, BUN 9 mg/dl, creatinine 0.8 mg/dl, calcium 10.3 mg/dl. Glucose 311 mg/dl. HgbAlc 12.0 mg/dl. TSH 1.0 µU/ml. Routine urinalysis: glucosuria.

Question: What clinical syndrome is this patient at an increased risk for developing in adulthood?

Answer: Dysmetabolic syndrome

Discussion: In the adult population, the constellation of clinical findings consisting of obesity, peripheral glucose resistance, hypertension, and hyperlipidemia is called dysmetabolic syndrome. These disorders significantly increase the risk for cardiovascular events. Although this patient's presentation is rather dramatic in terms of the extent of progression towards cardiovascular disease at such a young age, new clinical data now show that the presence of even one risk factor for cardiovascular disease should prompt investigation for additional potentially treatable disorders.

The relationships involving **obesity, insulin resistance, and hypertension** have been the subject of many investigations. Framingham and other studies have reported a strong association of weight gain with cardiovascular risk. These cardiovascular sequelae appear to have their origins in childhood, with a direct association between weight and insulin resistance being reported. The increased pigmentation described around the posterior neck of this girl is known as **acanthosis nigrans** and, when present in obese girls and young women, may be significant due to its association with impaired glucose tolerance and hyperandrogenism. The development of hypertension and hyperglycemia in obese patients represents progression of dysmetabolic syndrome. However, the possible mechanism involved in the pathogenesis of this triad of cardiovascular abnormalities is both biochemically and physiologically complex.

Secondary causes for hypertension should always be considered, especially in children and adolescents. The adolescent in the vignette was hypertensive, but this is not the case with all obese patients. There are most likely genetic components influencing both the development of hypertension and an individual's blood pressure responses to weight gain. In addition, there may be differences in individual baseline blood pressure, as most individuals do show an increase in blood pressure with weight gain, although some may not eventually reach the hypertensive range. There is evidence that, like obese adults, obese adolescents have an elevated blood pressure that is reduced with weight loss.

Further, there is the relationship of insulin resistance with lipids and blood pressure. Increasing evidence seems to indicate that increased insulin resistance occurring in the context of obesity, which leads to increased circulating insulin, serves to stimulate the sympathetic nervous system in an effort to restore energy homeostasis. As a result of this increased adrenergic activity, a pro-hypertensive effect may be generated through vasoconstriction, increases in cardiac output, and sodium reabsorption in the kidneys. There may also be an effect on the concentration of serum lipids as influence is exerted on hepatic lipid metabolism.

In many cases, the "gestalt" approach is all that is necessary to diagnose obesity. From a morphologic stand point, individuals often profoundly exhibit the results of excess caloric intake. A more useful means of accurately diagnosing and quantifying obesity is to calculate the **body mass index (BMI).** This weight-for-height index is clinically useful as an assessment of obesity that reflects excess body fat, and it is simple to use. The distribution of body fat is an important aspect to consider, as abdominal obesity is associated with a greater risk of metabolic and cardiovascular disorders. Recent recommendations are that children and adolescents with a BMI ≥95th percentile for age and sex should undergo an in-depth medical examination and should be evaluated for any complications of obesity such as hypertension, hyperglycemia, and hyperlipidemia. Clinicians should also be familiar with signs of rare complications of obesity, including genetic syndromes, endocrinologic disorders, renovascular abnormalities, and psychological disorders. Adolescents with complications are at increased risk for adult cardiovascular morbidity.

The mainstay of obesity treatment is alteration of energy balance by means of lifestyle change. Weight loss programs that incorporate exercise with caloric restriction produce the most desirable effects on blood pressure reduction. Another desirable effect of regular, aerobic exercise is the reduction of insulin resistance. An achievable goal of relatively modest weight loss, 5–10% of initial body weight (15 kg in the case of this adolescent), can result in decreased blood pressure. An abnormal lipid profile may also improve with such intervention. When significant medical morbidities are present, obese individuals have increased motivation for change. Diets rich in fruits, vegetables, and low-fat dairy products are appropriate in children and adults with all stages of hypertension, and have been shown to decrease both systolic and diastolic blood pressure in normotensive and hypertensive patients.

This patient was prescribed a simple dietary modification plan for the initial treatment. Counseling was given to avoid soft drinks, increase fruit and vegetable consumption, and to drink at least eight glasses of water per day. In addition, she was encouraged to begin light exercise such as walking or bicycling four to five times per week for 15–20 minutes. On her return to clinic 8 weeks later, the patient was clearly excited over her recent progress regarding her lifestyle modification. On physical examination her blood pressure had decreased to 128/80 mmHg and her weight was now reduced to 139.5 kg. Three weeks later, her weight and blood pressure were continuing to decrease. Given her good progress, and her clear determination to continue in a likewise manner, no medicinal antihypertensive therapy was initiated. She was accepted by referral as a patient in the local diabetic education program and was to be followed clinically by her primary care provider to monitor continued blood pressure and insulin resistance response to weight loss.

Clinical Pearls:

1. Calculating the body mass index (BMI) is a simple method to diagnose and quantify obesity.
2. Any child with a BMI ≥ 95th percentile for age and sex should be examined for hypertension, insulin resistance, and hyperlipidemia (collectively termed "dysmetabolic syndrome").
3. Even one cardiovascular risk factor diagnosed in childhood increases adult risk.
4. Modest weight loss of 5–10% of initial body weight can result in decreased blood pressure.

REFERENCES

1. Falkner B, Hassink S, Ross J, et al: Dysmetabolic syndrome: Multiple risk factors for premature adult disease in an adolescent girl. Pediatrics 14:110, 2002.
2. Bray GA: Pathogenesis of obesity. *UpToDate* online, 2002.
3. Kaplan NM: The metabolic syndrome (insulin resistance syndrome or syndrome x). *UpToDate* online, 2002.
4. Sacks FM, Svetkey LP, Vollmer WM, et al: Effects on blood pressure of reduced dietary sodium and the Dietary Approaches to Stop Hypertension (DASH) diet. DASH-Sodium Collaborative Research Group. N Engl J Med 344:3–10, 2001.
5. Landsberg L: Insulin-mediated sympathetic stimulation: Role in the pathogenesis of obesity-related hypertension (or, how insulin affects blood pressure, and why). J Hypertens 19:523–528, 2001.
6. Sinaiko AR, Donahue RP, Jacobs DR, et al: Relation of weight and rate of increase during childhood and adolescence to body size, blood pressure, fasting insulin, and lipids in young adults. Circulation 99:1471–1476, 1999.
7. Huang Z, Reddy A: Weight change, ideal weight, and hypertension. Curr Opinion in Nephrol Hyperten 8:343–346, 1999.
8. Barlor SE, Dietz WH: Obesity evaluation and treatment: Expert committee recommendations. Pediatrics 20:102, 1998.
9. National High Blood Pressure Education Program Working Group on Hypertension control in Children and Adolescents: Update on the 1987 task force report on high blood pressure in children and adolescents: A working group report from the National High Blood Pressure Education Program. Pediatrics 98:649–658, 1996.
10. Rocchini AP, Katch V, Anderson J: Blood pressure in obese adolescents: Effect of weight loss. Pediatrics 82:16–23, 1988.

Rebecca L. Wood, PharmD
Marion R. Wofford, MD, MPH

PATIENT 50

A 25-year-old graduate student taking licorice tablets for stomach pain and stress reduction

A 25-year-old graduate student was preparing to defend her master's thesis in botany. For the last 6 months she has been under tremendous pressure to complete her research. In addition to the feeling of anxiety, she had begun to notice abdominal pain for which she took Tums (calcium carbonate). Having read about the potential medicinal benefits of herbal supplements, she searched the Internet for therapies that might make her feel better. She had been taking licorice tablets twice a day as recommended on a website. Although her abdominal pain improved after 2 weeks, she developed headaches and palpitations, which she attributes to stress and lack of sleep. The review of systems was otherwise noncontributory. She has no prior medical problems. The family history is significant only for a maternal aunt with breast cancer.

Physical Examination: Temperature 98.0°F, blood pressure 170/100, pulse 80. General: well-developed, well nourished. Funduscopic examination: normal. Cardiac: normal rhythm. Chest: clear. Abdomen: soft, no bruits. Extremities: normal. Neurological: no tremors, reflexes normal.

Laboratory Findings: WBCs normal. Hgb 18 mg/dl. Electrolytes: potassium 2.8 mmol/dl, bicarbonate 30 mmol/dl, BUN 19 mg/dl, creatinine 0.9 mg/dl, magnesium 1.8 mg/dl. Thyroid-stimulating hormone normal.

Question: What is the etiology of hypokalemia in this patient?

Diagnosis: Licorice-associated hypertension and hypokalemia

Discussion: Licorice has been used throughout the world for many years to cure various ailments. Its healing properties include, but are not restricted to healing of gastric and duodenal ulcers, anti-inflammatory effects on the upper respiratory tract mucous membranes, laxative, throat soother, thirst quencher, antitussive, pain reduction in arthritis, and correction of primary adrenocortical insufficiency. These healing properties can be attributed to glycyrrhizinic acid, the active component in licorice. Glycyrrhiza is derived from the Greek root words "glukus," meaning "sweet," and "riza" meaning "root." Glycyrrhizinic acid is 50 times sweeter than sugar cane and is used in many products including various chewing gums, cough drops and syrups, candy, and chewing tobacco. Natural licorice is more readily available in European countries but may be purchased worldwide via the Internet.

For many years it has been established that products containing glycyrrhizinic acid, such as licorice, exogenously induce hypermineralocorticoidism. This excess is characterized by hypertension, hypokalemia, peripheral edema, headache, and metabolic alkalosis. Hypermineralocorticoidism is the result of glycyrrhizinic acid inhibition of 11ß-hydroxysteroid dehydrogenase. The enzymatic action of 11ß-hydroxysteroid dehydrogenase promotes the conversion of cortisol to cortisone. In the healthy individual, cortisol binds as readily as aldosterone to the mineralocorticoid receptor. However, because of the early conversion to cortisone, which does not have mineralocorticoid activity, aldosterone has little competition from cortisol. Excessive ingestion of licorice will cause an increased level of cortisol, which will compete with aldosterone for binding sites on the mineralocorticoid receptors. This process promotes an increase in sodium and water retention with increased potassium excretion and suppression of renin-angiotension-aldosterone activities.

Although licorice is not a prescription medication, it does have the potential to interact with various medications. Clinicians may see a decrease in the effectiveness of antihypertensives due to licorice ingestion. Concomitant use of licorice products and potassium-depleting agents may potentiate potassium loss and increase the risk of hypokalemia. In addition, estrogens may react with mineralocorticoid receptors or inhibit 11ß-hydroxysteroid dehydrogenase activity, which may explain why women using oral contraceptives tend to be more susceptible to the effects of glycyrrhizinic acid. On the positive side, because of its gastrointestinal mucosa protective properties, glycyrrhizinic acid may protect against mucosal damage related to aspirin and nonsteroidal anti-inflammatory agent use.

The most appropriate treatment for people who present with pseudoaldosteronism related to ingestion of glycyrrhizinic acid is termination of the use of the products. It is important to note that inhibition of 11ß-hydroxysteroid dehydrogenase continues for approximately 2 weeks after removal of the glycyrrhizinic acid–containing agent. However, suppression of the renin-angiotensin-aldosterone axis may persist anywhere from 2–4 months.

This patient exhibited the classic symptoms of exogenously induced hypermineralocorticoidism due to licorice ingestion. She complained of headaches, which started after the initiation of ingestion of licorice tablets. Her physical examination showed an elevation in her blood pressure, along with laboratory findings of hypokalemia and a high-normal bicarbonate level. The patient was instructed to stop taking the licorice tablets, and within 3 weeks her headaches and palpitations had resolved. Within the next 2 months her blood pressure returned to 107/78 mmHg.

Clinical Pearls

1. In patients with resistant hypertension and hypokalemia, the use of licorice-containing products such as chewing gum, chewing tobacco, sore-throat preparations, or candies should be considered.
2. Women who are taking oral contraceptives are more susceptible to the effects of glycyrrhizinic acid.
3. Licorice ingestion can interact with some prescription medications.
4. Licorice, which contains glycyrrhizinic acid, may result in pseudoaldosteronism by inhibition of 11ß-hydroxysteroid dehydrogenase.

REFERENCES

1. Jellin JM, Gregory PJ, Batz F, et al: Pharmacist's Letter/Prescriber's Letter Natural Medicines Comprehensive Database, 4th ed. Stockton, California, Therapeutic Research Faculty, 2002, pp 807–810.
2. Kaplan NM, Rose BD: Licorice and the syndrome of apparent mineralocorticoid excess. UpToDate, 2002.
3. Mansoor GA: Herbs and alternative therapies in the hypertension clinic. *Am J Hyperten* 14:971–975, 2001.
4. Stolpman D, Benner K, Flora K: A cautionary note regarding glycyrrhiza (licorice root). Am J Gastroenterol 94 (2):540–541, 1999.
5. Klerk GJ, Nieuwenhuis MG, Beutler JJ: Lesson of the week: Hypokalaemia and hypertension associated with use of liquorice flavoured chewing gum. B Med J 314:731, 1997.
6. Richason J: The Little Herb Encyclopedia: The Handbook of Natures Remedies for Healthier Life. 1st ed. Jack Ritchason N.D. Woodland Health Books: Pleasant Grove, UT, 1997, pp 134–135.

154

PATIENT 51

A 47-year-old man with severe back pain and nausea

A 47-year-old man with a history of uncontrolled hypertension presents to the emergency department with acute onset of severe back pain and associated nausea that began approximately 30 minutes prior to admission. He describes the pain as "tearing" in quality and unrelieved with positional change. He denies any recent trauma or any prior history of back pain. His only medication is an occasional over-the-counter nonsteroidal anti-inflammatory drug (NSAID), which he takes for headaches. Family history is significant for coronary artery disease in his father, who sustained a myocardial infarction at age 52. Social history is significant for a 60 pack/year history of cigarette smoking.

Physical Examination: Temperature 98°F, pulse 110, respirations 20, blood pressure 160/96. Weight 240 pounds, BMI 36. General: diaphoretic and anxious. Skin: cool lower extremities with decreased dorsalis pedis pulses at 1$^+$ bilaterally. Cardiac: regular rhythm, tachycardic, without murmurs. Abdomen: obese, diminished bowel sounds, nondistended, without guarding.

Laboratory Findings: Hemogram: WBC count 11,000/µl, with normal differential; Hgb 17g/dl. Serum chemistries: electrolytes, BUN, creatinine normal. Chest radiograph: widened mediastinum with small left pleural effusion. Computed tomographic (CT) scan of thorax with contrast: see figure.

Questions: What diagnosis best explains this constellation of symptoms? What is the most appropriate initial treatment?

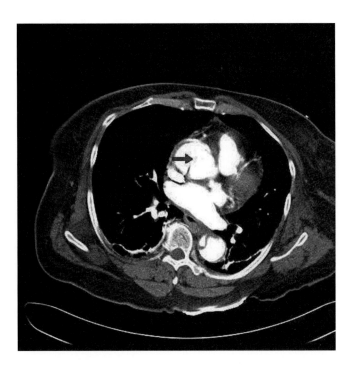

Diagnosis: Acute distal aortic dissection, which should be treated initially with intravenous beta-blockers and nitroprusside for emergent blood pressure reduction

Discussion: This patient's back pain is caused by acute aortic dissection as seen by "false lumen" on CT scan of the thorax. Aortic dissection is a severe and potentially life-threatening disease that requires early diagnosis and treatment. Aortic dissections involve a tear in the intima of the vessel with subsequent splitting of the media, creating a false lumen. This can have numerous consequences including aortic rupture (leading to cardiac tamponade or exsanguination), incompetence of the aortic valve, or obstruction of aortic branches. Autopsy studies reveal that 74% of deaths in dissection cases occur during the initial 2 weeks. For this reason, the first 14 days of an aortic dissection are labeled as the acute period.

Dissections of the aorta have classically been described by two systems, or classifications. The first, the DeBakey system, consists of type I dissections, which involve the ascending and descending aorta; type II, which involve the ascending aorta only; and type III, which are confined to the descending aorta. The second system, the Daily system, simplifies classification into two types of lesions: either type A, any lesion involving the ascending aorta, or type B, those lesions confined to the descending aorta. Most dissections (65%) begin in the ascending aorta, a few centimeters distal to the aortic valve. Because of their proximity to the coronary vessels, aortic valve, and the pericardial space, type A dissections are associated with the greatest mortality.

Risk factors for dissection include hypertension and diseases of the aortic media. Proximal dissections are classically associated with connective tissue diseases, such as Marfan's syndrome, and this is typically the picture seen in younger patients with dissection. Hypertension is usually associated with long-term disease and is more often a factor in distal aortic disease. Dissections are more commonly seen in male patients than in female patients, with a ratio of 3:1.

Patients with acute dissections often describe pain that is rapid in onset, has maximal intensity at onset (as opposed to myocardial infarction, which has crescendo-type quality), and has a tearing or ripping quality. The pain of ascending dissections is usually in the anterior chest, whereas the pain of the dissections in the descending aorta is most frequently localized to the back. The location can be movable, with the pain initially anterior and then progressing to the back as the dissection extends. Physical examination findings in dissection may include a significant difference in blood pressure between the upper extremities or between the lower extremities (depending on the location of the dissection), or signs of cardiac tamponade (pulsus paradoxus, etc.). Chest x-ray findings include a widened mediastinum, enlarged cardiac silhouette, and/or left pleural effusion. Diagnosis is confirmed with transesophageal echocardiogram, aortogram, contrasted CT scan, or ultrasonogram.

In this patient, as is the case for all acute dissections, treatment requires strict control of blood pressure regardless of the location of the dissection (i.e., proximal versus distal). It has been shown that the crucial factor is to limit the velocity of the blood flow. Both intravenous beta-blockers and nitroprusside are used to control both the heart rate and blood pressure. Generally, an intravenous beta-blocker (propranolol or labetalol) is given initially, and if the diastolic blood pressure is > 100–110 mmHg, intravenous nitroprusside is added. Nitroprusside is a potent vasodilator, and, therefore, should not be used alone due to the associated risk of reflexive tachycardia. The goal of therapy is to maintain the systolic pressure at < 110–120 mmHg. Because consensus reveals a far greater mortality associated with proximal or ascending lesions, patients with these lesions should be taken for emergent surgical correction, whereas patients with distal lesions can be managed medically.

This patient was initially stabilized with medical therapy but was taken to surgery several days later despite blood pressure control, for surgical repair secondary to concerns of further dissection.

Clinical Pearls

1. Patients with acute onset of intense chest or back pain that is "tearing" in quality and of maximal intensity should have aortic dissection included in their differential diagnosis.
2. Dissections involving the proximal aorta are associated with a much greater mortality and typically require emergent surgical intervention, whereas distal dissections can be managed medically in most cases.
3. Blood pressure should be controlled with intravenous beta-blockers initially and intravenous nitroprusside, with the goal of maintaining a systolic blood pressure of < 120 mmHg, or as low as possible while maintaining cerebral, renal, and cardiac perfusion.

REFERENCES

1. Nienaber CA, Eagle KA: Aortic dissection: new frontiers in diagnosis and management: Part I: trometiology to diagnostic strategies. Circ 108(5):628–635, 2003.
2. Nienaber CA, Eagle KA: Aortic dissection: new frontiers in diagnosis and management: Part II: therapeutic management and follow-up. Circ 108(6):772–778, 2003.
3. Crawford ES: The diagnosis and management of aortic dissection. JAMA 264:2537–2541, 1990.
4. DeSanctis RW, Doroghazi RM, Austen WG, Buckley MJ: Aortic dissection. N Engl J Med 317:1060–1067, 1987.

Marion R. Wofford, MD, MPH

PATIENT 52

**A 78-year old woman who states that the "top number is high
and the bottom number is low"**

An elderly women was advised to have her blood pressure rechecked after finding that it was elevated at a senior citizens' health fair. She reports that her home blood pressure readings are "normal," but "the top number is high and the bottom, low." She believed that this was a good blood pressure given her age of 78. She says she has recently moved to the area, and was followed by an internist in her former home town. She had been told that her blood pressure was elevated during prior clinic visits because of stress. The patient takes no prescription medications, exercises regularly, and has no known medical problems. Her family medical history is noncontributory.

Physical Examination: Temperature 97.9°F, pulse 75, respirations 15, blood pressure sitting 155/78, standing 152/80. Height 5 feet 4 inches, weight 122 pounds, BMI 21. General: very thin, good posture. HEENT: slight hearing loss, neck with no masses or bruits. Cardiac: regular rate and rhythm with no murmur. Chest: clear. Abdomen: nontender, nondistended, no bruits. Extremities: no edema.

Laboratory Findings: CBC and chemistry values: normal. Electrocardiography: left ventricular hypertrophy.

Question: Is this patient's blood pressure appropriate for her age?

Answer: Isolated systolic hypertension should be treated regardless of age.

Discussion: There are many different ideas today among the public and healthcare providers as to what constitutes hypertension. The Joint National Committee (JNC) provides guidelines to aid in diagnoses and treatment strategies. According to the JNC VII guidelines, blood pressure should be classified as normal, prehypertension, or stage 1 or 2 hypertension. Normal blood pressure is considered to be a systolic blood pressure (SBP) of < 120 mmHg and a diastolic blood pressure (DBP) of < 80 mmHg. Prehypertension includes a SBP of 120–139 or a DBP of 80–89 mmHg; stage 1 hypertension is defined as a SBP of 140–159 or a DBP of 90–99 mmHg and stage 2 as > 160/100 mmHg.

A patient's average blood pressure may be difficult to assess, based on the many factors that may influence in-office measurement. Stress, amount of sleep, caffeine intake, tobacco, time of day, dietary sodium intake, and posture are just a few examples of factors that affect blood pressure. New patients should have their blood pressure taken in both arms in a sitting position, as well as supine and standing. It is important that blood pressure be measured with a cuff that is an appropriate size for the patient. If the cuff is too small, the reading may be elevated; if it is too large, the reading could be depressed. Two readings should always be taken after the patient has been seated quietly for 5 minutes. Home blood pressure monitoring should be encouraged for most patients and advice on appropriate devices should be given. Ambulatory blood pressure monitoring provides blood pressure readings over a 24-hour period. These instruments, although not widely used clinically, are recommended to evaluate a number of conditions including white-coat hypertension, resistant hypertension, autonomic dysfunction, hypotension, and response to antihypertensive medications.

Proper recording of blood pressure becomes increasingly important as the problem of hypertension grows in our society. The size of the elderly population continues to grow rapidly and so does the number of medical conditions with which this population struggles. Systolic blood pressure tends to increase with age, whereas diastolic pressure decreases. Therefore, isolated systolic hypertension (ISH) and elevated pulse pressure are growing concerns in the treatment of hypertension.

Mild increases in blood pressure can substantially increase risk factors for stroke, end-stage renal disease, congestive heart failure, coronary heart disease, and even dementia. In the elderly, the occurrence of ISH or elevated pulse pressure is even more problematic than in the younger population, as in the elderly these phenomena are also associated with increased risk of left ventricular hypertrophy as well as other cardiovascular problems. In fact, systolic blood pressure is a better indicator for cardiovascular risk than is diastolic blood pressure in patients older than 50 years.

Elevated pulse pressure (systolic minus diastolic) has importance in cardiovascular mortality, as it points toward the loss of elastin, decrease in vessel compliance, and increase in aortic pressure, all of which may promote atherosclerosis. Because of the relationship between age and increase in systolic blood pressure, the problems of ISH and elevated pulse pressure, as well as other forms of hypertension, should be seriously evaluated. As the size of the elderly population grows, it becomes increasingly evident that early prevention and early intervention in this group will help to prevent problems on a larger scale, as well as to allow these members of society to maintain their independence and quality of life.

One of the issues in treating hypertension, especially in the elderly, does not come from lifestyle or natural progression of blood pressure with age, but rather from the awareness of the population concerning their blood pressure. As in this patient, common misperceptions about hypertension include: systolic blood pressure should be the age plus 100, elevated blood pressure with age is normal and acceptable, and increases in systolic blood pressure are not as dangerous as those in diastolic blood pressure. In addition to having these misperceptions, many members of society do not know what their blood pressure numbers are and do not associate high blood pressure and hypertension with future health issues.

Healthcare providers play an extremely important role in the education about and awareness of hypertension. Clinicians should first ensure that their own knowledge is current on blood pressure guidelines and treatments. They should then take responsibility for educating their patients. Patients should be encouraged to monitor their blood pressure at home on a regular basis, and they should be educated accordingly. Even slight sustained increases in blood pressure warrant consideration, especially as the age of the patient increases. All individuals should attempt to keep their blood pressure under 140/90 and possibly lower depending on other medical complications, such as diabetes and renal disease. Educational materials should be provided to patients and to the general population. Hypertension is the most common chronic medical problem, yet the risk associated with untreated hypertension in all age groups is generally not appreciated by most patients.

As patients take a greater responsibility for knowing their own health information (i.e., blood pressure, glucose, and cholesterol levels, etc.) they will have the ability to take a more proactive role in their treatment. Awareness of guidelines and personal information may increase their willingness to seek treatment early if problems begin to arise.

This patient who presented with ISH was counseled on the current information concerning her blood pressure. She was also counseled on the effects that elevated blood pressure could have on other aspects of her health and encouraged to come in for regular follow-up visits. After a period of dietary modification she remained hypertensive, so hydrochlorothiazide 12.5 mg daily was recommended. She was advised to monitor her blood pressure regularly at home and to continue healthy eating habits and an exercise regimen. The patient left the health fair more knowledgable about her blood pressure and encouraged that this chronic disease was manageable with lifestyle interventions and medication use.

Clinical Pearls

1. Knowledge of current guidelines for hypertension is important for proper treatment.
2. Hypertension in the elderly, especially ISH and elevated pulse pressure, are common and difficult to manage.
3. Increased awareness among patients is needed to aid in the prevention of future medical complications associated with hypertension.
4. Patients should be encouraged to know their own health information and take a proactive role in their treatment.

REFERENCES

1. Chobanian AV, Bakris GL, Black HR, et al: National Heart, Lung, and Blood Institute Joint National Committee on Prevention, Detection, Evaluation, and Treatment of High Blood Pressure; National High Blood Pressure Education: The Seventh Report of the Joint National Committee on Prevention, Detection, Evaluation, and Treatment of High Blood Pressure: the JNC VII report. JAMA 289(19):2560–2572, 2003.
2. Egan BM, Lackland DT, Cutler NE: Awareness, knowledge, and attitudes of older americans about high blood pressure implications for health care policy, education, and research. Arch Intern Med 163:681–687, 2003.
3. Moser M: No surprises in blood pressure awareness study findings—We Can Do a better job. Arch Intern Med 163:654–656, 2003.
4. Wizner B, Gryglewska B, Gasowski J, et al: Normal blood pressure values as perceived by normotensive and hypertensive subjects. J Hum Hypertens 17:87–91, 2003.
5. Kaplan NM, Rose BD: Treatment of hypertension in the elderly. In Rose BD (ed): UptoDate, June 2002.
6. NM Kaplan: Kaplan's Clinical Hypertension. 8th ed. Philadelphia, Lippincott Williams & Wilkins, 2002, pp 25–55.
7. Nemade SS, Ciocon JO, The Cleveland Clinic Florida, Naples, University of Miami, et al: Blood pressure therapy in the elderly: An observation in octogenarians. J Clin Hypertens 2(4):263–266, 2000.
8. Pavlik VN, Hyman DJ, Vallbona C, et al: Hypertension awareness and control in an inner-city African-American sample. J Hum Hyperten 11:277–283, 1997.

PATIENT 53

A 14-year-old girl with refractory hypertension

An adolescent girl was found during an annual physical examination to have a blood pressure of 160/100 mmHg. Her brother was diagnosed with hypertension at age 12, her mother's hypertension responded only to triamterene, and her maternal grandfather had hypertension that resolved completely after he received a kidney transplant. She has no significant medical history and her review of systems is negative.

Physical Examination: Temperature 98.4°F, pulse 68, blood pressure 166/104, respirations 16. General: well-developed, well-nourished, appears stated age; no apparent distress. Chest: clear. Cardiac: no heave, point of maximum intensity not displaced, normal S_1 and S_2, no S_3 or S_4, no murmurs, no thrill, no jugular venous distension. Abdomen: normal bowel sounds, no organomegaly. Extremities: no edema. Skin: normal facial and axillary hair. Genitourinary: Tanner Stage V.

Laboratory Findings: WBC 7200 with normal differential. Hct 42%; sodium 131 mmol/L, chloride 105 mmol/L, bicarbonate 22 mmol/L, potassium 3.1 mmol/L, BUN 11 mg/dl, creatinine 0.8 mg/dl, glucose 100 mg/dl. After sodium restriction her upright plasma aldosterone level was 236 pmol/L (normal, 140 to 1110 pmol/L). Urine levels of 18-hydroxycortisol and 18-oxocortisol: normal.

Question: What is the genetic defect causing this patient's hypertension?

Diagnosis: Liddle's syndrome (pseudoaldosteronism)

Discussion: Liddle's syndrome (LS) a rare, autosomal dominant cause of early-onset hypertension, was first described in a young girl with severe hypertension similar to the patient in this case. Hypokalemia, metabolic alkalosis, decreased aldosterone secretion, and low plasma renin activity are characteristic of the syndrome. Spironolactone, an antagonist of the mineralocorticoid receptor, has no effect on this condition. The blood pressure may be improved by a low-sodium diet combined with antagonists of the epithelial sodium channel (ENaC) in the distal nephron.

This patient has electrolyte abnormalities and a significant family history suggestive of LS. Low serum aldosterone and renin levels and a normal 18-hydroxycortisol level do not support the diagnosis of primary aldosteronism, another possible etiology in this patient. The patient's brother was affected similarly, and several similar families have been investigated subsequently. In this family, three generations are affected by early-onset or refractory hypertension. Her mother's hypertension responded only to triamterene, an antagonist of the epithelial sodium channel (ENaC), which controls sodium reabsorption. A renal transplant cured her maternal grandfather's disease.

Liddle's syndrome has been mapped to chromosome 16 with linkage studies in affected families. Subsequent work revealing the structure of ENaC included three subunits with similar structures, each of which spanned the plasma membrane twice with N-terminus and C-terminus, both located intracellularly. The three subunits were coded for by three genes, and the genes for the beta and gamma subunits were mapped to chromosome 16 in the region where LS had been mapped. Family studies showing mutations in either the beta subunit or the gamma subunit produced the same phenotype. The first mutations that were found all had the effect of eliminating the last 45 to 75 amino acids from the C-terminus of the subunits. In vitro expression studies identified a critical sequence of six amino acid residues that is necessary for normal sodium current through the membrane.

DNA testing has allowed studies of families with hypertension resulting from LS. Mutation carriers have also been shown to have increased transnasal potential differences, similar to the increase found in the renal distal tubules, but this test is not used widely to establish the diagnosis.

Salt restriction and ENaC inhibition are the major treatments for LS. Triamterene and amiloride are the drugs usually used. If not treated, prolonged hypertension can lead to a fixed hypertension due to changes in renal function. This patient also responded to treatment with triamterene.

Clinical Pearls

1. A family history of early-onset hypertension and hypertension responsive to ENaC antagonists such as triamterene are essential clues for Liddle's syndrome (LS).
2. In addition to salt restriction, treatment for LS should focus on inhibiting ENaC with amiloride or triamterene.
3. DNA testing can identify presymptomatic family members with LS who are at high risk of developing refractory hypertension.

REFERENCES

1. Baker E, Jeunemaitre X, Portal AJ, et al: Abnormalities of nasal potential difference measurement in Liddle's syndrome. J Clin Invest 102:10–14, 1998.
2. Hansson JH, Nelson-Williams C, Suzuki H, et al: Hypertension caused by a truncated epithelial sodium channel gamma subunit: genetic heterogeneity of Liddle syndrome. Nature Genet 11:76–82, 1995.
3. Snyder PM, Price MP, McDonald FJ, et al: Mechanisms by which Liddle's syndrome mutations increase activity of a human epithelial Na(+) channel. Cell 83:969–978, 1995.
4. Hansson JH, Schild L, Lu Y, et al: A de novo missense mutation of the B subunit of the epithelial sodium channel causes hypertension and Liddle syndrome, identifying a proline-rich segment critical for regulation of channel activity. Proc Nat Acad Sci USA 92:11495–11499, 1995.
5. Shimkets RA, Warnock DG, Bositis CM, et al: Liddle's syndrome: heritable human hypertension caused by mutations in the beta subunit of the epithelial sodium channel. Cell 79:407–414, 1994.
6. Rodriguez JA, Biglieri EG, Schambelan M: Pseudohyperaldosteronism with renal tubular resistance to mineralocorticoid hormones. Trans Assoc Am Phys 94:172–182, 1981.
7. Wang C, Chan TK, Yeung RTT, et al: The effect of triamterene and sodium intake on renin, aldosterone, and erythrocyte sodium transport in Liddle's syndrome. J Clin Endocr Metab 52:1027–1032, 1981.
8. Liddle GW, Bledsoe T, Coppage WS Jr: A familial renal disorder simulating primary aldosteronism but with negligible aldosterone secretion. Trans Assoc Am Phys 76:199–213, 1963.

Sharon B. Wyatt, RN, CANP, PhD
Audwin Fletcher, RN, CFNP, MSN

PATIENT 54

A 30-year-old African-American man with untreated high blood pressure

A man presents to a nurse practitioner for an occupational physical examination as a city police-man. He appears anxious as he enters the examining room and notes that he usually relies on home remedies recommended by his grandmother for most healthcare problems. He has not been to a health-care provider since a visit to an emergency department following an automobile accident as a teenager. He vaguely recalls being told that his blood pressure was "a little high" at that time, but he did not think the degree of elevation was significant. The patient lives with his wife and three children. His wife's salary as an elementary teacher's assistant has supported the family while he completed his police training at the local junior college. His childhood was marked by poverty and family conflict, and he admits to having a "quick temper." He is determined to overcome these odds through hard work as a policeman. His father has high blood pressure and had a stroke at age 58.

Physical Examination: Temperature 98.7°F, pulse 96, respirations 24, blood pressure 168/100 sitting, 160/98 standing. Body mass index 27. General: appears anxious. Neurological: normal. Cardiac: normal heart sounds, jugular venous pressure normal, pulses intact in all extremities. Respiratory: normal. Abdomen: normal. Extremities: no edema.

Laboratory Findings: Chemistries: normal, BUN 19 mg/dl, creatinine 1.3 mg/dl. Urinalysis: microalbuminuria 30 mg/dl. EKG, 12-lead: nonspecific ST-T wave abnormalities. Chest x-ray: normal.

Question: How should this patient's blood pressure elevation be defined?

Diagnosis: Primary hypertension with microalbuminuria

Discussion: Hypertension is a well-recognized risk factor for stroke, heart failure, and renal failure, particularly among African Americans, many of whom have high blood pressure and are unaware of its presence. African Americans experience more rapid progression of end-organ damage from this "silent" killer. African American men are at a particularly high risk because they are often unaware of the disease and therefore do not receive treatment, and/or may not adhere to the regimen prescribed. African American men between the ages of 18 and 49 have the lowest rates of awareness, treatment, and control of high blood pressure of all age, ethnic, and gender groups in the United States. Failure of healthcare providers to treat high blood pressure early and aggressively in this population is a key obstacle to reducing the disparities in blood pressure awareness and control in young African-American men. The misperception that it is medically more difficult to lower blood pressure in African Americans likely contributes to inadequate treatment. Management of hypertension in African-American men is complex and requires attention to the unique attributes of this population.

Assessment of cardiovascular risk, including unique psychosocial markers, should be recognized as an important part of the entire clinical picture. Risk-assessment models based on Framingham data have been validated in African American populations and include attention to the traditional risk factors of family history, total and low-density lipoprotein cholesterol levels, diabetes mellitus, obesity, tobacco use, and physical inactivity. Microalbuminuria has been shown to be an independent risk factor for cardiovascular and renal disease, even in persons without hypertension or diabetes. Furthermore, microalbuminuria has been shown to predict left ventricular hypertrophy in young hypertensive black men. In this patient, there are early signs of both microalbuminuria and mild ST-T wave changes on the ECG. These two abnormalities point to the need for intensive therapy to prevent overt target-organ damage. Angiotensin-converting enzyme inhibitors (ACEIs) offer an important benefit in target-organ protection and in arresting disease progression in African Americans.

The precursors of elevated blood pressure begin in youth. Reviews of the pediatric and adolescent literature suggest that family-process factors, particularly family conflict, predict changes in blood pressure, independent of the effects of age, gender, and body mass index. Although findings are preliminary, this relationship highlights the importance of exploring environmental processes that

may influence physiologic outcomes in later life. Another psychosocial process has been named "John Henryism" for the black, steel-driving folk character who refused to be deterred in his aspirations despite insurmountable odds. This kind of tenacious and active coping style in the face of few socioeconomic resources for achieving life goals has been associated with increasing systolic blood pressure in African-American men.

New guidelines for treatment of blood pressure in African Americans focus on persistent and intensive management of blood pressure at all stages of life, with a reduced blood pressure target of < 130/80 mmHg for those with nondiabetic insulin impairment or overt diabetes mellitus. Achieving this target depends on individually tailored lifestyle and multidrug pharmacologic regimens that include counseling and effective patient education. In this patient, health beliefs and few experiences with healthcare providers increase the challenge of establishing a therapeutic alliance. Assisting patients in engaging in lifestyle alterations such as sodium restriction, weight loss, and smoking cessation depends on assuring an adequate understanding of the causes and consequences of high blood pressure. Emphasizing realistic and appropriate lifestyle changes and providing ongoing education and support is crucial to successful lifestyle change. For example, the Dietary Approaches to Stop Hypertension (DASH) diet was most effective in African Americans with high blood pressure.

To reach blood pressure goals, most young black men will need pharmacological therapy. The Hypertension in African Americans Working Group of the International Society of Hypertension in Blacks has recently recommended initiating therapy early and persistently in African Americans by using a combination agent when systolic blood pressure readings are 15 mmHg above their target or diastolic blood pressure readings are 10 mmHg above their target. Combination agents may include a beta-blocker/diuretic, ACEI/diuretic, ACEI/calcium-channel blocker (CCB), or an angiotensin receptor blocker (ARB)/diuretic. All antihypertensive agents are associated with blood pressure lowering efficacy in African Americans, although, as monotherapy or in the absence of a diuretic, beta-blockers, ACEIs, or ARBs are not as effective as they are in Caucasians. Thiazide diuretics and CCBs have greater blood-pressure lowering efficacy in African Americans than do ACEIs when used as monotherapy. Centrally acting alpha-agonists should not be a first-line agent in primary hypertension. This is a potent antihypertensive class that can cause significant rebound hypertension in withdrawal states of poorly compliant patients. If monotherapy is begun, then a diuretic is a recommended first step. When blood pressure cannot be controlled with a single agent, it is preferable to add another class. If blood pressure goals cannot be achieved with a combination of two agents, either the dose of one agent can be increased or a third agent can be added. Factors of compliance, side-effect profiles, risk stratification, and the potential for end-organ damage help the clinician in selecting the most efficacious agent for each patient. For example, current data clearly support the use of the afore-mentioned agents in African Americans with renal impairment, left ventricular hypertrophy, and with or without diabetes mellitus. African Americans may be more prone to the typical prostaglandin-mediated side effects of ACEIs and may find it beneficial to take a low-dose aspirin in combination to reduce the potential for ACEI-associated cough. Compelling indications for beta-blockers are their usefulness in persons with angina and/or those who are post myocardial infarction. Two to four agents may be required to achieve optimal control.

Lifestyle changes including sodium restriction and weight loss, along with combination therapy of oral lisinopril/hydrocholorothiazide 10/12.5 mg daily were initiated in this patient. He was referred to a group education and counseling session conducted by the nurse practitioner with other African American men to discuss approaches to stress, anger management, and coping. After 6 weeks, his blood pressure was 140/90 mmHg. He reported a regular physical activity program with friends, an increase in fruits and vegetables in his diet, and a weight loss of 2 pounds. The medication dosage was increased to oral lisinopril/hydrochlorothiazide 20/12.5 mg daily. In 6 months, a repeated spot urine showed a microalbuminuria level of 25 mg/dl. No further changes were made in his medication regimen. Ongoing educational/support sessions were continued and routine follow-up was scheduled for 3-month intervals.

Clinical Pearls

1. African Americans are at higher risk than the general population for negative consequences of hypertension, necessitating lower blood pressure goals to prevent untoward sequelae.
2. Blood pressure control can be achieved in African Americans (despite old myths) with a combination of intensive and persistent lifestyle and pharmaco-therapeutic options.
3. Exploring environmental processes that may influence physiological outcomes is an important component of therapy.
4. All classes of antihypertensives are appropriate for use in African Americans.
5. Combination therapy including a diuretic is recommended, and compelling indications for use of either beta-blockers (angina, myocardial infarction), or ACEIs or ARBs (renal impairment, diabetes) are applied to treatment in African Americans and the general population.

REFERENCES

1. Douglas JG, Bakris GL, Epstein M, et al: Management of high blood pressure in African Americans: Consensus statement of the Hypertension in African Americans Working Group of the International Society of Hypertension in Blacks. Arch Intern Med 163:525–541, 2003.
2. Clark R, Armstead C: Family conflict predicts blood pressure changes in African American adolescents: A preliminary examination. J Adolesc 23(3):355–358, 2000.
3. Post WS, Blumenthal RS, Weiss JL, et al: Spot urinary albumin-creatinine ratio predicts left ventricular hypertrophy in young hypertensive African-American men. Am J Hypertens 13(11):1168–1172, 2000.
4. Rose LE, Kim MT, Dennison DR, Hill MN: The contexts of adherence for African-Americans with high blood pressure. J Adv Nursing 32(3):587–594, 2000.
5. Dressler WW, Bindon JR, Neggers YH: John Henryism, gender and arterial blood pressure in an African-American community. Psychosom Med 60(5):620–624, 1998.

James T. Samuel, PharmD
George E. Habeeb, Jr., MD

PATIENT 55

A 39-year-old female smoker with hypertension

A woman with hypertension and a history of type 2 diabetes mellitus, both of which have been controlled with medication, presents to a clinic for a 3-month follow-up visit. She insists that she has been compliant with both her lisinopril and her metformin. However, her home blood pressure is 160/92 mmHg, which is considerably higher than her blood pressure taken at her last clinic visit. When asked about changes in diet and exercise habits, she states vaguely that she is not eating any differently, and that her exercise level has dropped due to a loss in stamina. Upon further investigation, she admitted to restarting her cigarette smoking at one pack per day after her divorce 2 months ago. She has a family history of coronary artery disease.

Physical Examination: Temperature 98.7°F, pulse 85, respirations 18, blood pressure 160/96. General: overweight, smells of cigarette smoke. Cardiac: normal S_1, prominent S_2, no S_3 and no S_4 gallops, no murmurs. Chest: clear. Abdomen: no mass, no bruits. Extremities: no cyanosis, clubbing, or edema; however, there is mild yellow discoloration around the fingernail beds.

Laboratory Findings: Hemogram: WBC 4.5 th/cmm, Hct 39%. Chemistry: glucose, electrolytes, BUN, and creatinine normal. Lipids: normal except HDL for level of 30 mg/dl.

Question: Based on the history and physical, what could explain the patient's recent rise in blood pressure?

Diagnosis: A recent increase in blood pressure due to cigarette smoking

Discussion: There are several potential mechanisms for the rise in blood pressure in cigarette smokers. Some are related to the nicotine contained in cigarettes, and others are related to the byproducts of smoking. During smoking, the alpha-adrenergic effect predominates, leading to a rise in systemic vascular resistance and, subsequently, in arterial blood pressure. An increase in heart rate can be seen as early as one minute after the onset of smoking. Nicotine stimulates catecholamine and vasopressin release which causes tachycardia, increased systolic and diastolic blood pressure, and cutaneous vasoconstriction. Chemoreceptors in the carotid arteries and aortic arch are stimulated by nicotine. Hypertensive patients who smoke may have a fivefold increase in risk of malignant hypertension. Carbon monoxide content of cigarette smoke is 2.7–6%, which can injure the vascular endothelium and lead to thrombotic episodes. Carbon monoxide also reduces oxygen delivery to the tissues leading to a lowering of the anginal threshold in patients with coronary artery disease.

The effects of smoking on the cardiovascular system can be described temporally as acute and chronic. Acutely, smoking causes a transient elevation in blood pressure lasting 15–30 minutes after smoking. A smoker may not necessarily present as having high blood pressure in the clinic because of the acute variable regarding the time of the last cigarette and the chronic variable regarding body weight. At low doses of nicotine, the excitation of the central nervous system causes symptoms such as tremor, suppression of emotions, and increased concentration. Chronically, smoking can cause arterial rigidity leading to atherosclerosis. In addition, chronic smokers exhibit a reduction in thrombocyte lifespan. Hemostasis is generally exhibited due to higher levels of fibrinogen in smokers than in nonsmokers, which seems to be dose-dependent and which increases with age. Smoking has been shown to decrease high-density lipoprotein (HDL) levels, thereby adding another risk factor for cardiovascular disease. Smoking has also been associated with the development of accelerated-malignant hypertension.

In basic triage before taking a blood pressure, the history should reveal whether a patient uses cigarettes. If the patient reveals cigarette use, then determine the time of the most recent usage. Cigarette smoking within the previous 30 minutes can raise the blood pressure reading. It is also important to inform and instruct the patient about the effects of smoking upon blood pressure. Ideally, ambulatory blood pressure would be the most accurate tool for assessing this patient's blood pressure. However, if not readily available, other measures could be employed. If a patient continues to use cigarettes against medical advice, one suggestion includes having the patient take a blood pressure reading at home 30 minutes before and 30 minutes after smoking. Some smokers may have low-to-normal blood pressures in the intervals between cigarettes. The above-mentioned self-measurement allows the patient to discover the impact of smoking on blood pressure and reinforces the need for smoking cessation.

In this patient, with her hypertension and type 2 diabetes mellitus treatment options may include use of a selective beta-blocker, diuretics, angiotensin-converting enzyme (ACE) inhibitors, or angiotensin receptor blockers (ARBs). In smokers with hypertension and/or comorbid conditions, the recommendations for pharmacologic therapy as outlined in JNC VII apply. The only exception is to consider not using a nonselective beta-blocker, which could theoretically and indirectly potentiate the vascular effects of nicotine. Many smokers may develop comorbid vascular conditions such as atherosclerotic heart disease, myocardial infarction, left ventricular hypertrophy, arrhythmias, congestive heart failure, pulmonary hypertension, right heart failure, cerebrovascular disease, cerebrovascular accident, renal artery stenosis, peripheral vascular disease, and more. Many smokers also develop comorbid nonvascular conditions such as chronic obstructive pulmonary disease, frequent infections, gastrointestinal disturbance, neoplasms, and more.

All patients who smoke should be strongly advised to quit and should be offered treatment for smoking cessation. From another perspective, healthcare providers need to be very supportive of those patients trying to quit because relapse rates are high, and withdrawal from nicotine can be a tough obstacle to overcome. It may take several attempts for cessation, but it is important for the patient and physician to persevere. There have been numerous success stories in patients who have used nicotine replacement therapy, including the options of nicotine patch, gum, inhaler, or lozenges. Bupropion has also been employed in smoking cessation therapy with great results. Smoking cessation clinics and support groups are becoming increasingly available and may be of some benefit to patients who require constant reinforcement.

This patient may have smoked one or more cigarettes just before the office visit, thus explaining the rise in blood pressure. For the sake of accuracy, it would be wise to recheck the blood pressure after 30 minutes in a calm environment. The patient needs to understand the harmful effects of smoking on her body, and these points must be continually reinforced. Smoking cessation would reduce her risk for a cardiovascular event, and, in addition, exercise could raise her HDL level. Smoking may also be a source of her perceived drop in stamina during exercise due to its effect on lowering oxygen-carrying capacity. The patient was presented with information about smoking cessation and was referred to a smoking cessation clinic to assist her in her efforts to quit.

The adverse health consequences related to tobacco apply to cigarettes, chewing tobacco, pipes, cigars, and any other tobacco-related products. Therefore, instructions to a patient should include information about cessation of all forms of tobacco products.

Clinical Pearls

1. Smokers may actually have low-to-normal blood pressure for intervals between smoking.
2. Pharmacologic therapy includes the usual Joint National Committee (JNC) VII recommendations and treatment for comorbid conditions.
3. The only potential exception in drug selection would be nonselective beta-blockers.
4. Twenty-four hour ambulatory blood pressure monitoring is the most accurate assessment of blood pressure in smokers.
5. An absolute requirement in providing adequate care to patients is the unambiguous reinforcement that all forms of tobacco products are detrimental to overall health.

REFERENCES
1. Kaplan NM: Kaplan's Clinical Hypertension, 8th ed. Philadelphia, Lippincott Williams & Wilkins, 2002, pp 211.
2. Lee DH, Ha MH, Kim JR, Jacobs DR: Effects of smoking cessation on changes in blood pressure and incidence of hypertension. Hypertension 37:194–198, 2001.
3. Primatesta P, Falaschetti E, Gupta S, et al: Association between smoking and blood pressure. Hypertension 37:187–193, 2001.
4. Haustein KO: Smoking tobacco, microcirculatory changes and the role of nicotine. Int J Clin Pharmacol Ther 37:2:76–85, 1999.
5. Chobanian AV, Bakris GL, Black HR, et al: National Heart, Lung, and Blood Institute Joint National Committee on Prevention, Detection, Evaluation, and Treatment of Blood Pressure; National High Blood Pressure Education: The Seventh Report of the Joint National Committee on Prevention, Detection, Evaluation, and Treatment of High Blood Pressure: the JNC VII report, JAMA 289(19):2560–2572, 2003.
6. Kochar MS, Bindra RS: The additive effects of smoking and hypertension. Postgrad Med 100:5:147–160, 1996.

PATIENT 56

An 18-year-old man with exertional leg fatigue

A young man presents to his physician with complaints of bilateral leg fatigue when jogging or running. He is unable to complete games of football, basketball, or tennis due to exertional dyspnea and leg cramps. Sometimes he feels a "second wind," which allows him to play in short consecutive games with intervals of rest. He was told not to play varsity sports last year when a school physician discovered an elevated blood pressure in his left arm. He has headaches, occasional nosebleeds, and relative weakness of the right arm compared to the left arm.

Physical Examination: Temperature 98.6°F; pulse 90; respiratory rate 18; blood pressures right brachial 100/70, left brachial 164/104, right popliteal 90/60, left popliteal 90/60. Neurological: normal. HEENT: normal. Cardiac: regular rhythm, audible S_1, loud S_2, S_4 gallop, palpable ventricular heave; no jugular venous distention. Arterial pulses: left arm 3^+, right arm, right leg, and left leg 1^+ *parvus et tardus* (diminished and delayed). Lungs: clear. Abdomen: soft, nontender, no organomegaly, no bruits. Extremities: right arm slightly smaller than left, no cyanosis, no clubbing, no edema.

Laboratory Findings: Hemogram: normal. Serum chemistries: normal. BUN 22 mg/dl, creatinine 1.2 mg/dl. Liver panel: normal. Urine chemistries and microscopic examination: normal.

Additional Tests: EKG, 12-lead: normal sinus mechanism, suggestive of left ventricular overload/hypertrophy. Chest x-ray anteroposterior and lateral: cardiomegaly, proximal descending aorta dilated with figure "3" indentation, subcostal rib notching, mild pulmonary venous congestion.

Question: What syndrome is impairing this young patient's exercise tolerance?

Diagnosis: Coarctation of the aorta with anomalous origin of the right subclavian artery distal to the coarctation

Discussion: Native coarctation of the aorta is a stenosis of the lumen within the aortic isthmus, occurring in up to 10% of all congenital cardiac anomalies. Coarctation is most commonly distal to the origin of the left subclavian artery near the insertion of the ligamentum arteriosum.

Native coarctation of the aorta occurs both as a single anomaly and in association with other cerebrovascular and cardiovascular anomalies such as ventricular septal defect, aortic stenosis with or without bicuspid aortic valve, left-sided hypoplasia, aneurysm of the left subclavian artery, anomalous origin of the right subclavian artery distal to the coarctation (as in this patient), coarctation between the left subclavian and carotid arteries, aneurysm of the proximal descending aorta, and cerebral aneurysm.

The pathophysiology of hypertension in patients with coarctation of the aorta involves global hypoperfusion distal to the coarctation. Downstream renal hypoperfusion activates the renin-angiotensin-aldosterone system, leading to severe, persistent hypertension. Patients may present with headaches, epistaxis, leg claudication, and muscle weakness; this patient exhibited all of these symptoms. His hypertension was detectable only in the left arm, with a normal left subclavian artery origin upstream from the coarctation. The blood pressures downstream from the coarctation are relatively lower.

Beyond the neonatal period, normal leg systolic blood pressures are 5–20 mmHg higher than arm blood pressures. A systolic blood pressure gradient of at least 20 mmHg in upper versus lower extremities supports a diagnosis of coarctation of the aorta. In this patient, the estimated noninvasive peak systolic blood pressure gradient comparing left arm to left leg is 74 mmHg. Physical examination also revealed a developmentally reduced size of the right arm, and arterial pulses *parvus et tardus* (diminished and delayed) in all extremities, with arterial origin distal to the coarctation. The pulse strength and timing are compared to those of the left upper extremity in this case.

The 12-lead EKG may suggest chamber enlargement and/or hypertrophy with overload patterns. This patient's findings on chest x-rays are strongly suggestive of coarctation of the aorta. Transthoracic echocardiogram (TTE) with aortic windows in multiple planes can suggest the diagnosis. Contrasted computed tomography (CT), magnetic resonance imaging (MRI), and magnetic resonance angiography (MRA) with multiplane three-dimensional imaging reconstruction can further delineate the anatomy of the aortic coarctation and associated vascular anomalies. Invasive catheterization is the gold standard diagnostic test for defining anatomy of the coarctation, potential anomalies of aortic branches, cardiac anomalies, and the direction of blood flow with pressure gradients.

Untreated, most patients with coarctation of the aorta will die before 50 years of age. After diagnostic angiography defines the anatomy of the coarctation and/or co-existing anomalies, the therapeutic approach to repair must consider the age of the patient and any prior attempts at repair. Primary surgical repair is recommended for neonates, infants, and young children with native coarctation of the aorta. An older child with a near adult-sized aorta may be a candidate for balloon angioplasty and stenting. Primary balloon angioplasty with or without stent placement is widely accepted for adults with native coarctation of the aorta.

The goal of intervention is to achieve a residual peak systolic gradient of < 10 mmHg across the newly dilated and stented coarctation. Balloon angioplasty alone may relapse into re-coarctation with a residual gradient of > 10 mmHg, necessitating stent or surgical correction. Primary stenting is associated with a low re-coarctation rate. Patients may be followed postcatheter intervention by physical examination gradients, Doppler gradients, echocardiogram, CT, MRI, and/or MRA.

The pathophysiology of hypertension postsuccessful repair of coarctation is postulated to relate to abnormal upstream vascular structure and function (small and large vessels), which is not reversible. Hypertension persists in 27–68% of patients, requiring chronic therapy; after repair, fewer medications are generally required. A systolic blood pressure of > 165 mmHg predilation may correlate with an increased risk of chronic hypertension postdilation.

Treatment criteria may include a resting blood pressure of > 140/90 mmHg, or exercise systolic blood pressure of 200 mmHg in those normotensive at rest. Pharmacologic choices primarily include beta-blockers. Even after successful repair, postoperative late complications include a high incidence of accelerated coronary artery disease and acute myocardial infarction. Cerebrovascular accidents occur either from the hypertension or an aneurysm at the circle of Willis. Early diagnosis and intervention are critical for improving survival and for preventing co-morbid conditions.

Clinical Pearls

1. Coarctation of the aorta may present at any age, with isolated findings or with co-existing cardiovascular anomalies.
2. Physical examination findings include *parvus et tardus* pulses distal to the coarctation, arterial hypertension proximal to the coarctation, relative hypotension distal to the coarctation, and a pathophysiologic gradient (peak systolic blood pressure difference) of > 5 to 20 mmHg.
3. The goal of treatment (balloon angioplasty and stent or surgery) is to achieve a postprocedure peak systolic blood pressure gradient of < 10 mmHg.
4. Post successful repair, the hypertension may persist, requiring long-term drug therapy.

REFERENCES

1. Zabal C, Attie F, Rosas M, et al: The adult patient with native coarctation of the aorta: Balloon angioplasty or primary stenting? Heart 89 (1):77–83, 2003.
2. Goudevenos JA, Papathanasiou A, Michalis LK: Coarctation of the aorta with lower blood pressure at the right upper extremity. Heart 88 (5):498, 2002.
3. Godart F, Labrot G, Devos P, et al: Coarctation of the aorta: Comparison of aortic dimensions between conventional MR imaging, 3D MR angiography, and conventional angiography. *Eur Radiol* 12:2034–2039, 2002.
4. Greenberg SB, Marks LA, Eshaghpour EE: Evaluation of magnetic resonance imaging in coarctation of the aorta: The importance of multiple imaging planes. Pediatr Cardiol 18:345–349, 1997.
5. Weber HS, Mosher RM, Baylen BS: Magnetic resonance imaging demonstration of "remodeling" of the aorta following balloon angioplasty of discrete native coarctation. Pediatr Cardiol 17:184–188, 1996.

George E. Habeeb, Jr., MD
Marion R. Wofford, MD, MPH

PATIENT 57

A 44-year-old female hemodialysis patient in hypertensive crisis

A woman presents to the emergency department with intermittent generalized tonic-clonic seizures. Witnesses at home report that the patient became disoriented prior to the seizure activity. The patient has end-stage renal disease (ESRD) and has been receiving chronic hemodialysis for 4 years. She has a 17-year history of hypertension. She recently has been intermittently compliant with her medications, including labetalol and minoxidil, and she missed her last hemodialysis session. She has had seizures only during hypertensive crises. She receives Epogen shots once a week.

Physical Examination: Temperature 99.2°F, pulse 90, respirations 18, blood pressure 240/130. General: obese, postictal. Neurological: somnolent, but arousable, able to communicate, cranial nerves II–XII intact, no motor or sensory deficits. Skin: diaphoretic, no rash. HEENT: pupils are equal, round, and reactive to light, no papilledema. Neck/thyroid: no goiter, no mass. Cardiac: regular rhythm with S_4 gallop and left ventricular heave. Chest: clear. Abdomen: soft, nontender, no mass, no organomegaly. Extremities: no cyanosis, no clubbing, 2^+ edema both legs and feet.

Laboratory Findings: Hemogram: Hct 34%. Serum chemistries: glucose 123 mg/dl, calcium 8.2 mg/dl, magnesium 2.0 mg/dl, phosphate 5.5 mg/dl, sodium 136 mmol/L, potassium 4.2 mmol/L, chloride 106 mmol/L carbon dioxide 18 mmol/L, BUN 45 mg/dl, creatinine 3.7 mg/dl.

Additional Tests: EKG, 12-lead: normal sinus mechanism with suggestion of left ventricular hypertrophy and left ventricular overload pattern. Chest x-ray, anteroposterior portable: suggests mild pulmonary venous congestion. Computed tomographic scan of head without contrast: normal.

Question: What is the main contributor to this patient's acute hypertensive crisis, pulmonary venous congestion, and edema?

Diagnosis: Volume overload

Discussion: ESRD is a worldwide health problem. It is predicted that the total number of patients with ESRD will double from 1997 to 2010. The most common causes of ESRD are diabetes mellitus, hypertension, and glomerulonephritis. The majority of patients with ESRD have hypertension even after initiation of dialysis, and an estimated 60% continue to have poor blood pressure control.

The factors contributing to hypertension associated with ESRD are multiple. The expansion of extracellular fluid volume is the primary factor complicating blood pressure control and variation, and is likely related to the development of seizure and hypertensive emergency in the current patient. Vascular autoregulation is affected by increased angiotensin II, increased vascular sensitivity to endogenous pressors, increased cardiac output with elevated peripheral vascular resistance, and failure to suppress vasoconstrictor systems. Volume sensitivity is greater in hypertensive versus normotensive dialysis patients. Other factors that affect blood pressure regulation in ESRD include increased sympathetic nerve activity, alteration of nitric oxide synthesis, activation of neurohormones, secondary hyperparathyroidism associated with hypercalemia, and the use of erythropoietin used to treat anemia.

Blood pressure measurement in ESRD should be based on manual home readings, physician office readings, and hemodialysis unit readings. Home blood pressure monitoring is highly recommended. Twenty-four-hour ambulatory blood pressure monitoring (24-hr ABPM) is useful in the evaluation of circadian variations.

The definition of systolic-diastolic hypertension in ESRD is a pre-dialysis blood pressure of > 140/90 mmHg. The pre-dialysis blood pressure goal is similar to the blood pressure goal of the general population. The recommended target for systolic blood pressure (SBP) is < 130, diastolic blood pressure (DBP) of < 80 mmHg, and pre-dialysis mean arterial pressure of < 99 mmHg. In isolated systolic hypertension, some authors propose pre-dialysis SBP target ranges of 150 to 160 mmHg.

Abnormal circadian blood pressures are found in 75% of patients with creatinine levels > 6.8 mg/dl, 80% of dialysis patients, and many kidney transplantation patients. Chronic hemodialysis patients do not have nocturnal dipping of blood pressure. Pre-dialysis DBP compared to pre-dialysis SBP correlates best with the overall 24-hr ABPM.

Sleep disorder is common among patients with ESRD. If obstructive sleep apnea (OSA) is present, a change in dialysis time from morning to night may decrease night time blood pressure by reducing extracellular fluid volume which, in turn, reduces airway obstruction. Of course, complete diagnostic and therapeutic polysomnography is still necessary to confirm the OSA and to prescribe necessary treatment of supplemental oxygen and positive airway pressure machines.

Cardiovascular disease is the most common cause of mortality in long-term dialysis patients. Left ventricular hypertrophy (LVH) is an independent predictor of cardiovascular disease and mortality in dialysis patients. Hypertension usually contributes to concentric LVH, whereas anemia contributes to eccentric LVH. Left ventricular dysfunction occurs in 80% of patients with ESRD and correlates with coronary artery disease, congestive heart failure, and mortality. For each 10-mmHg rise in mean arterial pressure, the risk of LVH, congestive heart failure, and coronary artery disease increases. Hypertension in ESRD is associated with an increased risk for stroke and cerebral atrophy.

The primary treatment of hypertension in ESRD is to correct excess volume gradually to a dry stable weight. Hemodialysis (HD) strategies may include the following options: slower HD, daily HD, nocturnal HD, lower sodium in the dialysate, and dietary sodium and volume restrictions. These methods are shown to reduce blood pressure and total peripheral vascular resistance, LVH, and cardiovascular complications. Peritoneal dialysis has been shown to improve blood pressure control. Regulation of osmolality of the dialysate, dietary sodium restriction, and dietary volume restriction are also required to achieve optimal control in patients who are undergoing peritoneal dialysis. These methods have been shown to reduce blood pressure and total peripheral vascular resistance.

The pharmacological options in the treatment of hypertension in ESRD include most classes of antihypertensive drugs except diuretics. An adjustment in standard dose and regimen is often required, depending on the degree of renal failure and the type of dialysis employed. Dose and frequency will depend upon dry weight estimation, volume of distribution, concomitant hepatic dysfunction, half life, and whether the drug is cleared by the dialysate. The use of angiotensin-converting enzyme inhibitors (ACEIs) or angiotensin receptor blockers (ARBs) have been shown to reverse LVH and improve diastolic function in ESRD. Beta-blockers, ACEIs, or ARBs may be used in patients with congestive heart failure and coronary artery disease.

In conclusion, the control of hypertension in ESRD depends predominantly on the control of sodium, volume, and extracellular fluid volume with dialysis. In the majority of patients with ESRD, antihypertensive drugs are also required to achieve blood pressure control. This patient underwent emergent dialysis on the first 2 days of admission. Intravenous labetolol was initiated but discontinued after her mental status improved. The patient and her family were counseled on the importance of regular dialysis and adherence to recommendations regarding dietary sodium and volume intake and the consistent use of antihypertensive medications. She was discharged on labetolol and resumed hemodialysis 3 times a week.

Clinical Pearls

1. The etiology of hypertension in ESRD is predominantly sodium and volume dependent.
2. Circadian rhythms are abnormal in dialysis patients with daytime hemodialysis patients being nondippers.
3. Sleep disorders are common in patients with ESRD and may improve with nocturnal dialysis regimens.
4. Blood pressure goals in dialysis patients are the same as those of the general population, with treatment decisions being based upon the pre-dialysis blood pressures.
5. Proper and efficient dialysis regimens are the mainstay of therapy and are critical for the success of pharmacologic therapy.

REFERENCES
1. Horl MP, Horl WH: Hemodialysis-associated hypertension: Pathophysiology and therapy. Am J Kidney Dis 39(2):227–244, 2002.
2. Rahman M, Smith MC: Hypertension in hemodialysis patients. Curr Hypertens Rep 3:496–502, 2001.

PATIENT 58

A 14-year-old boy presents for a pre-sports physical

A family physician is asked to evaluate a male adolescent for an elevated blood pressure on a pre-sports screen. The student was noted to have two separate blood pressure readings of 132/84 and 134/86 mmHg. He is an avid soccer player and has participated in multiple team and individual sports since the age of 10. He reports no symptoms of syncope, shortness of breath, or chest pain during exercise. His family history is significant for a father who developed hypertension in his late 30s and a mother with hypertension in her early 40s. The patient denies taking over-the-counter medications or herbal supplements and he denies illicit drug use. Medical history is pertinent for tympanostomy tubes secondary to frequent otitis media during early childhood.

Physical Examination: Temperature 98.5°F, pulse 60, respiratory rate 16,   blood pressure 136/84 mmHg (right arm), 136/84 mmHg (left arm), 138/86 mmHg (left leg). Height 5 feet 5 inches, weight 150 pounds, BMI 24.9. Neurological: normal. Cardiac: normal heart sounds, no peripheral edema, jugular venous pressure normal, pulses intact in all extremities. Respiratory: normal.

Laboratory Findings: Hemogram: hematocrit 47%. Serum chemistries, glucose: normal. Urinalysis: normal. 12-lead EKG: sinus mechanism, rate 60, left axis deviation.

Question: What issues should this physician consider in diagnosing and treating this patient's elevated blood pressure?

Answer: In the evaluation of an adolescent patient with elevated blood pressure, a basic knowledge of age-specific parameters for hypertension is required.

Discussion: Whereas elevations in the adult population are based on arbitrary cutoff points, pediatric and adolescent blood pressures are based on percentiles matched to gender and height. A percentile of < 90% is considered normal, 90–95% high normal, and > 95% high blood pressure. Generally speaking, both systolic and diastolic pressures increase as height increases. The percentiles correlate very well with an increased risk of adult hypertension as well as with other cardiovascular risk factors. An appropriate-sized cuff should always be used in the measurement of blood pressure. The cuff bladder width should be at least 40% of the arm circumference and should encircle at least 80% of the arm. As in adults, multiple readings should be taken to ensure a regression toward the mean blood pressure. A referral for 24-hour ambulatory blood pressure monitoring may be required to eliminate the possibility of "white coat" hypertension or secondary causes.

Appropriate screening questions are necessary to look for evidence of secondary hypertension and end-organ damage. Exogenous medications, many of which are either over-the-counter or herbal supplements, should be sought out as potential causes. The potential for illicit drug use is high in this population and should also be considered. Performance-enhancing drugs are becoming increasingly popular among junior high and high school athletes and are associated with hypertensive side effects. Primary or secondary renal disease is the most common cause of secondary hypertension in this age group. The review of systems or family history may suggest endocrine or genetic forms of secondary hypertension. Premature birth and low birth weight are now considered to be independent risk factors for hypertension later in life. In addition, as the incidence of obesity in the adolescent population is increasing, attention to BMI percentiles (matched for age and gender) is extremely important as an additional cause of hypertension in adolescence. The physical examination should be thorough and focused on findings related to secondary hypertension such as coarctation of the aorta, endocrine disorders including Cushing syndrome, congenital adrenal hyperplasia, and pheochromocytoma, or renal disease.

Appropriate screening laboratory testing should include a complete blood count, electrolytes, serum BUN and creatinine, glucose, routine urinalysis, and an EKG. As with the history, the focus should be on identifying secondary causes and end-organ damage. Concomitant risk factors such as hyperlipidemia should be considered if the patient's history is suggestive of these. Indiscriminant laboratory evaluation or tests such as plasma renin, aldosterone, or renal imaging are not routinely necessary, unless the suspicion is high for secondary causes.

The treatment of hypertension in pediatric and adolescent patients should begin with family education about dietary factors that affect blood pressure control. Caloric restriction in overweight and obese children and modification of sodium intake should be discussed. Participation in aerobic activities should be encouraged for all patients without evidence of continuing end-organ damage. The choice of antihypertensive agent for essential hypertension in this age group is largely at the discretion of the primary care physician. After a 3- to 6-month period of lifestyle changes, medications may be necessary to lower the blood pressure below the 90th percentile. Although there is generally a lack of prospective data involving the efficacy of many of the medication classes in adolescents, observational data are supportive of ACE inhibitors, angiotensin receptor blockers, beta-blockers, calcium channel blockers, and diuretics in adolescents. Close attention to side-effect profiles should be considered before initiating therapy. Compliance issues with multiple daily dosing, cost issues, risk of teratogenic effects during pregnancy, and negative effects on exercise should all be considered. When in doubt about assessment or treatment of hypertension, consultation with a specialist in pediatric hypertension should be initiated.

The parents of this patient were queried further regarding the family history of hypertension, although there was no apparent etiology. The patient and his parents attended a meeting with a nutritionist who encouraged an increase in fresh fruits and vegetables and a reduction in sodium intake. Home blood pressure measurements showed an average blood pressure of 128/78 mmHg over subsequent months.

Clinical Pearls

1. Percentiles based on height and gender are necessary for in classifying blood pressure in pediatric and adolescent patients. A percentile of > 90% is considered hypertensive.
2. Secondary causes of hypertension should be carefully considered when taking the medical and family history, review of systems, and performing the physical examination.
3. Indiscriminant laboratory and renal imaging studies are not necessary in most patients.
4. The choice of hypertensive agent should be dictated by a thorough understanding of side-effect profiles and compliance issues.

REFERENCES

1. Doyle LW: Blood pressure in late adolescence and very low birth weight. Pediatrics 111(2):252–257, 2003.
2. Wuhl E: Distribution of 24-h ambulatory blood pressure in children: normalized reference values and role of body dimensions. J Hyperten 20(10):1995–2007, 2002.
3. Nehal US. Pediatric hypertension: Recent literature. Curr Opin Pediatr 14:189–196, 2002.
4. Washington RL, Bernhardt, DT, Gomez J, et al. for Committee on Sports Medicine and Fitness. Medical conditions affecting sports participation. Pediatrics 107(5):1205–1209, 2001.
5. Sinaiko A. Hypertension in children. N Engl J Med 375(26):1968–1973, 1996.

Rebecca L. Wood, PharmD
Kimberly G. Harkins, MD

PATIENT 59

A 46-year-old woman with anxiety

A woman with anxiety presents for evaluation of hypertension. At her last routine gynecological examination, her blood pressure was elevated at 152/94 mmHg. She has no prior history of hypertension and exercises fairly regularly. She takes alprazolam on occasion for severe anxiety; she is careful not to use it often as she does not wish to "become addicted." She does not use tobacco. She works at a local bank as an account representative and describes herself as a "high-strung" personality. Her father had a stroke at age 70 and is now in a long-term nursing care facility. She reports episodes of waking from sleep with chest discomfort associated with palpitations, dyspnea, and extreme anxiety. She never has chest pain while exercising. She recently purchased a home blood pressure monitor, and has a journal of readings that average 133/83 mmHg.

Physical Examination: Temperature 98.0°F, pulse 88, respiratory rate 14, blood pressure 148/94. General: anxious, appears nervous. Funduscopic examination: normal. Cardiac: normal. Chest: clear. Abdomen: soft, no bruits. Extremities: normal. Neurological: no tremors, reflexes normal.

Laboratory Findings: Hemogram: normal. Serum chemistries, glucose: normal. Thyroid stimulating hormone: normal.

Question: What could explain the discrepancy between this patient's home and physician's office blood pressure readings?

Diagnosis: White coat hypertension

Discussion: White coat hypertension is diagnosed when a patient demonstrates a persistently elevated blood pressure (> 140/90 mmHg) measured by conventional techniques in the office or clinic, with daytime ambulatory blood pressure measurements below 135/85 mmHg. White coat hypertension is common, accounting for up to 20% of newly diagnosed hypertensive patients. To diagnose white coat hypertension, patients should demonstrate office readings > 140/90 mmHg on at least three occasions, with at least two ambulatory blood pressure readings < 140/90 while not receiving antihypertensive therapy. White coat hypertension should be distinguished from white coat effect, which is the difference between the average clinic blood pressure and the daytime ambulatory blood pressure. Patients with white coat *hypertension* have elevated office blood pressures but are not truly hypertensive and do not require medical therapy. Patients with white coat *effect* are being treated for hypertension and demonstrate higher blood pressure readings in clinic than in ambulatory settings. A degree of white coat effect is seen in most hypertensive patients.

Factors contributing to white coat hypertension include unfamiliarity with a particular healthcare provider, conversation before or during blood pressure measurement, patient concern regarding a possible abnormal blood pressure, an uncomfortable environment, and improper measurement of blood pressure. This patient was known to be anxious, was concerned about a stroke after witnessing her father's illness, and was new to the clinic. These sources of anxiety stimulated increased sympathetic activity, which, in turn, led to an elevated blood pressure.

In order to diagnoses white coat hypertension, blood pressure must be measured outside the physician office setting. Some providers have patients check their own blood pressure at home where they can feel relaxed with less anxiety. The First International Consensus Conference on Self-Measured Home Blood Pressure recommends an upper limit of normal home blood pressure of 135/85 mmHg, based on the average of two measurements in the morning and in the evening for at least three work days. With properly calibrated instruments and a well-informed patient, these readings can be reliable.

An ambulatory blood pressure monitor is an excellent tool for diagnosing white coat hypertension. Twenty-four-hour blood pressure profiles have been shown to correlate better with target-organ damage than have casual office measurements. Although not yet proven in clinical trials, patients with white coat hypertension may have increased cardiovascular risk compared to normotensive individuals.

Identification of patients who may have white coat hypertension is important to avoid unnecessary cost and risk of treating those patients with antihypertensive agents. The American Society of Hypertension suggests 24-hour blood pressure monitoring in patients with persistently elevated office blood pressure but no target-organ damage. Patients are encouraged to purchase a self-monitoring device and monitor their blood pressure at home. If home readings confirm hypertension, it should be treated; if home recordings are normal, an ambulatory blood pressure monitor can be obtained.

This patient was instructed to bring her home blood pressure monitor into the office for comparison to a mercury manometer. Readings from her instrument correlated well with those of the mercury manometer and were thought to be reliable. The patient continued home monitoring of blood pressure and found that her average reading was approximately 133/83 mmHg, but that many of her readings were above 140/90, particularly when she awakened at night with palpitations and chest discomfort.

Often patients with inadequately treated anxiety, panic disorder, or depression can demonstrate labile blood pressure. Many patients have an evaluation for pheochromocytoma as a result of these episodic blood pressure elevations, which may be accompanied by symptoms that mimic catecholamine excess. Although this patient's nocturnal episodes prompted concern for a possible catecholamine-secreting tumor, a careful psychiatric review demonstrated several classic features of anxiety. Rather than intermittent therapy with benzodiazepines, she was treated with a selective serotonin reuptake inhibitor. After 3 months of therapy she reported no nocturnal symptoms and very rare need for alprazolam. Her blood pressure fluctuations resolved with anxiety therapy and her average home readings dropped to 127/79 mmHg. Clinic readings improved as well, although she continues to demonstrate white coat hypertension.

Clinical Pearls

1. White coat hypertension can be defined by office blood pressures exceeding 140/90 mmHg with daytime ambulatory blood pressure measurements below 135/85 mmHg.
2. Patients with white coat hypertension may be at increased risk for adverse outcomes as compared to normotensive patients, but antihypertensive drug therapy is not recommended for patients with white coat hypertension.
3. Home monitoring or ambulatory monitoring should be considered in patients with uncontrolled hypertension but no evidence of target-organ damage.
4. Patients with anxiety or untreated depression will often exhibit labile blood pressures, white coat hypertension, or significant white coat effect, all of which respond to treatment of the underlying disorder.

REFERENCES

1. Hond ED, Celis H, Fagard R, et al: Self-measured versus ambulatory blood pressure in the diagnosis of hypertension. J Hypertens 21:717–722, 2003.
2. Verdecchia P, O'Brien E, Pickering T, et al: When can the practicing physician suspect white coat hypertension? Statement from the Working Group on Blood Pressure Monitoring of the European Society of Hypertension. Am J Hypertens 16:87–91, 2003.
3. Myers MG, Valdivieso MA: Use of an automated blood pressure recording device, the BpTRU, to reduce the "white coat effect" in routine practice. Am J Hypertens 16:494–497, 2002.
4. Mann SJ: Severe paroxysmal hypertension (pseudopheochromocytoma): Understanding the cause and treatment. Arch Intern Med 159:670–674, 1999.

PATIENT 60

A 67-year-old man with a broken hip and ankle

A family physician is asked to evaluate the operative risk for a man with a broken hip and ankle. The fractures were sustained in a fall from a ladder, and the patient presented to the emergency department late in the evening. Because of the nature of the injuries, the orthopedic surgeon desires repair as quickly as possible. The patient reports good health, and takes medication only for hypertension (hydrochlorothiazide 25 mg daily). He has no history of cardiac, cerebrovascular, or renal disease. He is active, working part-time in a garden store and tending to his cattle and horses daily. He has no previous surgeries or hospitalizations.

Physical Examination: Temperature 99.0°F, pulse 86, respiratory rate 18, blood pressure 183/105. General: appears uncomfortable from pain. Neurological: normal. Cardiac: normal heart sounds, no peripheral edema, jugular venous pressure normal, pulses intact in all extremities. Respiratory: normal.

Laboratory Findings: Hemogram: hematocrit 39%, WBC count 14,500 with 80% neutrophils. Chemistry: electrolytes normal. Urinalysis: normal. 12-Lead EKG: nonspecific ST-T wave abnormalities. Chest x-ray: normal.

Question: What should the physician advise about this patient's surgical risk?

Answer: This patient requires surgery and has uncontrolled hypertension.

Discussion: Primary care physicians are frequently asked to evaluate surgical risk, particularly in older patients. Hypertension is one of the most common diagnoses in the United States, and is frequently seen in patients who are undergoing surgery.

Hypertension is a risk factor for coronary artery disease, left ventricular hypertrophy, congestive heart failure, and renal insufficiency. All of these conditions represent target-organ damage from the effects of hypertension and can contribute to adverse outcomes in patients who are undergoing surgery, including myocardial infarction and death. Few studies focus on hypertension alone as a risk factor for perioperative morbidity and mortality. Early studies of severe hypertension (≥ 180 mmHg systolic, ≥ 110 mmHg diastolic) demonstrated increased lability of blood pressure during anesthesia and an increased risk of adverse outcomes in patients with severe uncontrolled hypertension who are undergoing surgery. Less-severe hypertension does not predict adverse outcomes in these patients. The American College of Cardiology (ACC) and the American Heart Association (AHA) consider hypertension a minor risk factor for perioperative morbidity and mortality, whereas the presence of target-organ damage from hypertension is a significant predictor of adverse outcomes.

Many patients who undergo surgery will be taking antihypertensive therapy, as in this patient. Nearly every antihypertensive medication can be continued during the perioperative period; most medications can be taken the morning of surgery. Patients who are taking diuretics require special consideration, as hypokalemia and volume depletion may potentiate the effects of anesthesia. Angiotensin-converting enzyme inhibitors and angiotensin receptor blockers may lead to prolonged hypotension following anesthesia by blunting the renin-angiotensin-aldosterone compensatory response to sympathetic blockade. Some experts advocate withholding these medications the morning of surgery. Beta-blocking agents and centrally acting sympatholytic drugs such as clonidine may cause rebound hypertension after abrupt cessation and should not be stopped during the perioperative period. Patients who are using herbal products such as garlic for hypertension may be at increased risk of bleeding due to that agent's anticoagulant properties.

Patients who have uncontrolled hypertension or risk factors for adverse cardiac outcomes should be treated before, during, and after surgery with beta blockers. Beta blockers reduce myocardial ischemia and decrease perioperative morbidity and mortality in patients at risk for adverse outcomes. Very low-risk patients do not benefit from perioperative beta blockade.

This patient's uncontrolled hypertension at the time of evaluation was likely due, in part, to his discomfort from his fractures and to anxiety regarding the procedure. He reported adequate control of blood pressure in the outpatient setting. Given his advanced age and pre-existing hypertension, he was treated with perioperative beta blockers. Surgery was not delayed; he underwent successful repair of his fractures and had an uneventful postoperative course.

Clinical Pearls

1. Severe uncontrolled hypertension is a risk factor for perioperative morbidity. In patients with systolic blood pressure of ≥ 180 and/or diastolic blood pressure of ≥ 110, elective surgery should be delayed.
2. Patients with severe hypertension who require immediate surgery should be treated with parenteral therapy to lower blood pressure.
3. Caution is required for patients who are taking diuretics, ACE inhibitors, or angiotensin receptor blockers, but all may be continued up to the time of surgery.
4. Perioperative beta-blocker therapy reduces morbidity and mortality in patients at risk for cardiac or vascular disease.

REFERENCES

1. Fleisher LA: Preoperative evaluation of the patient with hypertension. JAMA 287(16):2043–2046, 2002.
2. Eagle K, Berger P, Calkins H, et al: ACC/AHA guideline update for perioperative cardiovascular evaluation for noncardiac surgery—executive summary: A report of the American College of Cardiology/American Heart Association Task Force on Practice Guidelines (Committee to Update the 1996 Guidelines on Perioperative Cardiovascular Evaluation for Noncardiac Surgery). J Am Coll Cardiol 39:542–553, 2002.
3. Poldermans D, Boersma E, Bax JJ, et al: The effect of bisoprolol on perioperative mortality and myocardial infarction in high risk patients undergoing vascular surgery. N Engl J Med 341:1789–1794, 1999.
4. Wallace A, Layug B, Tateo I, et al: Prophylactic atenolol reduces postoperative myocardial ischemia. Anesthesiology 88:7–17, 1998.

Sharon Dickey, PharmD
Deborah S. King, PharmD

PATIENT 61

A 38-year-old man who cannot afford his medications

A man presents to the emergency department for a blood pressure check. He has recently been diagnosed with hypertension but has been off medications for 3 weeks. He completed the samples of amlodipine 5 mg and trandolopril 2 mg once daily, but could not afford the $80.00 required to get a 1-month supply of these medications. He recently lost his job as a construction worker and has no medical insurance. His wife is employed as a nurse's aid.

Physical Examination: Temperature 98.8°F, pulse 89, respirations 18, blood pressure sitting 176/96. General: well-nourished, moderately obese. HEENT: neck, no masses or bruits; eyes, arteriovenous nicking. Cardiac: regular rate and rhythm. Chest: clear bilaterally. Abdomen: nontender, nondistended. Neurological: normal.

Laboratory Findings: CBC and chemistry values normal.

Question: What choices are available to assist patients who have financial constraints with medications?

Answer: Several options are available to aid patients in selecting affordable medication regimens.

Discussion: When initiating medical management of hypertension, several factors play an important role in selecting therapy such as concomitant diseases, adverse events, regimen complexity, and cost of therapy to ensure medication adherence. Healthcare providers are diligent at addressing these issues when formulating a plan for patients, but many times the cost of therapy plays a minor role in selecting the optimal treatment. Although providers may be cognizant of the financial burden to patients, the actual cost of medications and the patient's ability to pay for monthly medical expenses may not be realized.

In developing a plan with the patient, financial issues must be addressed to select the therapy. If a patient cannot afford the recommended medications, the adherence to the overall health plan may not be achieved, resulting in the expenditure of additional healthcare dollars related to unnecessary visits, tests, and, most importantly, to adverse events. This patient presented to a local emergency department rather than to his primary physician. Addressing the cost of care with patients may result in a more empathetic physician–patient relationship. The patient needs to be made aware, within a few dollars, of the cost of the prescribed regimen when developing the therapeutic plan.

Financial issues are most often addressed with uninsured patients, but should be considered for all groups. Currently, the elderly may be covered by Medicare, but this plan does not cover outpatient prescriptions. The elderly are usually on fixed incomes and complex multidrug regimens that are often cost prohibitive. Patients who have Medicaid coverage or coverage from some similar state program often have a fixed formulary and a limitation on the number of prescriptions filled per month. Furthermore, even though the co-pay for these medications may seem minimal, some patients do not have the resources available to cover this expense.

The Joint National Committee (JNC) on Prevention, Detection, Evaluation, and Treatment of High Blood Pressure has concurred that a diuretic is a very good initial medication. The Antihypertensive and Lipid-Lowering Treatment to Prevent Heart Attack Trial (ALLHAT) showed that diuretics are effective in decreasing the cardiovascular complications of hypertension and should, therefore, be recommended as first-line therapy for most patients with hypertension. This patient was prescribed hydrochlorothiazide 12.5 mg daily and advised to return to his primary care physician for follow-up. The emergency department pharmacists informed the patient that his cost would be approximately $3.00 per month if he purchased the medication from a local discount pharmacy.

During clinic visits, the healthcare team should address the financial concerns of patients. Considerations for decreasing the cost of medications to patients include the following:

1. Inexpensive diuretics should be considered as an initial choice for most patients.

2. Consider prescribing generic brands of medications.

3. A full-stock bottle of medications may be more economical. For example, it would be more cost-effective to prescribe 100 tablets of hydrocholorothiazide rather than 30 tablets per month.

4. Prescribing higher-dose pills that can be safely divided to achieve the recommended daily dose may decrease costs.

5. Request prior authorization for extension of benefits for Medicaid recipients.

6. Fixed-dosed combination medications may improve adherence and cost, but the generic equivalent may be more affordable.

7. Application to pharmaceutical patient-assistance programs is time-consuming, but improved adherence and healthcare outcomes may result.

8. Pharmacists, case managers, and social workers may need to assist in acquisition of medications.

9. Sample medications are useful for initiating therapy but should not dictate prescribing patterns.

The optimal long-term management of hypertension requires an empathetic and multidisciplinary approach to achieve effective care. Addressing the financial concerns of a patient may improve adherence and clinical outcomes. This patient was seen 1 month later for follow-up by his primary care provider. His blood pressure was reduced but not at target, so lisinopril/hydrochlorothiazide 20/25 mg was prescribed. The pharmacist informed the patient that a 30-day supply would cost $14.50, whereas a 100-day supply cost $29.50.

Clinical Pearls

1. Awareness of actual medication costs will ensure that the most cost-effective regimen is prescribed.
2. Awareness of patient financial situations and prescription coverage is vital to prescribing a regimen that can improve patient adherence.
3. Hydrochlorothiazide is an appropriate initial therapy for patients with financial constraints and no contraindications. The agent has been proven to prevent cardiovascular disease.
4. Consider patient-assistance programs, when available, for the uninsured or for fixed-income patients.
5. If a state-funded plan provides for additional medication, prior authorization may be required.

REFERENCES

1. Chobanian AV, Bakris GL, Black HR, et.al: National Heart, Lung, and Blood Institute Joint National Committee on Prevention, Detection, Evaluation, and Treatment of High Blood Pressure; National High Blood Pressure Education Council. The Seventh Report of the Joint National Committee on Prevention, Detection, Evaluation, and Treatment of High Blood Pressure: the JNC VII report. JAMA 289(19):2560–2572, 2003.
2. Korn LM, Reichert S, Simon T, Halm EA: Improving physician's knowledge of the actual costs of common medications and willingness to consider costs when prescribing. J Gen Intern Med 18:31–37, 2003.
3. The ALLHAT Officers and Coordinators for the ALLHAT Collaborative Research Group: The Antihypertensive and Lipid-Lowering Treatment to Prevent Heart Attack Trial (ALLHAT). JAMA 288(23):2981–2997, 2002.
4. McDonald HP, Garg AX, Haynes RB: Interventions to enhance patient adherence to medication prescriptions. JAMA 288:2868–2879, 2002.

Christopher Christensen, MD
Marion R. Wofford, MD, MPH

PATIENT 62

A 40-year-old woman post liver transplantation

An obese women with a medical history significant for hypertension, diabetes, hyperlipidemia, and end-stage liver disease, status post successful liver transplantation, presents to your clinic for management of increasing blood pressure. The patient states that she was first diagnosed with hypertension at age 29 and that her blood pressure was well controlled on a medication, the name of which she cannot recall. Likewise, her diabetes has always been controlled by diet alone. She became pregnant at age 32, and her antihypertensive regimen was changed to methyldopa 250 mg twice a day for the duration of the pregnancy and continued postpartum for several years. She states that at age 35 she "developed cirrhosis from her medication." She became normotensive and no longer required antihypertensive medication. Her liver disease progressed and she required transplantation which she underwent 3 years ago. She denies any history of ethanol intake or family history of liver disease, and her viral hepatitis panel was negative. Her current medications include cyclosporine 250 mg twice daily, prednisone 25 mg daily, and atorvastatin 10 mg daily.

Physical Examination: Temperature 98.3°F, pulse 85, respiratory rate 14, blood pressure 165/88. General: well nourished, well developed, slight moon facies. Mild supraclavicular and dorsocervical fat pads are present. Skin: a few spider angiomas on chest. Funduscopic: normal. Cardiac: regular rate and rhythm, no murmurs; pulses equal throughout, 1^+ bilateral lower extremity edema. Abdomen: obese, nontender, nondistended; flesh-colored striae are present.

Laboratory Findings: Hemogram normal. Serum potassium 3.3 mg/dl, BUN 17 mg/dl, creatinine 1.3 mg/dl, glucose 285 mg/dl, LDL 165 mg/dl, hemoglobin A1c 9%. Urinalysis: 3^+ protein. Pretransplantation Liver Biopsy: marked fatty infiltration, ballooning degeneration of hepatocytes, polymorphonuclear cell infiltration, and moderate fibrosis.

Question: What is the mechanism causing this patient's rise in blood pressure?

Diagnosis: Hypertension secondary to the effects of steroids and calcineurin inhibitors

Discussion: Adverse antihypertensive drug reaction, hypertension in cirrhosis, and the effects of various immunosuppressive/anti-rejection agents on blood pressure are important aspects of the pathophysiology of liver disease related to hypertension. This patient's history demonstrates a number of important issues.

Her negative history of alcohol intake and viral hepatitis serology, and a history of exposure to methyldopa make nonalcoholic steatohepatitis the most likely cause of her end-stage liver disease. This diagnosis is supported by the findings seen on this patient's pretransplantation liver biopsy.

Nonalcoholic steatohepatitis (NASH) is uncommon but usually occurs in obese women with insulin resistance or metabolic syndrome, as in this patient. Methyldopa has been reported in association with NASH and cirrhosis in obese middle-aged women, but this association may have been fortuitous because some recent studies have identified equal numbers of affected men at ideal body weight.

Methyldopa was one of the first drugs described to cause immunoallergic drug hepatitis. Hepatic reactions to methyldopa vary from abnormal results of liver function tests, severe acute hepatitis, to chronic hepatitis with bridging necrosis and cirrhosis. Methyldopa is generally reserved for use in pregnant patients because of its safety profile on the fetus, and currently the agent is rarely used outside of the scope of pregnancy. A recent review of the current literature reveals that several antihypertensive medications, including calcium-channel blockers, angiotensin-converting enzyme (ACE) inhibitors, angiotensin receptor blockers, and beta-blockers can cause hepatocyte destruction through this and other mechanisms. Reports suggest that up to 40% of cases of NASH progress to fibrosis or cirrhosis. The primary goal of treatment is to stop the offending agent once elevated transaminases are noted, and to emphasize weight reduction and management of hyperglycemia and dyslipidemia.

As mentioned previously, this patient became normotensive at the time her liver disease progressed to cirrhosis. Cirrhosis has a unique effect on the systemic circulation. Portal systemic shunting occurs, and endotoxins and cytokines are released into the systemic circulation. These agents stimulate synthesis and release of nitric oxide in the vascular endothelium, thereby causing a decrease in both splanchnic and peripheral vascular resistance, with pooling and vasodilation leading to a lower effective arterial blood volume, thus hyperdynamic circulation. This phenomenon is further accentuated by the response of the kidneys, sympathetic nervous system, and various hormones that displace fluid volume into the abdomen in the form of ascites. The systemic arterial blood pressure is thus substantially lowered, and many patients with cirrhosis no longer require antihypertensive medications to maintain ideal blood pressure.

Systemic hypertension is a frequent complication seen in patients who have undergone organ transplantation. The endogenous process of vasodilation elicited by the cirrhotic liver is no longer occurring, and the underlying essential hypertension can again emerge. The rise in blood pressure may be related to the effects of glucocorticoids and calcineurin inhibitor–induced renal vasoconstriction. This patient is receiving a large dose of prednisone to prevent rejection, and consequently she has become cushingoid. This condition is evident by the moon facies, buffalo-hump, abdominal striae, low potassium level, and elevated blood pressure, and glucose and LDL levels. She is retaining extracellular fluid and sodium as a result.

Cyclosporine is a calcineurin inhibitor that also prevents organ rejection, but has the side effect of constricting renal blood flow, thereby elevating systemic blood pressure through extracellular volume expansion and sodium retention. The renin system is minimally affected, and thus ACE inhibitors have little effect on lowering the blood pressure. Cyclosporine is also known to cause nephrotoxicity. Several retrospective studies have shown that > 60% of patients who are receiving a combination of cyclosporine and prednisone develop hypertension.

Generally, calcium-channel blockers are the drugs of choice for hypertension associated with post-transplantation hypertension. Cyclosporine and tacrolimus levels are increased by verapamil and diltiazem; therefore, nifedipine is usually the first-line agent. Beta-blockers are the second-line agents that are recommended if the hypertension remains uncontrolled. Calcineurin inhibitors may cause hyperkalemia secondary to renal tubular acidosis. For this reason, ACE inhibitors and potassium-sparing diuretics are relatively contraindicated. However, in this patient, given her low serum potassium level and co-morbid diabetes and proteinurea, an ACE inhibitor should be considered. Diuretics are used with caution, as they may result in renal insufficiency and electrolyte imbalances in transplant recipients. If fluid overload is present, furosemide is the diuretic of choice. For patients in whom hypertension is not controlled, clonidine is a suitable agent to add to the regimen. In the minority of patients with intractable hypertension who are receiving cyclosporine-based immunosuppression, tacrolimus may be substituted for cyclosporine. Although tacrolimus is associated with hypertension, it is not as potent a renal vasoconstrictor as cyclosporine, so blood pressure control may improve.

This patient was placed on nifedipine SR 60 mg once daily, lisinopril 20 mg once daily, low-dose aspirin, a strict diabetic diet, and an insulin regimen. Her atorvastatin was increased to 40 mg once daily and her prednisone was decreased to 15 mg daily. She was maintained on her current dose of cyclosporine with frequent blood level checks along with routine chemistry and liver panels. The patient returned for follow-up 3 months after initiation of therapy and had lost 5 pounds; her blood pressure was 130/82 mmHg, potassium 4.0, creatinine 1.3, LDL 103 mg/dl, hemoglobin A1c 7.0%. The urinalysis showed no proteinuria, and ALT/AST and cyclosporine levels were normal. The patient stated that she felt well and that a recent liver biopsy by her hepatologist revealed the liver to be in good standing with minimal rejection.

Clinical Pearls

1. Nonalcoholic steatohepatitis (NASH) is an uncommon disorder associated with the metabolic syndrome and certain antihypertensives including methyldopa. NASH may progress to cirrhosis. Discontinuation of the offending agent is the primary treatment.
2. Cirrhosis effectively lowers blood pressure through the effects of endotoxins, cytokines, and nitric oxide, causing peripheral vasodilation.
3. Transplant recipients often develop hypertension secondary to calcineurin inhibitor (cyclosporine and tacrolimus)–induced renal vasoconstriction and the effects of glucocorticoids.
4. The treatment of choice for post-transplantation hypertension is calcium-channel blockers; beta-blockers and clonidine may be added for additional control.
5. Renal insufficiency, renal tubular acidosis, and electrolyte imbalances are common in transplant recipients; therefore, ACE inhibitors, potassium-sparing diuretics, and diuretics are relatively contraindicated.

REFERENCES

1. Diehl AM, Poordad F: Nonalcoholic fatty liver disease. In Feldman M, Friedman LS, Sleisenger MH (eds): Sleisenger and Fordtran's Gastrointestinal and Liver Disease, 7th ed. Philadelphia, Saunders, 2002, pp 1403–1405.
2. Farrel C: Diseases caused by drugs, anesthetics, and toxins. In Feldman M, Friedman LS, Sleisenger MH (eds): Sleisenger and Fordtran's Gastrointestinal and Liver Disease, 7th ed. Philadelphia, Saunders, 2002, p. 1420.
3. Martin P, Rosen HR: Liver transplantation. In Feldman M, Friedman LS, Sleisenger MH (eds): Sleisenger and Fordtran's Gastrointestinal and Liver Disease, 7th ed. Philadelphia, Saunders, 2002, p. 1636.
4. Curtis JJ: Cyclosporine induced hypertension. In Laragh JH, Brenner BM (eds): Hypertension: Pathophysiology, Diagnosis, and Management, Vol 2. New York, Raven Press, 1990, pp 1829–1833.

Kristi W. Kelley, PharmD, BCPS
Marion R. Wofford, MD, MPH

PATIENT 63

A 57-year-old woman with chronic renal insufficiency

A middle-aged woman with a long-standing history of hypertension is referred to a hypertension specialty clinic for consultation. In the last several months she has noted an increase in home blood pressures. The primary care provider had advised her to decrease salt intake and increase diltiazem to 420 mg daily. One month before the referral, furosemide 40 mg once a day was added to reduce blood pressure and to reduce edema that was progressively bothersome. The patient's medical history includes hypothyroidism and gastroesophageal reflux.

Physical Examination: Temperature 98.2°F, pulse 72, respirations 16, blood pressure 158/84 seated, 160/92 standing. BMI 23. General: no acute distress. Chest: clear to auscultation with symmetrical respirations; Cardiac: regular rate, 2/6 systolic murmur at the left upper sternal border. Abdomen: soft, nontender, and no masses or organomegaly. Extremities: 2+ edema; no clubbing or cyanosis.

Laboratory Findings: WBC 7950/µl Hct 37.7%. Electrolytes normal, BUN 27 mg/dl, creatinine 1.6 mg/dl. TSH normal EKG: normal sinus rhythm.

Question: What changes should be made in the antihypertensive regimen?

Answer: Alteration in diuretic use

Discussion: Diuretics are widely used in the treatment of hypertension. Clinical trials have shown significant reduction in the risk of stroke, coronary heart disease, congestive heart failure, cardiovascular mortality, and all-cause mortality. Most diuretics, particularly thiazides, are relatively inexpensive compared to many antihypertensive agents, making them desirable as first-line, therapy or as add-on therapy to a multidrug regimen. The appropriate choice of diuretics improves adherence, and blood pressure reduction, and reduces risk of co-morbid conditions.

Thiazide diuretics (hydrochlorothiazide, chlorthalidone) result in acute renal changes and chronic vascular effects. Thiazide diuretics inhibit the Na^+/Cl^- co-transporter in the distal convoluted tubule, resulting in a reduction of extracellular volume. Long-term use of thiazides lowers the peripheral vascular resistance. A reduction of systolic blood pressure by 15–20 mmHg and diastolic blood pressure by 8–15 mmHg can be expected with thiazide diuretics. These agents can be used safely in combination with other antihypertensive agents, including diuretics of another type, and with many agents provide a synergistic response in blood pressure reduction.

Thiazides are well-tolerated by most patients when used in the currently recommended low doses (12.5–25 mg of hydrochlorothiazide). Hypokalemia and hyponatremia are dose-dependent and uncommon effects. Although hyperuricemia, hyperlipidemia, and impairment of glucose control have been observed in patients on thiazides, large clinical trials have shown that these adverse effects are not significant when a low-dose diuretic is used.

Patients who are not responding adequately to diuretic therapy should be evaluated for causes of diuretic resistance as well as for adequate doses and regimen. Excessive sodium intake may decrease the potential effect of a diuretic response. In general, patients with hypertension should reduce dietary sodium intake to reduce blood pressure levels and to increase the response of blood pressure to medications. The use of nonsteroidal anti-inflammatory drugs (NSAIDs) may blunt the antihypertensive effect of diuretics.

Thiazide diuretics may not be effective in the presence of renal disease. In this patient, a creatinine of 1.6 mg/dl is a reflection of renal impairment and should be further evaluated with a measure for creatinine clearance, such as a 24-hour urine collection. Thiazides are not the best diuretic choice in the context of a creatinine clearance of < 30 mL/min. In those patients with this degree of renal dysfunction, loop diuretics should be used.

Loop diuretics (furosemide, bumetanide, torsemide) inhibit the $Na^+/K^+/Cl^-$ co-transporter in the ascending loop of Henle. Water resorption is decreased, ultimately resulting in increased excretion of solute, water, and electrolytes (Na^+, K^+, Mg^{++}, Cl^-). Loop diuretics provide a more rapid and more potent diuretic effect, thereby contributing to a greater reduction in extracellular volume, a desirable effect in patients with pedal or pulmonary edema. However, the blood pressure response is no more effective than that to thiazide diuretics, particularly if the loop diuretic dose is inadequate. Loop diuretics with short half-lives such as furosemide should be administered two to three times a day to achieve consistent blood pressure lowering throughout the day. Once-daily use of furosemide causes a rapid diuresis-naturesis effect, followed by a period of sodium and volume retention. The net result is a neutral effect on volume and blood pressure.

Loop diuretics may be used in combination with other diuretic classes. Failure to achieve adequate diuresis may be the result of ineffective blockade of the $Na^+/K^+/Cl^-$ co-transporter in the ascending loop of Henle. Thiazide diuretics, such as chlorthalidone or hydrochlorothiazide (HCTZ), or thiazide-like diuretics, such as indapamide or metolazone, are beneficial because they can block the Na^+ from being reabsorbed in the distal tubule and allow diuresis to continue. When diuretics are administered in combination, electrolyte abnormalities are more likely, so monitoring should be initiated.

Aldosterone-blockers including spironolactone and eplerenone are effective in lowering mild-to-moderate hypertension in black, white, and elderly patients. The recognition of benefits in congestive heart failure and a higher prevalence of primary aldosteronism than previously known has increased the use of spironolactone. Potassium-sparing diuretics are often used in combination with thiazide-type diuretics. Amiloride and triamterene are less effective as monotherapy but are available in combination preparations with thiazides.

This patient had been receiving increasing doses of a diltiazem that likely caused the pedal edema. A better strategy for treatment might have been the addition of a thiazide diuretic or twice-daily dosing of furosemide. Her creatinine clearance measured on a 24-hour urine collection was 70 mL/min. Hydrochlorothiazide 12.5 mg daily was added and diltiazem was decreased to 240 mg once a day. The pedal edema resolved and furosemide was discontinued.

Clinical Pearls

1. Thiazide diuretics have been shown to be effective in lowering blood pressure and reducing risk of coronary and cerebrovascular disease and congestive heart failure.
2. Loop diuretics may provide a more pronounced diuresis than thiazide diuretics, but are not as potent blood-pressure-lowering agents as thiazides.
3. Patients who are not responding adequately to diuretic therapy should be evaluated for causes of diuretic resistance and for adequate doses and regimens.
4. When diuretics are used in combination, patients should be monitored closely for electrolyte abnormalities and provided with supplementation as needed.

REFERENCES

1. Chobanian AV, Bakris GL, Black HR, et al. National Heart, Lung, and Blood Institute. Joint National Committee on Prevention, Detection, Evaluation, and Treatment of High Blood Pressure; National High Blood Pressure Education. The Seventh Report of the Joint National Committee on Prevention, Detection, Evaluation, and Treatment of High Blood Pressure: the JNC VII report. JAMA 289(19):2560–2572, 2003.
2. The ALLHAT Officers and Coordinators for the ALLHAT Collaborative Research Group: Major outcomes in high-risk hypertensive patients randomized to angiotensin-converting enzyme inhibitor or calcium channel blocker vs. diuretic. JAMA 288:2981–2997, 2002.
3. Kaplan NM: Treatment of hypertension: Drug therapy. In: Kaplan NM (ed): Clinical Hypertension. 8th ed. Baltimore, Lippincott Williams & Wilkins, 2002, pp. 237–337.
4. Pruschett JB: Diuretics. In: Izzo JL, Black HR (eds): Hypertension Primer. 2nd ed. Dallas, American Heart Association, 1999, pp. 358–361.
5. Brater DC: Diuretic therapy. N Engl J Med 339:387–395, 1998.

PATIENT 64

A 48-year-old man with diabetes and swollen ankles

A middle-aged man with type 2 diabetes presents to a clinic for evaluation of hypertension. He reports ankle swelling, which worsens throughout the day and resolves over night. His medications include amlodipine, metoprolol, hydrochlorothiazide, metformin, and glyburide. He does not use tobacco. He is fairly active, although he does not have a specific exercise program, and he tries to adhere to a diabetic diet. He has no heart disease, but he has been told that his kidneys are not normal. He has been taking medications for diabetes and hypertension for about 10 years.

Physical Examination: Temperature 97.8°F, pulse 72, respiratory rate 12, blood pressure 179/99. Funduscopic: arteriovenous nicking, soft exudates, no papilledema. Cardiac: normal heart sounds, no gallop, 2+ bilateral pedal edema to knees. Respiratory: normal. Neurological: decreased sensation in both feet.

Laboratory Findings: Hemogram: normal. Chemistry: electrolytes normal, BUN 18 mg/dl, creatinine 1.1 mg/dl. Total cholesterol 359 mg/dl, HDL cholesterol 45 mg/dl, triglycerides 312 mg/dl, LDL cholesterol 252 mg/dl. Timed urine collection: protein 3729 mg/24 hours, creatinine clearance 53 mL/min.

Question: What single diagnosis explains this patient's physical examination and laboratory abnormalities?

Diagnosis: Nephrotic syndrome from diabetic nephropathy

Discussion: Nephrotic syndrome is defined by a urinary protein excretion > 3.5 g in 24 hours, hypoalbuminemia, and peripheral edema. Diabetes is a common cause of nephrotic syndrome, with glomerular diseases accounting for most cases in nondiabetic patients. Risk factors for diabetic nephropathy include hypertension, poorly controlled diabetes, smoking, and dyslipidemia.

Pathologic changes in diabetic nephropathy include mesangial expansion, glomerular basement-membrane thickening, and glomerular sclerosis. Hyperglycemia and resultant glycosylation of tissues are postulated mechanisms of injury. Diabetic patients with renal disease may have nonspecific interstitial or vascular lesions without glomerular changes. Some patients with diabetes develop ischemic nephropathy as a result of renal artery atherosclerosis.

Proteinuria and edema, both present in this patient, are the predominant clinical manifestations of nephrotic syndrome. Patients often exhibit sodium retention, dyslipidemia, infectious complications, and venous thromboembolic disease. The dyslipidemia is most often hypercholesterolemia and hypertriglyceridemia. Nephrotic syndrome patients with severe hypoalbuminemia (< 1.5 g/dl) are prone to hypovolemia, usually as a result of aggressive diuresis.

Management of nephrotic syndrome in diabetic patients is multifaceted. Blood pressure control is essential. Numerous clinical trials have demonstrated the value of angiotensin-converting enzyme (ACE) inhibitors and angiotensin receptor blockers (ARBs) in slowing the progression of renal disease and decreasing proteinuria in patients with diabetes. Most patients will also require diuretic therapy and may need three, four, or even more medications to achieve blood pressure control. Lifestyle modifications including regular aerobic exercise and weight loss are an important adjunct to medical therapy. The fall in blood pressure with intensive therapy may decrease the glomerular filtration rate; however, unless the serum creatinine rises more than 30%, therapy should not be altered.

In addition to blood pressure lowering, tight glycemic control is essential in the management of diabetic nephropathy. Whether control is achieved through the use of oral agents, insulin, or a combination, the glycosylated hemoglobin concentration should be maintained below 6.5% or 7%. Combination therapy may also be required to achieve lipid goals of LDL cholesterol levels of < 100 mg/dl and triglycerides levels of < 150 mg/dl. Patients should be strongly advised to stop smoking. Prophylactic aspirin should be used in all patients with diabetes unless contraindications exist. Routine use of warfarin is not recommended, except in patients who have experienced thromboembolism.

This patient achieved blood pressure goals through intensive lifestyle modifications and an ARB-based three-drug antihypertensive regimen. Metformin was discontinued. He is receiving combination therapy for both his diabetes and dyslipidemia. He requires seven daily prescription medications plus aspirin to achieve his goals. His proteinuria and renal function have not only stabilized, but have shown modest improvements.

Clinical Pearls

1. Diabetes frequently causes nephropathy, which may manifest as nephrotic syndrome.
2. Nephrotic syndrome includes heavy proteinuria, hypoalbuminemia, edema, dyslipidemia, and risk for thromboembolism.
3. Patients with nephrotic syndrome require aggressive blood pressure lowering using ARB-based or ACE inhibitor–based antihypertensive regimens.
4. Tight glycemic control, aggressive lipid lowering, lifestyle modifications, and smoking cessation are imperative in patients with nephrotic syndrome from diabetes.

REFERENCES

1. Sowers JR: Diabetic nephropathy and concomitant hypertension: A review of recent ADA recommendations. Am J Clin Proc 3:27–33, 2002.
2. Lewis EJ, Hunsicker LG, Clarke WR, et al: Renoprotective effects of the angiotensin receptor antagonist irbesartan in patients with nephropathy due to type 2 diabetes. The Collaborative Study Group. N Engl J Med 345:851–860, 2001.
3. Brenner BM, Cooper ME, de Zeeuw D, et al: Effects of losartan on renal and cardiovascular outcomes in patients with type 2 diabetes and nephropathy. The RENAAL Study Investigators. N Engl J Med 345:861–869, 2001.
4. Ritz E, Orth SR: Nephropathy in patients with type 2 diabetes mellitus. N Engl J Med 341:1127–1133, 1999.
5. Orth SR, Ritz E: The nephrotic syndrome. N Engl J Med 338:1202–1211, 1998.
6. Lazarus JM, Bourgoignie JJ, Buckalew VM, et al: Achievement and safety of a low blood pressure goal in chronic renal disease. The modification of diet in renal disease study group. Hypertension 29:641–650, 1997.

Bryan N. Batson, MD
Jimmy L. Stewart, MD

PATIENT 65

A 16-year-old boy with hypertensive encephalopathy

A male adolescent presented to the local emergency department with a 4-day history of intermittent headaches, nausea, vomiting, and blurring of vision. Review of systems includes a history of fever, sore throat, and conjunctivitis that occurred 2 weeks prior to presentation, for which his local doctor prescribed ophthalmic drops, and these symptoms resolved. Family history is significant for essential hypertension in both parents. The patient reported occasional marijuana use but none in over a month.

In the emergency department, his blood pressure was 178/79 mmHg. A computed tomographic (CT) scan of the head was normal. He was discharged on an analgesic with a follow-up scheduled. He returned to the emergency department the following day with vomiting and lethargy and was found to have a blood pressure of 195/90 mmHg. A complete blood count, chemistry panel, and urinalysis were normal. He was admitted with a diagnosis of hypertensive encephalopathy.

Initially the antihypertensive agents chosen for this patient were timolol and clonidine, but his blood pressure continued to be labile. On hospital day 4, his blood pressure was 196/111 mmHg, and he was transferred to a local pediatric intensive care unit. Parenteral labetolol was initiated and he was given 1.2 million units of long-acting for presumed poststreptococcal glomerulonephritis (PSGN). Three days later he was discharged on nifedipine and hydrochlorothiazide with a BP of 123/63 mmHg.

Physical Examination: Blood pressure 162/82 right arm, 170/90 left arm, 198/82 right leg, and 177/78 left leg, pulse 70, temperature 99°F. Funduscopic: no arterio venous nicking, papilledema, or hemorrhages. Oropharynx: healing ulcer on lip, no erythema or exudate. Cardiovascular: regular rate, no heart murmur or abdominal bruit, distal pulses palpable and equal.

Laboratory Findings: BUN 21 mg/dl, creatinine 1.0 mg/dl. WBC 10,900/µl, Hgb 11.8 g/dl, platelets 233,000/µL. Total protein 5.9, albumin of 2.8 g/dL. Toxicology and anti-nuclear antibody negative. Urinalysis specific gravity 1.008, pH 6.0, trace blood, no protein. Random plasma renin level 0.4 (normal, 0.4–0.8 ng/ml/hr), urine catecholamines normal. Lumbar puncture: cerebrospinal fluid clear with glucose 58 mg/dl, protein 26 mg/dl, a negative cryptococcal antigen, and negative culture. Streptozyme test positive (titer 1:200 STZ units); C3 level 35 (88–201 mg/dl). Throat culture: heavy group A streptococcus. CT of head: normal. Magnetic resonance imaging of head: changes consistent with hypertensive encephalopathy. CT of the abdomen and renal ultrasonography with Doppler flow imaging: normal. Magnetic resonance angiography of kidney: normal.

Question: What is the most likely cause of this hypertensive emergency?

Answer: Streptococcal glomerulonephritis

Discussion: The evaluation of hypertension in the pediatric and adolescent populations necessitates a clear understanding of a higher prevalence of secondary causes for the elevated blood pressure. An abrupt onset of hypertension, recent infection, or evidence of target-organ damage in this age group suggests the presence of secondary causes. In the pediatric age group, renal vascular, renal parenchymal, and vascular causes are most common. Although an increase in obesity in the adolescent group is becoming a major cause of elevated blood pressure, secondary causes should be entertained on the basis of the history and screening laboratory test results.

This adolescent initially presented with severe hypertension and encephalopathy, but no urine abnormalities or physical examination findings suggestive of nephrotic syndrome, which made the evaluation very confusing and difficult. Typically, with postinfectious glomerulonephritis (PSGN), patients report discolored urine and insidious edema, and are found to be hypoalbuminemic with proteinuria and to have at least microscopic hematuria. There is usually a latent period, which can range from 10 days to 3 weeks, between the streptococcal infection and the first manifestations of nephritis. Hypertension is found in ~75% of PSGN cases. Proteinuria is almost uniformly present, but the amount is < 3 g/day in > 75% and < 500 mg/day in > 50% of cases. Red cell casts are found in 60–85% of hospitalized children with acute glomerulonephritis. Urinalysis also commonly has a specific gravity of >1.02 and a low pH. The C3 level is almost always depressed to 50% of normal. Although complement levels are expected to return to normal after 8 weeks, proteinuria may persist for up to 6 months, and microscopic hematuria for up to 1 year.

As this case exhibits, however, PSGN can have an extremely broad range of presentation, varying from an entirely asymptomatic condition to one of oliguric acute renal failure. It has been reported that subclinical episodes occur about four times more frequently than does easily recognized disease; however, nearly all of these patients have abnormal urinalysis. Several cases of biopsy-proven PSGN with minimal urinary findings have been described, but it is still an extremely rare and easily overlooked entity. Furthermore, none of these reported cases were associated with hypertensive encephalopathy. Encephalopathy is an atypical manifestation of PSGN, but is seen more commonly in older pediatric patients. It is important for the physician to remember that PSGN with normal urinalysis does exist and can present as hypertensive encephalopathy, as seen in this patient. The diagnosis must be considered with a high degree of suspicion in any child with unexplained acute hypertension, edema, oliguria, or encephalopathy. It is a diagnosis that can be made quickly, noninvasively, and inexpensively, and if the condition is discovered, it can be treated very easily.

Three months after discharge, the patient was off all blood pressure medications. His blood pressure was 115/63 mmHg. A urinalysis at that time showed a specific gravity of 1.020 with no protein or blood. Renal function tests included a BUN of 15 mg/dl and a serum creatinine level of 0.8 mg/dl. A C3 level was back to normal at 166 mg/dl.

Clinical Pearls

1. The evaluation of hypertension in the pediatric and adolescent populations necessitates a clear understanding of a higher prevalence of secondary causes for the elevated blood pressure.
2. Poststreptococcal glomerulonephritis (PSGN) should be considered in any child with unexplained acute hypertension, edema, oliguria, or encephalopathy.
3. A latent period ranging from 10 days to 3 weeks precedes the first manifestations of PSGN.
4. The most common presentation of PSGN includes hypertension, edema, proteinuria, hematuria, and a history a febrile illness

REFERENCES

1. Madaio MP, Harrington JT: The diagnosis of glomerular diseases: Acute glomerulonephritis and the nephrotic syndrome. Arch Intern Med 161(1):25–34, 2001.
2. Dodge WF, Spargo BH, Travis LB, et al: Poststreptococcal glomerulonephritis, a prospective study in children. N Engl J Med 286:273, 1972.
3. Albert MS, Lemming JM, Scaglione PR: Acute glomerulonephritis without abnormality of the urine. J Pediatr 68:525, 1966.

Keith Thorne, MD
Marion R. Wofford, MD, MPH

Patient 66

A 64-year-old man with claudication

A man with a history of hypertension and back pain presents for a scheduled clinic visit and describes progressive bilateral lower extremity pain with ambulation. He denies any prior myocardial infarctions, foot ulcers, or injury to his legs. He reports pain in both calves when walking; however, this discomfort resolves with rest. His medications include amlodipine, acetaminophen, and a multivitamin.

Physical Examination: Temperature 98°F, pulse 86, respirations 16, and blood pressure 156/94. Funduscopic: extensive arteriovenous nicking and copper wiring. Cardiac: regular rhythm with laterally displaced point of maximum intensity with no murmurs. Musculoskeletal: normal range of motion with normal strength. Extremities: paucity of hair on both lower extremities with diminished, < 1+, bilateral posterior tibial and dorsalis pedis pulses.

Laboratory Findings: Hemogram: WBC 8000/µl, Hgb 15 g/dl. Serum chemistries: electrolytes normal, BUN 28 mg/dl, creatinine 1.6 mg/dl. Bilateral lower extremity plain film radiographs: normal. Bilateral lower extremity angiogram: see figure.

Question: What is the most likely cause of this patient's lower extremity discomfort?

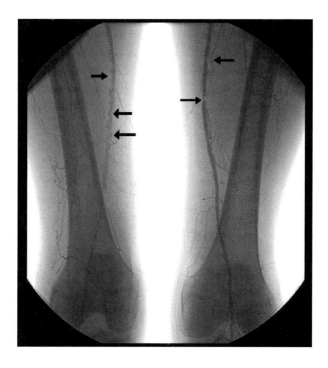

Diagnosis: Intermittent claudication with focal and diffuse peripheral vascular disease

Discussion: This patient's lower extremity discomfort is caused by peripheral arterial occlusive disease (PAOD). Intermittent claudication is the physical symptom produced when PAOD limits the blood flow to active muscles. PAOD is not only an indicator of systemic vascular disease, but it is also a prognostic indicator of future cardiovascular disease in otherwise asymptomatic patients. It is estimated that 28% of the population has PAOD at the age of 66 years. This value increases to 58% at 81 years of age.

The ankle-brachial index (ABI) is the most accurate tool to differentiate symptomatic PAOD from other musculoskeletal and neurologic causes of leg pain, as well as to find patients with otherwise asymptomatic disease. The ABI is a simple, noninvasive test that can be easily performed in the clinical setting. To calculate the ABI, divide the systolic blood pressure measured at the ankle by the systolic blood pressure measured in the arm. To measure the systolic pressure at the ankle, place the cuff just above the malleolus, inflate the cuff, and then record the first sound heard over the dorsalis pedis or posterior tibial artery as the cuff deflates. Similarly, measure the systolic pressure in the arm by placing the cuff above the elbow and recording the first sound heard over the brachial artery as the cuff deflates. Use an appropriately sized cuff to measure the systolic pressure in each location, and consider that a Doppler flowmeter may make determination of the first Korotkoff sound easier than auscultation with a stethoscope. For the most accurate results, evaluate the pressures on both the left and the right sides, and then use the side with highest pressure to calculate the ABI.

An ABI of 1.0 to 1.1 is considered normal. Values > 1.1 are associated with calcified vessels that do not compress normally and that therefore do not yield accurate blood pressure readings. Values between 0.4 and 0.9 are typically associated with PAOD that is severe enough to cause intermittent claudication, whereas those > 0.4 are usually found in patients with advanced ischemia and often with ulcerations. The area of concern occurs in patients with readings between 0.9 and 1.0. Studies have determined that an ABI of < 0.90 is 95% sensitive and 99% specific for peripheral arterial disease. An ABI in this range is associated with asymptomatic disease that may be amenable to intervention before permanent damage occurs. This may also be an indication that the patient may benefit from other cardiovascular testing. To increase the sensitivity of the ABI, evaluate the patient before and after walking on a treadmill or before and after calf raises.

Not only is the ABI useful in determining the etiology and extent of PAOD, but it has also been shown to have an inverse and independent relationship with cardiovascular mortality. Treatment of the known risk factors for cardiovascular disease such as hypertension, smoking, diabetes, and dyslipidemia in this patient population may prove to be even more beneficial than in the general population.

In this patient, the history is consistent with PAOD manifested by intermittent claudication. This patient's ABI was 0.7, and angiography revealed arterial disease that was amenable to percutaneous intervention. Another option for treatment is surgical bypass. Given this patient's history of uncontrolled hypertension and decreased ABI, he is at high risk for future cardiovascular mortality. His blood pressure should be more aggressively controlled, and he needs further evaluation for and treatment of other risk factors.

Clinical Pearls

1. The ankle-brachial index (ABI) is an inexpensive, noninvasive, reliable measure of the severity of peripheral arterial occlusive disease (PAOD) and is inversely related to cardiovascular mortality.
2. An ABI value of < 0.9 is diagnostic of PAOD.
3. Management of cardiac risk factors such as diabetes mellitus, hypertension, dyslipidemia, and smoking is required. Therapy should be maximized to limit the future morbidity and mortality of patients with PAOD.

REFERENCES

1. McDermott MM, Greenland P, Liu K, et al: The ankle-brachial index is associated with leg function and physical activity: The walking and leg circulation study. Ann Intern Med 136:873–883, 2002.
2. Hooi JD, Stoffers HE, Kester AD, et al: Peripheral arterial occlusive disease: Prognostic value of signs, symptoms, and the ankle-brachial pressure index. Med Decis Making 22: 99–107, 2002.
3. McPhail IR, Spittel PC, Weston SA, Bailey KR: Intermittent claudication: An objective office-based assessment. J Am Coll Cardiol 37:1381–1385, 2001.
4. Kuller LH, Shemanski L, Psaty BM, et al: Subclinical disease as an independent risk factor for cardiovascular disease. Circulation 92:720–726, 1995.
5. Vogt MT, Cauley JA, Newman AB, et al: Decreased ankle/arm blood pressure index and mortality in elderly women. JAMA 270:465–469, 1993.

Sharon Dickey, PharmD
Deborah S. King, PharmD

PATIENT 67

A 74-year-old woman with a cough

An elderly woman presents for her annual medical examination. Her only complaint at this visit is a nonproductive cough that she has had for the past 3–4 weeks. The cough "just will not go away." She reports having been seen at an after-hours clinic and treated with antibiotics several weeks ago. The cough is dry and nonproductive with tickling, and it is worse at night. She has no associated upper respiratory symptoms. She has a history of hypertension and has been treated with hydrochlorothiazide 25 mg once a day and trandolopril 4 mg once a day for the past several months. She has no other medical history. Her social history is significant for an occasional glass of red wine. Her family history is noncontributory.

Physical Examination: Temperature 98.8°F, pulse 82, respirations 18, blood pressure sitting 160/91. Height 5 feet 8 inches, weight 190 pounds. General: well nourished, slightly overweight. HEENT: slight hearing loss, neck with no masses or bruits, oropharynx normal with no postnasal drip or redness. Cardiac: regular rate and rhythm. Chest: clear bilaterally. Extremities: no edema.

Laboratory Findings: CBC and chemistry values: normal. ECG: no changes from previous; left ventricular hypertrophy.

Question: Given this patient's medical history and negative examination findings, what is the most likely cause of her cough?

Answer: Angiotensin-converting enzyme (ACE) inhibitors are associated with cough as an adverse event.

Discussion: In the management of hypertension, diet modification and exercise therapy may not be sufficient to control blood pressure. Pharmacologic management is often necessary. Agents utilized in the management of hypertension include diuretics, calcium-channel blockers, beta-blockers, alpha-blockers, ACE inhibitors, and angiotensin receptor blockers (ARBs). These agents are often effective, either alone or in combination. They are generally safe but can have adverse events associated with their use.

ACE inhibitors are widely prescribed agents used to control blood pressure and manage congestive heart failure. The side effects associated with ACE inhibitors range from minor to major. In this patient, the cough is an adverse event associated with the ACE inhibitor, trandolopril. ACE inhibitor-induced cough occurs at an incidence of 0.7–48% in a review of the literature from the 1980s. Post-marketing surveys have reported an incidence of up to 15%.

The ACE inhibitor-induced cough is usually a dry, nonproductive, tickling cough that is persistent and tends to be worse at night. Patients will often report sleep disturbances, sore throat, and voice changes. The cough onset may occur with the first dose, or it has been reported as late as 10 months after starting the drug. Many patients seek medical care for the cough. It is often treated with antibiotics as an upper respiratory infection. Despite antibiotic therapy, the cough tends to remain. Suspicion must be high for this adverse event. Any patient who presents, as this patient, with a chronic cough and no associated upper respiratory symptoms should receive a medication review to ascertain any association.

The pathophysiology associated with cough and ACE inhibitors is not fully understood. The proposed mechanism may be related to inhibition of both ACE and bradykininase. When kininase is inhibited bradykinin, substance P, and prostaglandin levels increase in respiratory tissue, resulting in a cough or bronchospasms. Another proposed mechanism involves the induction of nitrous oxide synthase, generating nitric oxide in the bronchial tissues, which induces cough. Prostaglandins may also be involved in the mechanism, since nonsteroidal anti-inflammatory agents have been found to be effective in eliminating cough. Because all ACE inhibitors may have cough associated with their use, one might ponder why not every patient exhibits cough as an adverse event. There may be a genetic association or a difference in levels of kininase activity.

The incidence of ACE inhibitor-induced cough has a 3:1 female-to-male preponderance, occurring more often in postmenopausal women. The incidence in patients 60 years or older is about 13–17%. There is also a higher incidence in non-Caucasians and persons who smoke cigarettes.

Several therapies have been attempted for management of patients with ACE inhibitor-induced cough, with varying success. Antitussives have proven to be ineffective. Supplemental elemental iron, which may suppress production of nitrous oxide, has been used with varying success. Nonsteroidal anti-inflammatory agents have had some success in eliminating ACE inhibitor cough, but their problems in hypertension are well recognized. Cromolyn sodium and topical anesthetics have both been successful but have associated adverse events. The cough may resolve on its own over several days to several weeks, even with continued therapy. If the ACE inhibitor-cough is not tolerated, the definitive therapy has been to discontinue therapy. Switching among the ACE inhibitors is not an option, since there may be cross-reactivity related to cough. If an ACE inhibitor is the preferred therapy, changing to an ARB would offer an appropriate alternative for most patients, since ARBs do not affect bradykinin levels and have a low incidence of associated cough. When the offending medication is discontinued, the patient needs to be made aware that the cough may not resolve for several days to 4 weeks.

Other side effects that occur with ACE inhibitors are hyperkalemia, angioedema, hypotension, and acute renal failure. ACE inhibitors as well as ARBs should be used cautiously in women of child-bearing potential. Angioneurotic edema with ACE inhibitors is rare but serious and potentially fatal. Angioedema may occur with the initial dose, during the first week, or as late as one or more years. In these patients with a history of angioedema, changing to an ARB is controversial, since the ARBs also have an associated angioedema adverse event.

All antihypertensive agents are associated with adverse events. Consider common adverse events of agents typically utilized in the management of hypertension. Adverse events of therapy with diuretics are hypokalemia, exacerbation of gout, and photosensitivity. Adverse events commonly associated with beta-blocker therapy are bradycardia, heart block, depression, and intermittent claudication. Adverse events associated with calcium-channel blockers are peripheral edema, constipation, and heart block. Therefore, it is important to assess each patient at each visit, not only for efficacy of therapy, but also for any adverse events that they may be experiencing.

Clinical Pearls

1. Consider assessment of adverse events as well as therapeutic efficacy in each patient at each visit.
2. A patient on an ACE inhibitor who presents with a nonproductive, persistent cough should be assessed for a possible relationship.
3. An ACE inhibitor-induced cough may occur within the first week of therapy or after 10 or more months of therapy.
4. If the cough is affecting the patient's quality of life, then the medication should be discontinued.
5. It may take several days to 4 weeks for the cough to resolve once the ACE inhibitor has been discontinued.

REFERENCES

1. Baker DE: ACE inhibitor–induced cough. Micromedex Healthcare Series Drug Consult Volume 116, accessed June 2003. http://www.micromedex.com.
2. Chobanian AV, Bakris GL, Black HR, et al: National Heart, Lung, and Blood Institute Joint National Committee on Prevention, Detection, Evaluation, and Treatment of High Blood Pressure; National High Blood Pressure Education. The Seventh Report of the Joint National Committee on Prevention, Detection, Evaluation, and Treatment of High Blood Pressure: the JNC VII Report. JAMA 289(19):2560–2572, 2003.
3. Kaplan NM: Clinical Hypertension, 8th edition. Baltimore, Lippincott Williams & Wilkins, 2002.

Christopher Christensen, MD
Marion R. Wofford, MD, MPH

PATIENT 68

A 27-year-old man with a spinal cord injury

Severe hypertension and tachycardia are detected by a home health nurse's vitals check in a man who sustained a T3-T4 spinal cord injury 8 weeks earlier in a motor vehicle collision. He denies headache, chest pain, shortness of breath, and visual changes. The patient denies a history of hypertension and states that he was in excellent health prior to the injury. Since discharge from the rehabilitation hospital, he admits to being noncompliant with his prescribed Colace, 100 mg twice a day, and Dulcolax, 5 mg once a day. His last bowel movement was 7 days ago. For convenience, he has also changed the frequency of his in-and-out bladder catheterizations from every 6 hours to twice a day.

Physical Examination: Temperature 98.7°F, pulse 120, respiratory rate 18, blood pressure 210/115. General: well nourished, well-developed in no acute distress. Funduscopic: normal. Cardiac: tachycardic, no murmurs; pulses equal throughout, no edema. Abdomen: nontender, tympanic, distended bladder, suprapubic dullness to percussion. Neurological: bilateral lower extremity flaccid paralysis with marked hyperreflexia; decreased anal spincter tone.

Laboratory Findings: Urinalysis, CBC, and chemistry profile: normal. Abdominal radiographs: a large amount of stool and gas throughout the large bowel and distension of the sigmoid colon.

Question: What is the correct diagnosis?

Diagnosis: Autonomic dysreflexia

Discussion: Disorders of the autonomic nervous system can manifest as acute or chronic disorders of virtually any organ system in the body. Severe hypotension during the early minutes or hours after spinal cord injury is a potentially life-threatening condition. Hypotension and bradycardia may follow cervical injury because the lesion interrupts the descending sympathetic pathways. Bradycardia distinguishes such neurogenic hypotension from hypovolemic shock, which is associated with tachycardia. Treatment of hypotension in either case involves elevation of the legs to improve venous return and generous fluid resuscitation.

Autonomic function remains a concern long after the initial insult, as severe hypertension can become a problem. Disconnected distal autonomic pathways can induce several symptoms. These symptoms include systemic hypertension, sweating, skin flushing, goose bumps, headache, spasms, blurry vision, stuffy or running nose, anxiety, angina, and other signs of vasomotor instability. Typically, a spinal cord injury at or cephalad to the sixth thoracic level is associated with these signs and symptoms.

Autonomic dysreflexia is a life-threatening condition that sometimes affects patients whose spinal cord injury lies above this thoracic root. The precise mechanisms that lead to the clinical manifestations of autonomic dysreflexia are not fully understood; however, pre-existing dysfunction of the sympathetic nervous system has been implicated as a possible contributing factor. The upper level of greater splanchnic flow is innervated at the thoracic level. The pathophysiology of autonomic dysreflexia is believed to involve an abnormal autonomic reflex that is initiated by noxious stimuli of hollow organs of the abdomen. The clinical presentation is highly variable and may include one or more of the previously described signs and symptoms. Acute uncontrolled hypertension causes the majority of the morbidity and mortality in this syndrome. Bladder distention or fecal impaction are frequent triggers of such acute-onset reflex dysautonomia; however, any noxious stimulus may be the cause, and urgent treatment is required. Systolic blood pressures can often exceed 200 mmHg and if untreated, the process can be complicated by seizures, stroke, subarachnoid hemorrhage, or death. The patient in this case became noncompliant with his bladder catheterizations and medications prescribed for bowel maintainance. Given this patient's history of spinal cord injury, abnormal physical examination finding of a distended bladder, and abdominal x-rays showing large amounts of retained stool and dilated bowel, autonomic dysreflexia must be considered.

Routine bladder catheterization and avoidance of constipation are preventive. Patients are often unaware of a change in urinary bladder function. Bladder catheterization should be performed every 4 to 6 hours. For reflex spasms, diazepam, 5 to 10 mg three times a day, or baclofen, 10 to 60 mg in divided doses given long-term may be useful. Good bowel regimens consisting of bulk-forming, high-fiber agents, stool softeners, routine enemas, and occasionally stimulant laxatives are of extreme importance in avoidance of autonomic dysreflexia.

Initial management of this potentially life-threatening syndrome includes raising the patient's head and loosening any tight clothing, binders, elastic stockings, or bandages. The supine position is known to exacerbate hypertension in victims of spinal cord injury. Markedly increased autonomic discharge can be elicited by pressure. In 85% of patients with a traumatic spinal cord injury above the C6 level and hypertension, the blood pressure can be decreased by tilting the head upward. The bladder should be catheterized immediately, and the patency of indwelling catheters should be ensured. Enemas should be administered, but blood pressure must be monitored diligently. Appropriate management may include admission to a hospital or transfer to an intensive care unit if the blood pressure does not return to baseline. Patients that are too sedated to report the subjective symptoms of autonomic dysreflexia, or those, such as this patient, who lack the additional symptoms, should be monitored more frequently. Vasodilators and clonidine can be used to treat hypertensive episodes.

In this patient, the head of the bed was elevated to 45 degrees, an indwelling Foley catheter was placed, clonidine 0.2 mg was given, and three soap-sud enemas were given with good result. The patient was placed on baclofen, and stool softeners and laxatives were resumed. His blood pressure improved markedly to 120/75 mmHg, heart rate 90, and he was monitored closely for signs of autonomic dysreflexia. No symptoms or episodes of hypertension developed.

Clinical Pearls

1. Autonomic dysreflexia is a life-threatening condition that can cause acute hypertensive crisis in patients with spinal cord lesions at or above the sixth thoracic level.
2. The clinical syndrome is marked by systemic hypertension and tachycardia. Other symptoms of vasomotor instability that may occur include diaphoresis, skin manifestations, headache, spasms, visual changes, rhinorrhea, and anxiety.
3. It is postulated that the syndrome is mediated by an abnormal autonomic reflex of the sympathetic nervous system in patients with spinal cord injury. This reflex is most commonly exacerbated by bladder or bowel distension.
4. Treatment is primarily preventative and consists of frequent bladder catheterizations, bowel preparations, avoidance of the supine position, antispasmodics, and vasodilators or clonidine in select cases.

REFERENCES

1. Han M, Hubert K: Chronic hip instability as a cause of autonomic dysreflexia: successful management by resection arthroplasty: A case report. J Bone Joint Surg Am 85:126–128, 2003.
2. Kim DD, Ryan JC: Gastrointestinal manifestations of systemic diseases. In Feldman M, Friedman LS, Sleisenger MH (eds): Sleisenger and Fordtran's Gastrointestinal and Liver Disease, 7th ed. Philadelphia, Saunders, 2002, pp 524.
3. Engstrom JW, Martin JB: Disorders of the autonomic nervous system. In Braunwald E, Fauci AS, Kasper LH, et al (eds): Harrison's Principles of Internal Medicine, 15th ed. New York, McGraw-Hill, 2001, pp 2419.
4. Morris GF, Taylor WR, Marshall CF: Spine and spinal cord injury. In Goldman L, Bennett JC, et al (eds): Cecil's Textbook of Medicine, 5th ed. Philadelphia, Saunders, 2001, pp 2183.

Peter N. Johnson
Deborah S. King, PharmD

PATIENT 69

A 31-year-old man with newly diagnosed hypertension

A 31-year-old man presents to his primary care physician for follow-up. At his last clinic visit, 2 months ago, his blood pressure was elevated, with an average reading of 156/92 mmHg. At that time, he elected a trial of lifestyle changes for blood pressure reduction and wished to avoid medications if possible.

This patient has a positive family history of hypertension, coronary artery disease, and diabetes. During the physical examination today, the patient becomes distraught and admits that since his last visit his father has died, at the age of 52. The patient stated, "I don't want to die of a heart attack like my dad. I have to get my pressure down." The patient is given a prescription for initial hypertension therapy, and lifestyle changes are reinforced. The patient also requests recommendation of a home blood pressure monitor but states, "I don't have much money."

Physical Examination: Temperature 98.4°F, pulse 90, respiratory rate 19, blood pressure 162/94 mmHg. BMI 29, arm circumference 15.5 inches. General: overweight, quite anxious about his health. Neurological: normal. Cardiac: normal heart sounds, no edema, pulses intact, no evidence of jugular-venous distention. Respiratory: normal.

Laboratory Findings: Hemogram: normal. Chemistry: normal. Urinalysis: normal. EKG, 12-lead: normal sinus mechanism with suggestion of left ventricular hypertrophy.

Questions: What types of home blood pressure monitors are available? What factors should be considered when making a recommendation?

Topic: Home blood pressure monitors

Discussion: Many patients request information about home blood pressure monitoring. Healthcare providers should not only be advocates for home blood pressure monitoring, but should also provide consistent education regarding proper blood pressure measurement and goals of therapy. For this patient, like others, home blood pressure monitoring can be an effective tool for increasing awareness, monitoring response, and achieving the goals of therapy. Perhaps most importantly, home blood pressure monitoring provides the opportunity for improving adherence and actively involves the patient in management of their disease. Home blood pressure monitors generally provide the same type of information as that obtained with ambulatory blood pressure monitoring, with the exception of blood pressure responses during sleep.

As a general rule, home blood pressure monitors should not be used routinely for the initial diagnosis of hypertension. Office sphygmomanometry remains the standard for diagnosis. However, the JNC 7 report suggests that a patient with average blood pressures >135/85 mmHg with home blood pressure monitoring should generally be diagnosed as hypertensive. Home blood pressure monitoring is also useful in the assessment of or to rule out stress-induced hypertension. Likewise, progression of cardiovascular disease, target-organ damage, and albuminuria have a greater correlation with home blood pressure readings than those obtained in the clinic setting.

There are three primary types of blood pressure monitor marketed for home use. *Consumer Report* has reviewed individual monitors to determine differences in consistency, convenience, and price between these types of monitors. In review, wrist monitors were reported as the most convenient monitors to use but the least consistent in blood pressure measurement. The wrist monitor may be more comfortable than an arm monitor for some patients. They also are the most expensive of the types reviewed, ranging in price from approximately $70 to $130. The manual arm monitors are the least expensive, ranging in price from $40 to $50. With these monitors, convenience is the major disadvantage because the patient must actually inflate the blood pressure cuff. Automatic arm monitors received the highest ratings and were judged superior to the other types of monitors because they provided the most consistent blood pressure readings and are of intermediate price, ranging from $50 to $90. These monitors also offer greater convenience than do the manual arm monitor because inflation is automatic and does not require a high inflation pressure for blood pressure determination.

Several factors should be considered when discussing or recommending a monitor for an individual patient. Obvious individual considerations are patient dexterity, both visual and hearing acuity, and proper cuff size. With any monitor, patients should be advised to compare their home blood pressure readings with those obtained by their healthcare provider. By bringing their monitor to clinic visits, the patient and provider can compare measurements, verify consistency of readings, and ensure proper use. Currently, no regulatory agency requires the validation of automated blood pressure measuring devices. An additional concern that this patient has expressed is monetary. Even for patients with third-party insurance coverage, the majority of plans do not reimburse for home blood pressure monitors.

Selection of the appropriate-sized arm cuff for blood pressure measurement is imperative for accurate assessment. Unfortunately, most blood pressure monitors come with only a regular sized cuff. Larger cuffs often need to be purchased separately, ranging in price from $10 to $20. Because the incidence of overweight and obesity reach epidemic levels, a regular adult cuff is not appropriate for proper blood pressure measurement for the majority of adults. This patient, with an arm circumference of 15.5 inches, will need a large sized cuff. A cuff that is too small tends to overestimate blood pressure and a cuff that is too large tends to underestimate blood pressure. To put this in perspective, a systematic error of underestimating true blood pressure by 5 mmHg would mean that 21 million persons who would benefit from drug treatment for hypertension could be mislabeled as having prehypertension rather than hypertension. A systematic error of 5 mmHg in the opposite direction could misclassify 27 million people as being in the hypertensive range rather than as having prehypertension. This would needlessly expose many of these persons to the expense and adverse effects of treatment. This issue is compounded by the challenge of the "white coat" or "office" effect, i.e., the tendency for blood pressure to increase when it is measured, particularly in the presence of a clinician.

Home blood pressure monitoring can be very helpful in the evaluation of drug therapy. Home monitoring can identify patients who appear resistant to drug therapy in a clinic setting, but who have controlled home blood pressures. An alternative scenario is the elderly patient who has well-controlled blood pressures on clinic assessment but extremely lower blood pressures at home. Home monitoring is also useful for evaluating blood pressure variability and maintenance of blood pressure control over the full 24-hour period. Optimal blood pressure control requires a consistent and sustained 24-hour reduction. Greater blood pressure variability is associated with more extensive carotid atherosclerosis and cardiovascular mortality. Most patients take their medications in the morning, and lack of sustained blood pressure reduction may result in significantly elevated morning blood pressures. Recognition of the increased incidence of cardiovascular events and blood pressure surge shortly after awakening has heightened awareness of both the chronopathology of cardiovascular disease and chronotherapeutic approaches for optimal blood pressure management. Home monitoring can effectively evaluate peak and trough blood pressure reductions associated with particular medication regimens. Many patients continue to have signs of white coat hypertension after purchasing a monitor and measuring blood pressures at home. However, most patients lose this anxiety and are eventually able to obtain nonstressed readings. Patients should understand the common fluctuations of as much as 20 mmHg in blood pressure and the need to report sustained elevations.

This patient received education regarding the proper technique for blood pressure monitoring. A manual arm blood pressure monitor with a large-sized cuff available by order was recommended. This highly motivated patient has adopted a health-promoting lifestyle, monitors his home blood pressures, and has his blood pressure controlled with the help of a generic combination product containing a beta-blocker and a diuretic.

Clinical Pearls

1. Home blood pressures may be useful in evaluating patients with white coat hypertension, assessing response to drug therapy, and improving patient adherence.
2. Home blood pressure monitors include wrist monitors, manual arm monitors, and automatic arm monitors.
3. Healthcare professionals should advise on the appropriate cuff size and the type of device to be purchased.
4. The consistency of blood pressure readings with a patient's monitor should be confirmed.

REFERENCES
1. Blood-pressure monitors. Consumer Reports June 2003.
2. Joint National Committee: The seventh report of the Joint National Committee on Prevention, Detection, Evaluation, and Treatment of High Blood Pressure (JNC 7). JAMA 289:2560–2572, 2003.
3. Jones DW, Appel LJ, Sheps SG: Measuring blood pressure accurately: new and persistent challenges. JAMA 289:1027–1030, 2003.
4. Kaplan NM: Kaplan's Clinical Hypertension. 8th ed. Philadelphia: Lippincott Williams & Wilkins, 2002.

Hal Dillon, PharmD
Karen Dillon

PATIENT 70

A 26-year-old man with a family history of heart disease and diabetes

A young man requests his first adult physical examination from a family physician who cared for him as a child. The patient is concerned about his risk for cardiovascular disease. He has gained 40 pounds in the last 3 years and exercises only occasionally. He does not use tobacco products and takes no medications. His father, age 50, has a 10-year history of hypertension and hyperlipidemia, had a coronary artery bypass graft 3 years ago, and was recently diagnosed with diabetes mellitus type 2.

Physical Examination: Temperature 98.2°F, pulse 87, respirations 14, blood pressure 138/88 (sitting). Height 76 inches, weight 127.3 kg, BMI 34, waist circumference 46 inches. General: visceral obesity. HEENT: normal. Cardiac: regular rate and rhythm with no murmurs, rubs, or gallops. Respiratory: normal.

Laboratory Findings: Hemogram: normal. Chemistry: normal. Total cholesterol 222 mg/dl, LDL-C 133 mg/dl, HDL-C 24 mg/dl, triglycerides 148 mg/dl.

Question: What is this patient's blood pressure classification?

Diagnosis: Prehypertension

Discussion: Prehypertension, as defined by the Joint National Committee (JNC) VII report, is a systolic blood pressure of between 120 and 139 mmHg and/or a diastolic blood pressure of between 80 and 89 mmHg. According to JNC VII, patients shown to have blood pressure readings in this range are twice as likely to develop hypertension as are individuals with lower values. This patient, on two separate office visits, had a blood pressure of 134/84 and 138/88 mmHg confirming the classification of prehypertension.

Lifestyle modifications, which are outlined in the table, are the only treatment measures recommended for patients age 18 and older with prehypertension. Antihypertensive drug therapy and a target blood pressure of < 130/80 mmHg is recommended for prehypertensive patients with concomitant kidney disease and/or diabetes mellitus. This patient's healthcare provider did not initiate drug therapy, but explained to his patient that even mildly elevated blood pressure increases the risks for the development of target-organ damage, such as myocardial infarction, heart failure, stroke, and kidney disease. Appropriately, the patient was advised to implement lifestyle changes to prevent the increase of blood pressure to stage 1 hypertension.

This patient also should adopt significant lifestyle changes to decrease his risk for cardiovascular disease. Excess weight (a BMI > 25), especially when associated with a visceral distribution identified by a waist circumference > 40 cm in men and > 35 cm in women, has been associated with an increase in risk of cardiovascular disease. Reduction of calories and an increase in physical activity should be discussed to achieve weight loss.

The patient should be advised to implement the nutritional approach known as DASH (Dietary Approaches to Stop Hypertension). This diet, although not designed for weight loss, stresses a reduction in total fats (namely saturated fats and cholesterol), red meat, sodium, and sweets, and emphasizes an increase in the amounts of vegetables, fruits, low-fat dairy products, whole grains, nuts, fish, and poultry consumed.

An increase in daily consumption of potassium-rich foods and a decrease in sodium, as in the DASH-sodium diet, have been proven to significantly lower blood pressure. Several studies have shown that increases in potassium intake result in a reduction of stroke-related mortalities. Potassium-rich foods should be recommended to patients who present with hypertension. Some good choices are bananas, oranges, cantaloupe, potatoes, spinach, beans, nuts, and avocados. Patients should be instructed in the use of food labels to evaluate sodium content. Most convenient and processed foods are very high in sodium, resulting in excessive sodium intake (> 2.4 g per day).

In addition, patients should be counseled about the importance of establishing a consistent

Lifestyle Modifications to Manage Hypertension

Modification	Recommendation	Approximate Systolic BP Reduction, Range
Weight reduction	Maintain normal body weight (BMI, 18.5–24.9)	5–20 mmHg/10-kg weight loss
Adopt DASH eating plan	Consume a diet rich in fruits, vegetables, and low-fat dairy products, with a reduced content of saturated and total fat	8–14 mmHg
Dietary sodium reduction	Reduce daily dietary sodium intake to no more than 100 mEq/L (2.4 g sodium or 6 g sodium chloride)	2–8 mmHg
Physical activity	Engage in regular aerobic physical activity such as brisk walking (at least 30 minutes per day, most days of the week)	4–9 mmHg
Moderation of alcohol consumption	Limit alcohol consumption to no more than 2 drinks per day (1 oz or 30 mL ethanol [eg, 24 oz beer, 10 oz wine, or 3 oz 80-proof whiskey]) in most men, and no more than 1 drink per day in women and lighter-weight persons	2–4 mmHg

BMI, body mass index; BP, blood pressure; DASH, Dietary Approaches to Stop Hypertension.

exercise regimen. Commitment to a minimum of 30 minutes of moderate-intensity aerobic exercise (e.g., brisk walking) on most days of the week is recommended for controlling elevated blood pressure. Physical activity has been shown to directly decrease blood pressure, independent of its effect body weight.

Tobacco use of any kind should be discouraged. Alcoholic beverages should be limited to 1 ounce of alcohol per day for men (the amount in 24 ounces of beer, 10 ounces of wine, or one mixed drink) and 0.5 ounces per day for women.

This patient should be advised that his cholesterol values are not optimal. According to the Adult Treatment Panel (ATP) III guidelines, the HDL-C value should be > 40 mg/dl, the total cholesterol < 200 mg/dl, and the LDL-C goal is < 130 mg/dl. Dietary modifications and exercise should be stressed to the patient in an attempt to bring these values to the recommended goals.

The epidemic of high blood pressure has been appropriately named "the silent killer." An estimated 50 million Americans have hypertension, making it the most prevalent primary diagnosis. More than one third of patients with hypertension are not aware of this diagnosis. Although the etiology of hypertension is multifactorial, it is clear that healthy lifestyle habits improve control. Public health initiatives to increase education, awareness, and motivation are needed. Healthcare providers should inform patients and the public of the risks associated with prehypertension. Early identification of those at risk for cardiovascular disease, and early adoption of healthy lifestyle habits are critical in decreasing the incidence of stroke, heart disease, and renal failure.

Clinical Pearls

1. Individuals with prehypertension (systolic blood pressure of 120–139 mmHg or diastolic blood pressure of 80–89 mmHg) are twice as likely to develop hypertension as are those with lower blood pressure.
2. Lifestyle modifications to lower blood pressure include increased physical activity, weight reduction, the DASH diet, and moderation of alcohol intake.
3. Small increases in blood pressure are associated with an increased risk of myocardial infarction, heart failure, stroke, and kidney disease.

REFERENCES

1. Chobanian AV, GL Bakris, et al: The Seventh Report of the Joint National Committee on Prevention, Detection, Evaluation, and Treatment of High Blood Pressure (JNC VII). JAMA 289(19):2560–2572, 2003.
2. Crawford M: Current Diagnosis & Treatment in Cardiology. Lange/McGraw-Hill Medical Publishing Division, New York, 2003, pp 19–25.
3. Izzo JL, Black HR: AHA Hypertension Primer, 3rd edition. Lippincott Williams & Wilkins, Philadelphia, 2003, pp 385–387.
4. Kaplan N: Kaplan's Clinical Hypertension, 8th edition. Lippincott Williams & Wilkins, Philadelphia, 2002, pp 206–228.
5. Third report of the National Cholesterol Education Program (NCEP) Expert Panel on Detection, Evaluation, and Treatment of High Blood Cholesterol in Adults (Adult Treatment Panel III): Final report. U.S. Department of Health and Human Services; Public Health Service; National Institutes of Health; National Heart, Lung, and Blood Institute. [NIH Publication No. 02–5215. September 2002.] Circulation 106:3143, 2002.

INDEX

Page numbers followed by "f" denote figures and
"t" denote tables

M

Magnesium sulfate, 66
Magnetic resonance angiography, 25
Magnetic resonance imaging
  intracerebral hemorrhage evaluations, 36
  renal artery stenosis evaluations, 46–47
Malignant hypertension, 121–123
Mannitol, 36
Marfan's syndrome, 156
Meditative prayer, 99
Metabolic syndrome
  case study of, 74–77
  dietary modifications for, 76
  dyslipidemia associated with, 74
  risk factors, 74t
Metanephrines, plasma-free, 30
Methimazole, 125
Methyldopa
  chronic hypertension in pregnancy treated with, 86–87
  description of, 33
  hepatic reactions to, 188
Metoprolol, 79
Metyrosine, 50
Microalbuminuria, 164
Migraine headaches, 45
Mineralocorticoids, 72
Mitral inflow, 2
Multiple endocrine neoplasms, 30
Multiple myeloma, 101–104

N

Nausea and vomiting, 98, 105, 121, 155
Nephropathy
  diabetic, 56–58, 193–195
  immunoglobulin A, 139–140
Nephrosclerosis, hypertensive, 78–80
Nephrotic syndrome, 193–195
New-onset hypertension, 5, 60, 95
Nitrates, 142
Nitroprusside, 156
Nocturia, 141
Nocturnal dipping, 145
Nonalcoholic steatohepatitis, 188–189
Noncompliance with treatment
  description of, 8–10, 89–92
  hypertensive urgency caused by, 128
Nondippers, 145
Nonsteroidal anti-inflammatory drugs
  angiotensin-converting enzyme inhibitor-related cough treated with, 202
  description of, 28
Norepinephrine, 114

O

Obesity
  body mass index calculations, 22, 150
  description of, 17
  lifestyle modifications for, 150
  pediatric, 21–23
  polycystic ovary syndrome and, 117
Obstructive sleep apnea, 62–64, 173

Oral contraceptives
  hirsutism treated with, 118
  hypertension caused by, 93–94
Organ transplantation, 187–189
OSA. *See* Obstructive sleep apnea
Overshoot hypertension, 105–106

P

Panic disorder, 29
Parathyroid hormone, 102
Parathyroid hormone-related peptide, 103
Patient noncompliance, 8–10, 89–92
Pediatric patients
  blood pressure screenings in, 175–177
  obesity in, 21–23
Percutaneous transluminal coronary angioplasty, 25
Peripheral arterial occlusive disease, 199
Phenoxybenzamine, 50
Pheochromocytoma, 29–31, 49–50
Pituitary tumors, 72
Plasma renin activity, 12
Plasma-free metanephrines, 30
Polycystic kidney disease, autosomal dominant, 81–83
Polycystic ovary syndrome, 116–118
Polysomnography, 63
Poststreptococcal glomerulonephritis, 197
Potassium supplementation, 39, 211
Prazosin, 50
Preeclampsia, 65–67, 85
Pregnancy
  acute fatty liver of, 67
  cardiovascular changes in, 85
  chronic hypertension in, 84–88
  compensatory and physiologic changes during, 66, 85
  glomerular filtration rate in, 85
  HELLP syndrome, 67
  preeclampsia during, 65–67, 85
Prehypertension, 210–212
Primary hyperaldosteronism
  antihypertensives effect, 12
  case study of, 11–14
  classification of, 12
  description of, 6
  imaging studies, 13
  lifestyle modifications for, 14
  prevalence of, 12
  screening for, 12–13
  treatment of, 13–14
Primary hyperparathyroidism, 103
Prochaska's stages of change model, 40t
Propranolol, 125
Propylthiouracil, 125
Prostacyclin, 28
Prostaglandins, 28
Proteinuria
  diabetic nephropathy and, 57
  hypertensive nephrosclerosis and, 79
  immunoglobulin A nephropathy and, 140
  preeclampsia and, 66
  renal cell carcinoma and, 107–109
Pseudoaldosteronism, 153

Other Titles in the Pearls Series®